ADOLESCENT PSYCHIATRY

DEVELOPMENTAL AND CLINICAL STUDIES

VOLUME IX

Annals of the American Society for Adolescent Psychiatry

ADOLESCENT PSYCHIATRY

DEVELOPMENTAL AND CLINICAL STUDIES

VOLUME IX

Edited by
SHERMAN C. FEINSTEIN
JOHN G. LOONEY
ALLAN Z. SCHWARTZBERG
ARTHUR D. SOROSKY

The University of Chicago Press
Chicago and London

The University of Chicago Press, Chicago 60637
The University of Chicago Press, Ltd., London

© 1981 by The University of Chicago
All rights reserved. Published 1981
Printed in the United States of America

International Standard Book Number: 0-226-24054-1
Library of Congress Catalog Card Number: 70-147017

CONTENTS

PART III. PSYCHOPATHOLOGICAL ASPECTS OF ADOLESCENT DEVELOPMENT

PART IV. ADOLESCENT SUICIDOLOGY
ARTHUR D. SOROSKY, Special Editor

PART V. PSYCHOTHERAPEUTIC ISSUES IN ADOLESCENT PSYCHIATRY

PREFACE

In a sense this volume is concerned with the extremes in our society. The adolescent, like the artist, may tell us in what direction society is moving. The themes of many chapters focus on violence, while others deal with creativity. A special section deals with suicide as a growing expression of adolescent struggle. Clinicians deal with these matters, and as the developmental vicissitudes of adolescents become more understood we see a pattern of experimentation and eventual resolution.

The recently published reflections of a political prisoner said that to consider suicide under stress does not necessarily mean that one attempts suicide. It may mean the introduction of thoughts on the same level as the surrounding violence. This self-imposed state functions as a compensatory mechanism and provides a potential solution, one that contains a certain amount of pride. Later, when one rejects the idea of suicide, there again comes the feeling of defeat and the threat of madness.

The adolescent process is directed toward eventual synthesis, but during the process an inner divisiveness, a split between reason and emotion, takes place. Both the efforts at violence and the products of creativity can be seen as adaptive attempts at mastery. If society can remain convinced that these extremes are directed toward the eventual synthesis required to resolve the adolescent process and to achieve the capacities for independence, intimacy, and generativity of the mature adult, adolescents would not be programmed for turmoil but would be seen as a rich source of hope, energy, and a reflection of the future.

SHERMAN C. FEINSTEIN
JOHN G. LOONEY
ALLAN Z. SCHWARTZBERG
ARTHUR D. SOROSKY

PART I

ADOLESCENCE: GENERAL CONSIDERATIONS

EDITORS' INTRODUCTION

Bertram Slaff traces the historical development of the concept of child-hood and adolescence over the past centuries and views child and adolescent psychiatry as twentieth-century phenomena. With delineation of adolescence as a social, cultural, and psychological stage of life, a special interest in the psychiatric problems of this period has emerged. Various psychiatric societies developed to provide communication among the psychiatric community, and Slaff reviews the history of these groups and recounts the founding and purpose of the American Society for Adolescent Psychiatry.

Vivian Rakoff views today's alienated, directionless adolescents as an entropic form of those generations previously freed from constricting sociohistorical contexts. He attributes this to the loss of history and culture, a state of affairs both soul destroying and life destructive. Rakoff contributes the concept that custom and history in personal psychological development is analogous to Winnicott's transitional object in facilitating adolescent separation and individuation. The author emphasizes the important role of the father in providing the necessary authority and external controls. Professor Rakoff sees our changing social patterns leaving young people with little to hold on to, aspire for, and, ultimately, in a state of confusion created by our "performance society." He is, nevertheless, hopeful that the next generation will produce a positive synthesis.

The creative adolescent presents a unique challenge to his family, society, and adolescent psychiatry. While simultaneously burdened and blessed with special gifts, the creative adolescent must struggle alone to develop his talents. Creativity involves the ability to oscillate between different conscious and unconscious states and levels of experience, operating at very high levels of abstraction and integration. An important task of the adolescent psychiatrist is to appreciate the uniqueness of each creative and gifted adolescent, to understand the interaction between creativity and the adolescent process, and to distinguish between normal and pathological defenses in the service of creativity. The following chapters illustrate this approach.

Peter L. Giovacchini compares the essence of the creative process—the production of something that did not heretofore exist and expands reality—with the psychic viewpoint. That perception is that what had been previously unconscious becomes sufficiently structured so that it can be recognized and viewed by studying adolescent development and the manner it becomes intertwined with creative activity. Giovacchini explores the mental mechanisms involved with ego developmental process and points out that during adolescence a mechanism essential for creativity may decompensate into a pathological defense or become involved in a disintegrative regression resulting in the loss of adaptive and creative capacities.

Jon A. Shaw discusses adolescence and creativity and notes that both processes manifest great fluidity in defensive operations. He compares both states with the mourning process and uses poetry from both established poets and adolescents that illustrates the theme of time, loss, death, and the transient nature of experiences to clarify his hypothesis. Shaw postulates that creativity may represent a synthetic attempt to complete the mourning process while prolonging the psychic life of object representation. Art not only represents instinctual liberation, the expression of the pleasure principle, the recovery of a childhood experience, and the making of the unconscious conscious, it also represents the elaborated product of the synthetic and integrative function of the ego.

Bertram Slaff, in this chapter, considers that the creative personality and the narcissistic character may resemble each other and describes considerable overlap between the commonly accepted symptoms of psychological disturbance and manifestations of the creative personality in ferment. He concludes that while major psychological burdens may accompany the gift of creativity he considers creativity to be a most important aspect of the health of the individual, and outlines the understanding necessary for the therapist to help the gifted adolescent to cope successfully with those special capacities.

Adele D. Hofmann and Nancy R. Lewis describe a new development in the care of young people, adolescent medicine. In the authors' examination of the dilemmas facing hospitalized adolescents, they utilize the creative writing of these teenagers to illustrate patient concerns as well as to describe an innovative program in their medical setting. Examples of writings dramatize attitudes toward the medical staff, feelings about pain, chronic illness, death, body image, other patients, and their families. Further, Hofmann and Lewis believe that experience with creative writing is a unique opportunity for the vulnerable, hospitalized adolescent as a cathartic device for raising thoughts and feelings to consciousness and results in a new resource for the teenager in health as well as illness.

The increasing frequency of divorce necessitates an understanding of its effects on the adolescent's development and his interaction with his family system. Divorce is a process which alters but does not end family relationships. These chapters were designed to familiarize the adolescent psychiatrist with recent research on the effects of divorce in children and adolescents.

Allan Z. Schwartzberg provides an overview of the divorce process and its effects on children and adolescents. He views divorce as a process in which the family system is altered but not terminated. A family perspective emphasizes continuity and mutuality with reciprocal obligations and responsibilities extending well beyond the legal act of divorce. Schwartzberg discusses the predivorce, separation, and postdivorce phases while describing the process of divorce, the stress of divorce, problems in the single-parent family, the after effects of divorce on children and adolescents, and therapeutic approaches. He advises early therapeutic intervention to facilitate the mourning process so that the crisis of divorce can develop into an opportunity for continued growth and development.

Joan B. Kelly explores the potential disruptive influences of divorce on normal adolescent development. She considers the areas of future dating and marital relationships of those young people who were adolescents when their parents divorced and presents selected observations of their postdivorce heterosexual relationships five years later. The author found that adolescents of divorce experienced an acceleration and intensification of crucial developmental processes, particularly in the area of decathexis of parents and the subsequent move toward significant heterosexual objects, along with deidealization of the parents and the achievement and consolidation of greater autonomy and moral integrity. Kelly found that the intrapsychic chaos had left a strong impression on heterosexual relations, resulting in interference with the establishment of enduring ties and the formation of impoverished, immature, and ungratifying relationships. A very negative view of marriage remained, sustaining persistent doubts about marriage in general. The author concludes that longer study will help clarify whether the attitudes revealed indicate delay in otherwise normal developmental process or a more permanent developmental arrest.

Lee H. Haller describes approaches to child-custody evaluation as an advocate for the child rather than as an advocate for either parent. He believes all interested parties should participate in the study and describes various strategies for the entry of mental health experts—by agreement of both parties, by court appointment, or through the guardian *ad litem*. Haller outlines preparation for the study and discusses questions of visitation, legal criteria, fee determination, collateral material collection, arriving at a decision, and communicating your findings.

1   THE HISTORY OF ADOLESCENT
PSYCHIATRY

BERTRAM SLAFF

Aries in his *Centuries of Childhood* (1962) examined the life cycle from the Middle Ages to the present and concluded that during the Middle Ages the concept of childhood as we know it today simply did not exist. A stage of infancy, lasting until about age seven, was generally acknowledged. Thereafter, what we would consider children were simply assimilated into the adult world. The art, literature, and social documents of these times show children and adults dressed similarly, sharing in similar pursuits, and undifferentiated with regard to status or psychological development. The great majority of children were totally unschooled. Those who obtained minimal schooling to become priests or clerks were taught in ungraded schools where individuals of various age groups were unself-consciously intermingled.

The concept of childhood as a separate stage of life slowly began to emerge during the seventeenth and eighteenth centuries. Theories of education concerned with promoting the moral and intellectual development of the child began to be promulgated. Schools became increasingly age graded, and the number of children receiving schooling increased markedly.

The concept of adolescence is of even more recent origin. Keniston (1971) considers that while puberty as a biological state had been recognized, adolescence, as we think of it today, was discovered only during the nineteenth and twentieth centuries, and the extension of adolescence as a stage of psychological growth is far from complete even today. He observes that three changes occurred during the last century:

> First, adolescence as a stage of life has been socially recognized and acknowledged. Second, society has begun to sanction and support adolescence, increasingly buttressing it with educational, familial, institutional, and economic resources. Third, these new resources, coupled with other changes in society, have opened up to an ever larger proportion of the thirteen to eighteen year old age group the possibility of continuing psychological growth during the adolescent years. A further protection from adult responsibilities has been granted, educational institutions have been created to fill this moratorium, and a positive image of a postchildhood, preadult stage of life, adolescence, is now almost universally held.

This discovery of adolescence is closely related to other social, economic, and historical changes. Increasing industrialization has freed postpubertal youngsters from the requirements of farm and factory labor. The rising standards of economic productivity make the adolescent, especially the uneducated adolescent, a burden on the labor market. Growing affluence enables families and society as a whole to support economically unproductive adolescents in school.

As the concept of childhood historically preceded the concept of adolescence, child psychiatry was delineated first, with adolescent psychiatry emerging later. There is a major exception to this, however, in the publication of Hall's (1904) study on adolescence.

Weiner (1970) considers that Hall, heavily influenced by Darwin's theory of biological evolution, formulated an evolutional theory of psychological development based on the "law of recapitulation." Individuals develop through predetermined stages from primitiveness to civilized behavior in a manner that paralleled the development of the human race. The adolescent era was considered specifically analogous to the turbulent period in man's history that heralded the beginning of modern civilization.

Child psychiatry and adolescent psychiatry are predominantly twentieth-century phenomena. Noshpitz (1979) has described the significant developments. In 1905 Binet published the first draft of his scale to measure intelligence; Henry Goddard, at the Vineland Training School, made the tests available to the United States in 1910. In 1909 William Healy founded the Chicago Juvenile Psychopathic Institute, now known as the Institute for Juvenile Research, making use of the professional services of a psychiatrist, clinical psychologist, and psychiatric social worker in attacking the emotional problems of children. In 1912 Healy moved to Boston as the director of the Judge Baker Foundation. That same year Southard at the Boston Psychopathic Hospital introduced the term "clinic team" to describe the collaborative efforts of these professional groups.

In 1922 eight demonstration child-guidance clinics were organized in different parts of the country by the National Committee for Mental Hygiene, supported by the Commonwealth Fund. Private philanthropies later funded these clinics and many additional clinics were subsequently founded on this model.

The American Orthopsychiatric Association came into existence in 1923 (Lowrey 1948). Although membership was at first limited to psychiatrists, subsequently full membership was extended to qualified psychologists, social workers, and members of other disciplines.

The first U.S. textbook on child psychiatry was written by Kanner in 1935; Allen wrote the first U.S. textbook on psychotherapy for children in 1942.

During the twentieth century, the influence of Freud and his followers has been outstanding in the development of child and adolescent psychiatry. Early Freudian theory postulated certain innate drives that unfolded in predetermined ways, expressing themselves in a sequence of universal psychosexual stages (oral, anal, phallic) with specific conflict areas, such as the Oedipus complex. Freud (1905) in his essays on the theory of sexuality wrote on the transformations of puberty. In Esman's (1975) review he stated:

> Freud's argument is couched in terms of his libido theory; i.e., that the sexual drive is powered by a type of energy which he calls "libido," and that it undergoes a developmental course in which, after a succession of childhood ("pregenital") stages, it achieves its mature culmination in "genital primacy." Freud analogizes this development to the flow of a great stream, in which the various pregenital aims of sexuality (oral pleasure, voyeurism, sadism, etc.) are tributaries which, flowing into the mainstream, make their contributions in the form of "foreplay" and some of the secondary aspects of the sexual act. Puberty is, he suggests, the critical point at which all these tributaries merge to form the great river of adult genital heterosexuality.

9

Freud himself did not extensively study postpubertal aspects of adolescent growth and development.

Jones (1922) presented an evolutionary view of adolescent development that was seen as a reexperiencing of the first five years of life. He propounded "the general law . . . that adolescence recapitulates infancy, and that the precise way in which a given person will pass through the necessary stages of development in adolescence is to a very great extent determined by the form of his infantile development." Bernfeld, Aichhorn, and Anna Freud were other pioneers in the psychoanalytic study of the adolescent.

With the publication of *The Ego and the Mechanisms of Defense* (1946) Anna Freud is acknowledged as having been instrumental in ushering in the era of "ego psychology." Here the impact of adolescence on ego organization received its first systematic treatment. In her paper on adolescence (Freud 1958), she described adolescence as a period of normative upheaval and turmoil:

> I take it that it is normal for an adolescent to behave for a considerable length of time in an inconsistent and unpredictable manner; to fight his impulses and to accept them; to ward them off successfully and to be overrun by them; to love his parents and to hate them; to revolt against them and to be dependent on them; to be deeply ashamed to acknowledge his mother before others and, unexpectedly, to desire heart-to-heart talks with her; to thrive on imitation of and identification with others while searching unceasingly for his own identity; to be more idealistic, artistic, generous, and unselfish than he will ever be again, but also the opposite—self-centered, egoistic, calculating. Such fluctuations between extreme opposites would be deemed highly abnormal at any other time of life. At this time they may signify no more than that an adult structure of personality takes a long time to emerge, that the ego of the individual in question does not cease to experiment and is in no hurry to close down on possibilities.

Erikson (1950) has been another powerful influence in enriching the field of developmental psychology with his emphasis on crucial stages in personality development as "normative crises"—critical points that determine the outcome of subsequent developmental stages. His concepts of identity formation and the experiences of adolescence in promoting the sense of personal identity have been widely accepted, as well as his formulation of a basic conflict area of this period as "identity vs. identity diffusion."

Piaget (1969) made a remarkable contribution to the developmental study of human cognition. He demonstrated that in adolescence the capacity for abstract thought is achieved as the highest level of intellectual development and gives its special quality to the adolescent mind. Among psychoanalytic investigators Peter Blos (1962, 1967, 1979) has been prominent in his long-term study of "the adolescent process."

In the past decade a challenge has arisen to Anna Freud's view of adolescence as a developmental disturbance. Offer (1969) states, "Studies of normal populations that exhibit little behavioral disequilibrium might eventually lead to the concept that adolescence as a period of growth can be undergone without serious disruptions between the generations or between the adolescent and his former identity. The transition to adulthood may be accomplished gradually, but accomplished all the same. Our findings emphatically suggest that a state of inner turmoil need not be the password of adolescence." Masterson (1968) too has questioned the ubiquity of adolescent turmoil. It is his view that when the adolescent appears to be disturbed, he is disturbed and treatment is indicated.

The American Society for Adolescent Psychiatry

Psychiatry achieved a more general recognition as a consequence of its services during the Second World War. The National Mental Health Act of 1946 provided funding for teaching, training stipends for mental health professionals, and the establishment of psychiatric facilities. Major issues of the post–World War II era included interdisciplinary relationships and the setting of standards. The development of the adolescent psychiatry movement occurred, in part, in response to the conflicting forces dealing with these issues.

In 1948 fifty-four clinics formally ratified plans for a national association, the American Association of Psychiatric Clinics for Children. One of the purposes of the association was to set up standards for the training of child psychiatrists. Two years of specialized training in child psychiatry were required after the completion of two years of general psychiatry. Anxiety arose in some psychiatric circles about the standards for training in child psychiatry being set by a nonmedical organization.

In 1949 George S. Stevenson, president of the American Psychiatric Association, set up a committee on child psychiatry. Over the next few years this committee offered resolutions to the Council of the APA requesting that it approve child psychiatry as a subspecialty and that specialized training be required. This request was repeatedly turned down. Finally in 1958 the APA Council did endorse a statement that child psychiatry was a subspecialty of psychiatry, that competence called for special training, and recommended to the American Board of Psychiatry and Neurology that the three-year curriculum in psychiatry include six months of experience in child psychiatry. Later the APA accepted in principle a statement on standards of training in child psychiatry that called for two years of specialized training in child psychiatry in addition to at least two years of training in general psychiatry, and in 1959 the American Board of Psychiatry and Neurology established a Committee on Certification in Child Psychiatry. The subspecialty of child psychiatry had been recognized.

In 1953, before organized psychiatry accepted child psychiatry as a subspecialty, several child psychiatrists who were active as members of the American Association of Psychiatric Clinics for Children established an independent national organization of child psychiatrists, the American Academy of Child Psychiatry (Josselyn 1962). Membership was by invitation. Requirements for Fellow Membership included membership in the APA, certification in psychiatry by the American Board of Psychiatry and Neurology or board eligibility, four years of specialized training in child and general psychiatry, five years of experience after completion of training, a chief professional interest and activity in the field of child psychiatry, and the making of an "outstandingly significant" contribution to activities within the field. These requirements were modified significantly in 1969 (Tarjan 1978), and membership was now to be by application rather than by invitation.

In 1958 I was one of several New York City psychiatrists interested in working with adolescents who were invited by James Masterson to consider forming a group. Included were child and adult psychiatrists who shared this interest, were aware of the increasing needs of this growing segment of the population, and recognized that child psychiatry as it existed would not in the foreseeable future come close to meeting those needs.

With enthusiasm we decided to form an organization. Paradigmatic of this fledgling undertaking was the discussion of the name. I pointed out that the acronym of the proposed Society for Adolescent Psychiatry would be SAP. Edward Hornick asserted that that was just right;

that a group devoted to working with adolescents should have a quality of humor and a capacity not to take itself too seriously. Marynia Farnham, author of *The Adolescent* (1951) was elected first president. James Masterson, Edward Hornick, William A. Schonfeld, and Bertram Slaff followed in that office.

The Society for Adolescent Psychiatry met a real need in New York and stimulated similar developments in other cities. Masterson and I met in Philadelphia with a like group who organized the Philadelphia Society for Adolescent Psychiatry in 1962 with Philip Escoll as first president. Shortly after, the Chicago Society for Adolescent Psychiatry was formed under the leadership of Sherman C. Feinstein and Daniel Offer, and the Southern California Society for Adolescent Psychiatry came into being with Sheldon Selesnick as president.

In 1967, under the leadership of William A. Schonfeld, these local societies confederated and established the American Society for Adolescent Psychiatry with aims of providing a national forum for adolescent psychiatry, initiating efforts and cooperating with other organizations on behalf of adolescents, and facilitating communication and cooperation among the constituent societies. William A. Schonfeld was elected first president, Sheldon Selesnick vice-president, Herman D. Staples secretary, and Sherman C. Feinstein treasurer.

During the late 1950s and 1960s, as the postwar "baby boom" children reached adolescence, there was an enormous increase in demand for psychiatric services for this population group (Slaff 1970). In 1969 the National Institute of Mental Health published the results of a broad survey of American psychiatrists based on statistical data collected in 1965. In this study 8.2 percent of the total reported a primary subfield interest in child psychiatry, and 1.9 percent reported a primary subfield interest in adolescent psychiatry or student mental health. Nevertheless 16.2 percent reported seeing children and 32.9 percent reported seeing adolescents. In the private practitioner population a limited conclusion could be stated as follows: among those who saw one or more patients per week, 31.1 percent saw children and 63.2 percent saw adolescents. Obviously many who had not been specifically trained for work with children and adolescents were doing so (NIMH 1969).

To the question, "Another Society! Why?" Feinstein and Slaff (1975) responded:

The essential function of an adolescent psychiatry society is to provide a forum for the encouragement and discussion of the psy-

13

chiatric needs of youth. Teenagers are treated by child psychiatrists and adult psychiatrists, as well as by those who limit their work to this age group. Therapists' conceptualizations and approaches vary greatly, depending on their training opportunities and experience. The forum approach encourages communications in a specific area among psychiatrists of diverse backgrounds. The purpose of the society is not to create a subspecialty but rather to stimulate interest in this phase of life. It does not compete with or duplicate the groups formed by child psychiatrists. In organizational terms adolescent psychiatry societies should cooperate with child psychiatry groups, while encouraging the participation of interested members from adult psychiatry. For special aspects of adolescence such as college mental health, delinquency, marital counseling, drug abuse and the hospital treatment of the late adolescent and young adult, psychiatrists of various backgrounds are likely to become involved. It is through such cooperative efforts that expanded areas of psychiatric practice will be utilized to provide adequate advocacy and improved consultation and treatment resources for adolescents.

With continuing growth, over 1,700 members now belong to one of the nineteen constituent societies of the American Society for Adolescent Psychiatry. The autonomy of the local society is an important cornerstone of ASAP. Each has its own organizational structure, format of meetings, and tradition. Each has equal voice and vote in the national Council of Delegates. Membership generally is available to psychiatrists eligible to belong to the American Psychiatric Association who express an interest in adolescent psychiatry. Some of the local societies have recently extended associate membership to members of allied professions.

Society publications include an annual volume, *Adolescent Psychiatry, Annals of the American Society for Adolescent Psychiatry*, published by the University of Chicago Press, the *Newsletter*, published three times a year, and the *ASAP Membership Directory*, which includes geographical as well as alphabetical listings to facilitate the identification of psychiatrists with an interest in adolescence throughout the country.

An annual meeting of the Society is held which traditionally takes place during the period preceding the meeting of the American Psychiatric Association. This meeting also consists of clinical conferences on subjects of current importance in the field of adolescent psychiatry. An outstanding contributor to knowledge in this field is selected annually to receive the William A. Schonfeld Distinguished Service Award, named after ASAP's late first president. Recipients of this award include Peter Blos, Irene Josselyn, Rudolf Ekstein, Dana Farnsworth, E. James Anthony, Fritz Redl, Phyllis Greenacre, Melvin Sabshin, Moses Laufer, Robert Coles, Hilde Bruch, Heinz Kohut, George Tarjan, and Selma Fraiberg. Continuing Medical Education credits are granted for attendance at the conference. In addition, regional meetings have taken place in the fall or winter, sponsored by the societies of the eastern seaboard, the central states, and the western states.

A number of meetings on special topics have been sponsored by the American Society for Adolescent Psychiatry. In 1969 a conference on training in adolescent psychiatry was held at the University of Chicago under the leadership of Daniel Offer. A position statement representing the ASAP point of view spoke against the establishment of a certifying board in adolescent psychiatry, urged that training in adolescent psychiatry be given to all psychiatric residents, recommended that special training in adolescence be made available to those with this specific interest, and asked the National Institute of Mental Health to support the establishment of career adolescent psychiatry training programs. It spoke also to the need for special training programs in college psychiatry. Offer and Masterson have reported this meeting in their volume, *Teaching and Learning Adolescent Psychiatry* (1971).

In 1977, a conference on "Critical Issues in Adolescent Mental Health: A Response to President Carter's Commission on Mental Health" took place in Washington, D.C., and a meeting on "Emerging Trends in the Treatment of Adolescents and College Youth" was held at Northwestern University.

Representatives of ASAP have served as delegates at the White House Conference on Children, held in Washington, D.C., in 1970 and at the White House Conference on Youth, held in Estes Park, Colorado, in 1971. Active liaison is maintained with the National Institute of Mental Health officials who are concerned with the problems of youth. NIMH funds supported the recent "Demographic Study of Adolescent Psychiatry," organized by Paul Weisberg.

The Development of Inpatient Services for Adolescents

Beskin (1962) in his review of psychiatric inpatient treatment of adolescents stresses that recognition of this need has been a fairly

15

recent development. Curran (1939, 1978) reported that a children's ward had been established at Bellevue Hospital in New York City in 1923, the first ward of its kind. He became its director in 1932. At that time young adolescents from twelve to sixteen were frequently referred for diagnostic evaluation from the juvenile courts. These young teenagers were generally admitted to the "Quiet, Adult Male Ward." Whenever there were more than three or four adolescents, fights ensued and assaults were frequently made against elderly patients. This resulted in the transfer of some of the teenagers to the "Semi-disturbed Ward." When similar quarrels ensued there, some young patients were sent to the "Disturbed Ward." Curran states:

> My work with these youngsters in the various wards led me to believe that we should have a special service just for young teenagers and that, with individual and group therapy, we could salvage a large number of these disturbed youths. . . . In 1937 I was able to open the Adolescent Ward and I was the Director of that service until 1945. This ward was, to my knowledge, the first of its kind under medical supervision in a psychiatric hospital dealing exclusively with the management of adolescents. . . . We had an average population of eighty boys, from ages twelve to sixteen. . . . I was able to obtain various personnel to help in the program. These included remedial reading teachers, art teachers, dramatic coaches, and athletic coaches.

Inpatient adolescent psychiatry achieved important recognition in the mid fifties with the opening of adolescent units at Hillside Hospital, New York (Stahl 1960), and at the Neuropsychiatric Institute of the University of Michigan (Hendrickson 1957). In contrast the Psychiatric and Psychosomatic Institute of Michael Reese Hospital in Chicago distributed its adolescent patients on five autonomous adult units, while offering a special adolescent care service with individual psychotherapy, schooling, and an occupational and recreational program designed to meet their special needs (Falstein, Feinstein, and Cohen 1960).

Slaff (1980) reviewed the more recent developments in inpatient adolescent psychiatry, and de Marneffe (1974), director of McLean Hospital, summarized the challenge in the early 1960s of the growing population of a new group of patients, the adolescents. Before then, most psychiatric institutions had traditionally treated adults; hospitalization of adolescents was relatively a limited phenomenon. During the 1950s his institution gradually began to lower its minimum age for admission. In 1955, 6 percent of the patients admitted were under twenty-one; by 1960 the adolescent population had tripled to 18 percent of admissions, and this trend of sharply increased percentages of adolescent admissions continued over the decade.

Many hospitals were reluctant to admit adolescents because of uncertainties about the most effective way of handling such patients. The number of adolescent psychiatrists experienced in inpatient treatment of adolescents was extremely limited. There was growing recognition that, as a group, these patients were often very difficult to treat. It was decided not to turn away from the difficulties involved but rather to attempt to develop a comprehensive treatment program specifically designed for the adolescents' needs.

The influx of young patients and the commitment to establish such a program raised many questions and issues. An immediate problem related to the training of psychiatrists who would be responsible for developing adolescent patient units. For example, should the psychiatrist be trained primarily in child psychiatry or should he be trained principally in hospital psychiatry, gathering adolescent experience as he works in the hospital? Because the number of adolescent psychiatrists with inpatient adolescent treatment experience was so limited, McLean sought to develop its own training programs. Eventually this led to the establishment of a residency in adolescent psychiatry, supported by the National Institute of Mental Health. Whether adolescents should be housed in special units or mixed with older patients was considered. Should the units be sexually integrated or segregated? Decisions about a treatment milieu best suited to adolescents continued to be discussed over a period of years.

International Developments in Adolescent Psychiatry

Similar developments were taking place in other nations. In 1965 in Porto Alegre, Brazil, a therapeutic community was created and named for Leo Kanner. Training in adolescent psychiatry was begun there in 1967. That year the Asociación Argentina de Psiquiatria y Psicologia de la Infancia y de la Adolescencia (ASAPPIA) was founded; its members included psychiatrists, psychologists, social workers, and members of other professions. Early liaison was established between ASAPPIA and colleagues in Brazil. In the United Kingdom, the Association for

17

the Psychiatric Study of Adolescents (APSA) was formed in 1969. Societies for adolescent psychiatry came into being in Mexico in 1973 and Colombia in 1976. All these are multidisciplinary organizations. Active in the adolescent psychiatry movement in France were Serge Lebovici and Michel Vincent, while Emanuel Chigier was a leader in Israel.

Katz (1978) has described the history of the Canadian Society for Youth Psychiatry, which was initiated in 1970. The founding members wanted a society to parallel the American Society for Adolescent Psychiatry, with which it would have liaison. Interested members of the Canadian Psychiatric Association would be invited to join. The formation of the Canadian Society for Youth Psychiatry was strongly opposed by the then president of the Canadian Psychiatric Association who felt it would be a divisive force and would split the CPA. He felt that any breaking away by any group would be destructive to the mother organization. The founding members of the CSYP strongly objected to this point of view, maintaining that they had no wish to split away from the CPA but purely wished to have an organization that could further the interests of adolescent psychiatry and in particular capitalize on the development of ASAP in the United States. As a compromise the CSYP was established but as a section on youth psychiatry within the Canadian Psychiatric Association.

William A. Schonfeld, first president of the American Society for Adolescent Psychiatry, visited Argentina in 1969 and made contact with adolescent psychiatry leaders there. Consequent to this, a Panamerican Congress on Adolescent Psychiatry, consponsored by ASAPPIA and ASAP was held in Buenos Aires in 1971. Eduardo Kalina and Sherman C. Feinstein were copresidents of the congress, with Mauricio Knobel and Bertram Slaff as honorary copresidents. In response to the success of this congress and the conceptualizations of Kalina and Feinstein, the Panamerican Forum for the Study of Adolescence was organized with the purpose of holding biennial meetings of the countries of the Americas on the subject of adolescence. In 1973 the second *Reunion* was held in New Orleans led by Max Sugar. In 1975 the third *Reunion* under the direction of José Carrera, Armando Barriguete, and Bertram Slaff met in Merida, Mexico City, and Acapulco. The fourth *Reunion* convened in Rio de Janeiro and Salvador da Bahia under the leadership of Maria Eugenia Vianna Nery, Carlos Cesar Castellar Pinto, and Herman D. Staples. The late Margaret Mead was a much beloved guest at the Brazil meetings. Gustavo

Lage and Francisco Cobos directed the fifth *Reunion,* meeting in San Francisco and New York in 1979.

Eduardo Kalina (1978) has described the spirit of the *Reuniones* as "the idea of creating a friendly and brotherly environment where scientific exchanges are produced, where we get to know the different ways of thinking of Latin and North Americans—so different in organization, scientific development, work, economic-socio-political possibilities."

International meetings on adolescent psychiatry took place in Jerusalem and in Edinburgh during 1976. A committee with representatives from France, the United Kingdom, Belgium, and the United States is now formulating the organization of an international society for adolescent psychiatry.

Conclusions

Where does the adolescent psychiatry movement go from here? We appear to have established ourselves as spokesmen for the needs of youth and for those who professionally serve in that area. We have provided a bridge between child psychiatrists who quite appropriately deal with adolescents and other psychiatrists who also treat them. Gradually we have invited members of allied professions who share our interest to join with us, a development which is clearly international in scope. We have established a cadre of colleagues over much of the globe who share an interest, a commitment, and an expertise in dealing with the psychiatric problems of troubled youth. We have done this in an open manner, which we believe is in the best tradition of receptivity to new ideas, while maintaining those traditional ideas which still command respect.

REFERENCES

Allen, F.H. 1942. *Psychotherapy with Children.* New York: Norton.
Aries, P. 1962. *Centuries of Childhood.* New York: Knopf.
Beskin, H. 1962. Psychiatric inpatient treatment of adolescents: a review of clinical experiences. *Comprehensive Psychiatry* 3:354–369.
Blos, P. 1962. *On Adolescence: A Psychoanalytic Interpretation.* New York: Free Press.
Blos, P. 1967. The second individuation process of adolescence. *Psychoanalytic Study of the Child* 22:162–186.

Blos, P. 1979. *The Adolescent Passage*. New York: International Universities Press.

Curran, F.J. 1939. Organization of a ward for adolescents in Bellevue Psychiatric Hospital. *American Journal of Psychiatry* 95:1365–1388.

Curran, F.J. 1978. Child psychiatry, USA 1928–1978 (one man's perspective). Read before the New York Council on Child Psychiatry, May 18, 1978.

de Marneffe, F. 1974. Introduction. In M.C. Grob and J.E. Singer, eds. *Adolescent Patients in Transition*. New York: Behavioral Publications.

Erikson, E. 1950. *Childhood and Society*. New York: Norton.

Esman, A.H. 1975. *The Psychology of Adolescence*. New York: International Universities Press.

Falstein, E.I.; Feinstein, S.C.; and Cohen, W.P. 1960. An integrated adolescent care program in a general psychiatric hospital. *American Journal of Orthopsychiatry* 30:276–291.

Farnham, M. 1951. *The Adolescent*. New York: Harper.

Feinstein, S.C., and Slaff, B. 1975. Another society! Why? *Newsletter of the American Society for Adolescent Psychiatry*. Wallingford, Pa.: American Society for Adolescent Psychiatry.

Freud, A. 1946. *The Ego and the Mechanisms of Defense*. New York: International Universities Press.

Freud, A. 1958. Adolescence. *Psychoanalytic Study of the Child* 13:255–278.

Freud, S. 1905. The transformations of puberty. In A.H. Esman, ed. *The Psychology of Adolescence*. International Unversities Press, 1975.

Hall, G.S. 1904. *Adolescence*. New York: Appleton.

Hendrickson, W.J. 1957. Adolescent service, Neuropsychiatric Institute, University of Michigan. *Bulletin of the Michigan Society for Mental Health*.

Jones, E. 1922. Some problems of adolescence. *Papers on Psychoanalysis*. London: Bailliere, Tindall & Cox, 1948.

Josselyn, I.M., ed. 1962. The history of the American Academy of Child Psychiatry. *Journal of the American Academy of Child Psychiatry* 1:196–202.

Kalina, E. 1978. Personal communication.

Kanner, L. 1935. *Child Psychiatry*. Springfield, Ill.: Thomas.

Katz, P. 1978. Personal communication.

Keniston, K. 1971. Youth as a stage of life. *Adolescent Psychiatry* 1:161–175.

Lowrey, L. 1948. *Orthopsychiatry 1923–1948, Retrospect and Prospect*. American Orthopsychiatric Association, George Bank Publishing Co.

Masterson, J.F. 1968. The psychiatric significance of adolescent turmoil. *American Journal of Psychiatry* 124:1549–1554.

National Institute of Mental Health. 1969. *The Nation's Psychiatrists*. Public Health Service Publication, no. 1885. Washington, D.C.: Government Printing Office.

Noshpitz, J.D. 1979. Personal communication.

Offer, D. 1969. *The Psychological World of the Teenager*. New York: Basic.

Offer, D., and Masterson, J.F. 1971. *Teaching and Learning Adolescent Psychiatry*. Springfield, Ill.: Thomas.

Piaget, J. 1969. The intellectual development of the adolescent. In G. Caplan and S. Lebovici, eds. *Adolescence: Psychosocial Perspectives*. New York: Basic.

Slaff, B. 1970. The manpower emergency in adolescent psychiatry. *Psychiatry—the Mount Sinai Experience*. New York: Dekker.

Slaff, B. 1980. The history of hospital adolescent psychiatry. In D.R. Heacock, ed. *A Psychodynamic Approach to Adolescent Psychiatry—the Mount Sinai Experience*. New York: Dekker.

Stahl, A.S. 1960. The first five years of the Israel Strauss adolescent pavilion program. *Journal of the Hillside Hospital* 9(5):5–14.

Tarjan, G. 1978. The American Academy of Child Psychiatry: our 25th anniversary. *Journal of the American Academy of Child Psychiatry* 17(4):561–564.

Weiner, I.B. 1970. *Psychological Disturbances in Adolescence*. New York: Wiley-Interscience.

2   A RECONSIDERATION OF IDENTITY

VIVIAN RAKOFF

The much talked about autonomy of the present-day individual is the by-product of powerful social forces that, at their beginning, allowed people to escape from constricting and oppressive sociohistorical contexts. Unfortunately, we are now in the situation of seeing the negative side of those forces that were the generative motor for the huge social, technological, and migratory developments of which we are almost all direct beneficiaries. But this is a process of historical dialectic and probably inevitable.

Things that begin by being essentially benign generate their negative antitheses. Contradictions and unresolved tensions observed during the initial energetic thrust eventually develop their own momentum to emerge as strong countervailing forces as the energy subsides. This should be no surprise to an old-time Marxist or even Hegelian, and should certainly not be a surprise to anyone with a psychoanalytic background; all things exist in a dynamic equilibrium with contrary and opposing forces.

It is the consideration of these opposing forces that brings me to this particular essay. To put it very briefly, the free energetic individuals who laboriously discovered the right to personality and self-determination were the grandparents and the parents of the alienated, frightened, directionless adolescents who today appear in the clinics. These young people represent the entropic form of those who were freed to become themselves by the rise of capitalism. As a way out of the lack of direction they either drop out into a drug culture or cherish dreams of a Rousseauistic escape to the woods in farming, the study of solar energy, vegetarianism, or religious cults. We are seeing a continuous and possibly growing use of drugs. In fact the only characteristic holding all these diverse forms of distress together is that they are denials of history; they represent both an escape from a poorly understood context and an attempt to repair the confusion in the daily world by frequently substituting an artificial and historically unvalidated alternative.

The loss of history produces chaos and personality disorganization and one must consider its roles in a psychic organization. In addition to the adolescents who present in the way I have just described, there are certain epidemiological facts suggesting that the discontinuity of culture and history may be not only soul destroying, but in the most concrete sense life destructive. The increased rates of suicide among alienated older men, young American Indians deprived of their culture, and urban adolescents who find themselves constantly displaced and without a cultural home suggest that history—in the sense of a network of mythical, personal, institutionalized patterns received from the past and contemporaneously meaningful—has an essential role to play in keeping people alive.

I propose a model for the role of custom and history in personal psychological development analogous to Winnicott's (1958) transitional objects. In Winnicott's original formulation, the transitional object allows the child to separate from the mother and to preserve her in objects which symbolically contain her. Subsequently (1967), he proposed that this "safe space" was the place in which culture developed, since this protected dimension provides the necessary safety for play and creativity which is the substrate for culture.

I suggest that one must think of a second transitional stage during which separation from the nurturant protective family is essential. During that phase the child needs to leave the family for the world in the same way that he had to leave the breast of the mother for the more generalized but still protected territory of the household and close family group. The objects, or structures, which need to be internalized to allow the move are the history and general culture common to the child and the receiving society. But this time it is the parental functions that allow the child to make the transition.

The father ("the first stranger") is a figure traditionally active both in the family and the world. He bridges the fundamental territories of intimacy and public life by having an emotional bond to both the child and work in the world. The two dimensions satisfy different needs and require different modes of action. The first of these, the intimate, the familial, the emotional, can be referred to as the needs of the "unclothed man," while societal structure, the world of public events,

23

work, history, received religion, and ethical structures, represents the "clothed" human being.

In familial structure the guidelines and internal framework for intimate behavior are established. It is in this context that one is "loved for one's self alone." One is accorded respect and relationship simply because one *is*. It derives from the nonrational bonding experience between mother and child—between adult and infant. The child is not loved because he performs but because he has been born and radiates a series of cues. The mother in turn is felt as necessary and nurturant (is loved because she is there, and constant, and in Winnicott's phrase is "good enough") and therefore generates sufficient internal confidence for the individual to believe that he or she is valuable.

These intimate relationships are the template for later intimacy; for sexuality, loving, and nurturing. They may be the source of altruism, almost certainly the origin of a sense of inner security. However, the societal structure operates essentially on the performance principle. One is not necessarily rewarded because one *is* but because of what one *does*. One is not loved for oneself alone; one is loved for the work performed, the value given to one's role, the respect one may command, one's power, money, or even an unearned fame or celebrity.

Erikson's "Identity"

It almost requires an apology to talk once again on such contemporary preoccupations as narcissism and the excessively announced social crises of our time. (Was there ever a time when people didn't live under some terrible threat or the other?) But this is one of our shared interests and preoccupations.

While the formal definitions of identity have probably changed very little, we would probably all agree to some formulation such as: the continuing sense of self experienced by the individual and recognized by society. However, the way in which the word is used implicitly and explicitly has undergone some dramatic changes; consider Erikson's "identity." In his formulation, the individual's sense of identity was the result of an interaction between the intimate infantile relationships of the individual characteristics and society at large. In *Childhood and Society* Erikson (1950) formulates identity in almost entirely societal terms. He writes:

We concluded that only a gradually accruing sense of identity, based on the experience of social health and cultural solidarity at the end of each major childhood crisis, promises that periodical balance in human life which—in integration of the ego stages—makes for a sense of humanity. But whatever the senses lost, wherever integrity yields to despair and disgust, wherever generativity yields to stagnation, intimacy to isolation, and identity to diffusion, an array of associated infantile fears are apt to become mobilized: for . . . only an ego identity can . . . produce a workable equilibrium safely anchored in the patrimony of a cultural identity can . . . produce a workable equilibrium. [P. 369]

In his footnote to this particular paragraph, he says that "no ego, it is true, can develop outside of social processes which offer workable prototypes and roles. The healthy and strong individual, however, adapts these roles to the further processes of this ego thus doing his share in keeping the social process alive." And typically in his elaboration of this theme in later years Erikson (1958, 1969) in his full-length portrait of Luther and Ghandi depicted these men as finding themselves, that is, expressing their identity in the domain of social or ethical action. In his earlier footnote, Erikson (1958) included Jesus of Nazareth and the same comment applies that these three men are not—even in an extreme stretch of the contemporary definition—in the remotest way adolescent.

What has happened in the practical application of Erikson's ideas seems to be, and I say this somewhat tentatively, a corruption of his original statement. The strong, societal emphasis he gave appears to have become lost in the clinic. In my own experience, and perhaps those of many of my colleagues, when an individual adolescent was considered, he was almost invariably described in terms of his personal adaptation, his personal loss of identity, or at best his relationship to his immediate family. The family was described in terms of its interactions, its patterns of alliances and roles, and its particular disorders of communication; although the family itself was as detached and alienated from the world at large as the alienated adolescent. The family in these formulations exists in the same species of directionless and autonomous bubble as the narcissistic individual—only a somewhat larger bubble. Rarely is there a full exploration of the social context and the social value systems of the family. A long and detailed cultural history of the kind that Erikson so carefully gives in his early case reports is in my experience a clinical rarity.

Certainly, during the 1960s identity versus role diffusion becomes a central topic of the clinical focus, but it was the identity of the intimate

25

man. It is as though the unclothed human being receives almost the total attention of the therapist and the clothed person, the recipient and participant in the elaborate culture of the time, seems to be curiously neglected. I looked at a random sample of family and individual case reports and found in none of them more than the most cursory examinations of the sociocultural background or the belief system of the patient. The clinical records reflect an apparently unwitting collusion with those narcissistic personalities who increasingly present for therapy.

If identity was the buzz word of the 1960s and early 1970s, it will be no news that "narcissism" is the buzz word of the 1970s and 1980s. In fact we are indebted to Kernberg for many of the careful clinical descriptions of this condition and therapeutic strategies. Further, in Kohut's (1977) description and in the more recent and complex formulations of Lasch (1978), the characteristics of this narcissist emerges: he is essentially insecure, his world view is solipsistic, he feels empty, self-hating, dependent upon a distrusted world for supplies of self-esteem, alienated both historically and spatially, without regard for the past, and without feeling any commitment to the future. The achievements of others are at no point any source of pleasure; there is a constant and pervading fear of death and old age; and lacking coherent value systems, he operates by charm and coercion, has little adherence to principles, and loves others with only minimal investment. Many therapists report that this person appears in ever increasing numbers in many different forms ranging from the relatively benign to the malignant personality disorder of the borderline patient.

The individual, it appears, has finally assimilated the great societal movements toward privatism—the individual free of context—the thrust and achievement of capitalism. Paradoxically, as society has moved more and more toward mirroring the family, the individual, or at least the clinically identified individual, feels less at home within it. The familial principles are those of nurturance derived from existence and not from doing. These have been valuable achievements; not one of us would want (I think) a return to a Hobbesian society—a war of all against all.

We value and respect the public institutions of altruism, public education, and welfare. Yet there is concern that the attitude toward these necessary benefits has become one of petulant distress; the complaints of children toward depriving parents. The concepts of reciprocal loyalty, adherence to the particular society or group, stoicism and pride of association, which are so essential for working in the world as opposed to being in the world, are vitiated and for many so suspect that the context of community is untenable. Custom, manners, and history are desired, but are not, for many, a natural possession. Disneyland attracts millions who come not only for the rides and thrills but for its presentation of places and times, cleaned up, trivialized, and rendered merely nostalgic. Even the great travel boom reflects a wish to experience places with well-established identities—the more exotic the better. People and places are assimilated to a show-biz notion of reality.

With regard to the corruption of the world, Lasch's examination of the culture of narcissism is a particularly cogent text to examine. He castigates the therapeutic approach to problems of all human experience. In particular, what he calls "the awareness movement" is seen as a corrupt, extension of the empty self's overweaning preoccupation with that emptiness and an attempt to make a career out of a hypochondriacal preoccupation with inner process. He feels that it is a corruption of what might have been a religious, ethical search in the past and has paradoxically little real regard for inner-knowledge ethics, only requiring validation and celebrity. The narcissistic personality he believes has essentially given up on the world. He writes:

> The concept of narcissism provides us not with a ready-made psychological determinism but with a way of understanding the psychological impact of recent social changes. Assuming that we bear in mind not only its clinical origins but the continuum between pathology and normality, it provides us in other words with a tolerably accurate portrait of the "liberated" personality of our time with his charm, his pseudo-awareness of his own condition, his promiscuous pan-sexuality, his fascination with oral sex, his fear of the castrating mother (Mrs. Portnoy), his hypochondria, his protective shallowness, his avoidance of dependence, his inability to mourn, his dreaded old age and death.

He goes on to say that the prevailing social conditions therefore tend to bring out narcissistic traits that are present in varying degrees in everyone. These conditions have also transformed the family, which in turn shapes the underlying structural personality. A society that fears it has no future is not likely to give much attention to the needs of the next generation. From this he draws the terrible conclusion:

> The ethic of self-preservation and psychic survival is rooted, then, not merely an object of conditions in economic warfare, rising

27

rates of crime, and social chaos but in the subjective experience of emptiness and isolation. It reflects the conviction as much a projection of inner anxiety as a perception of the way things are—that envy and exploitation dominate even the most intimate relation. The cult of personal relations, which becomes increasingly intense as the hope of political solution recedes, conceals a thorough going disenchantment with personal relations, just as the cult of sensuality implies a repudiation of sensuality in all but its most primitive form. The ideology of personal growth, superficially optimistic, radiates a profound despair, and resignation. It is the faith of those without faith.

In place of rugged individualism and religion there is now an excessive reliance on "therapy."

His sad, angry, and at times impressive book goes on to describe the loss of cultural values, the celebration of spurious fame, the show-biz mode of the entire society, the loss of true playfulness in sport in favor of any aggressive disregard for the opponent summed up in George Allan's phrase, "Winning isn't the most important thing, it's the only thing" (p. 117). Lasch characteristically squeezes significance from trivial phenomena: "The intrusion of the market into every corner of the sporting scene, however, recreates all the antagonisms characteristic of late capitalist society." Very little in the society escapes his particular focus on narcissism; it includes schooling and what he calls, "the new illiteracy, the atrophy of competence and the trivialization of higher education."

His most carefully articulated anger is directed at the loss of paternal authority in the family. It is curious that Lasch does not acknowledge a debt to Marcuse in this regard. For Marcuse, the loss of paternal authority removed an intimate component of the superego in favor of the values of a tyrannically oppressive society, so that the individual becomes a psychic puppet of the repressive powers of the state. And because he shares the state's values, he is incapable of rebellion and criticism of accepted norms and cannot know that he is angry and oppressed because he is confluently part of the forces of his oppression. While Lasch shares the distress at the loss of parental authority he differs seriously from Marcuse on the grounds that societal values—far from having been incorporated into the individual superego because there is no paternal mediation—are for Lasch absent or trivialized and hence do not enter into the formation of the superego. In the absence of received and respected values and the overwhelming sense of self-doubt and emptiness, people no longer trust their own competence or the competence of those close to them. As a result they hand over their problems to experts and other agents, in particular psychiatrists, social workers, and physicians. And with the loss of the father's authority, the relatively benign components of the superego are overwhelmed by the primitive, punitive, id-superego. The so-called free individual then, is actually the victim of much more severe and irrational control than that internalized within the more apparently authoritarian traditional family.

Having carefully followed Lasch through his criticism of numerous social structures, one waits for some solution—a way out. However, the concluding paragraph of his book is a disappointment:

> In a dying culture narcissism appears to embody—in the guise of personal "growth" and "awareness"—the highest attainment of spiritual enlightenment. The custodians of culture hope, at bottom, merely to survive its collapse. The will to build a better society, however, survives, along with traditions of localism, self-help, and community action that only need the vision of a new society, a decent society, to give them new vigor. The moral discipline formerly associated with the work ethic still retains a value independent of the role it once played in the defense of property rights. That discipline—indispensable to the task of building a new order—endures most of all in those who knew the old order only as a broken promise, yet who took the promise more seriously than those who merely took it for granted.

Lasch, then, mourns for many of the values which would be called traditional. He asks for, among others, the reappearance of both local and national tradition, for a respect for history, for the restoration of the authority of the father, for self-reliance and self-help, for a return of playfulness, the reintroduction of the work ethic into daily life, and for a suspicion of celebrity. Unfortunately, his elaboration of an alternative and potentially sustaining value system must be sensed between the lines of his book.

Many elements of Lasch's angry—and alas at times somewhat petulant—criticism of the society are to be found in Sennett's (1978) *The Fall of Public Man.* Sennett's book is an attack upon the corruptions that an overemphasis on the intimate life have produced in soci-

29

ety. People do not know how to behave, they no longer have the protection of codes of manners which would allow strangers to confront one another without terror, and their expectations are wheedling and sentimental. Sennett says that the mature ego "takes" what it wants rather than expressing only a desire.

Both Sennett and Lasch take out of the clinic and into the world the concern for the expression of the self as it has come to be understood in contemporary life. And they both express the need once again to see the individual as connected to and reflected by a society with which he can feel an organic connection. While Lasch and Sennett share a critical position, Lasch is concerned by Sennett's alternatives to the excess of intimacy. Lasch suggests that Sennett enshrines rapacity as an alternative to narcissism. And in this phrase Lasch signals his awareness of some of the dangers in the attack on the ascendant private person. That danger from the clinical and the social point of view is that the valuable aspects of socially validated personal identity and the rights to an intimate existence may be lost because of their corruption. In social terms it could become the benignly intentioned mask for the reappearance of authoritarianism, puritanical sexual values, a distrust of expertise, and the help of others. Waiting in the wings are the worst aspects of what, in shorthand, we like to call the Victorian. I am not suggesting that this is Lasch's intention, but the ideas that take root in the marketplace are corrupt versions of their scholarly expression. All ideas contain their implicit entropic forms. And the entropic form of public virtue is rigid authoritarianism; the triumph of the context over the person.

At a certain point both Sennett and Lasch—and I am aware that I am not being entirely fair to either of them—can be seen as very sophisticated variants of Riesman's (1961) examples. Their criticisms of the entire society and invasion of personalist narcissistic values is so extreme and so all-encompassing that it is almost as if they are giving voice to precisely that unbridled and primitive superego which Lasch so carefully describes when he points to the loss of the traditional authority of the father within the family and the effect that this has on the individual's psychic development. At one point Lasch quotes Novak (1971) in the phrase "the virulent passion for debunking in the land." Perhaps, in addition to all his cogent and valid criticisms, Lasch has added his voice to that of the debunkers. In his discontent with almost everything in the world, his fury with physicians and other authorities, there is an echo of precisely the relentless hatred the narcissist—as he describes him—feels for society.

After reading Lasch's more rhetorical passages that depict social disintegration, one wonders which values one can draw to the attention of the floundering adolescent. And then one has to look out of the window at the superficial but actual world of partial reality. Out there, there is a society which, being human, is of course corrupt in many ways. One does not see the condensed highly dramatized version of life in the city that comes to one in the evening news or in Lasch's prose, but, for the most part, a relatively orderly society with a history of some concern for individuals and a tradition of self-examination which only in its most extreme moments reaches the point of despair.

Conclusions

One has to remember that the society from which we all escaped did not generate entirely good things for people, since the authoritarian father and the ethically dominated context were prisons for many individuals. The period of bourgeois civility celebrated by Sennett was a time of infinitely greater social oppression than that which we now live in.

Like the narcissistic individual, Lasch expresses a rage against the context of the society at large. The capitalist revolutions succeeded by destroying the prerevolutionary context and produced a major discontinuity of the preceeding social structures—a discontinuity of authority from which some societies seem never to have recovered, lurching from one makeshift social accommodation to the other. And the individual, it seems, having been released from one oppressive context became terrified of all context. The state, an institutionalized ethical system, was to be seen as always coercive, always evil.

Only recently do we seem to be developing an awareness that without a context, a continuing history, a sense of the past and future, and shared rituals and myths the freed individual, far from knowing who he is, may feel he is nobody. His selfhood and identity have not been liberated, but truncated. He lacks pride and definition.

What is in this age of diminishing expectations for the therapist? Again there are no ten commandments, no profound awareness of God intervening in history, no universally shared history of ethical commitment to back him up. All that the therapist has to offer is a rather

31

feeble appeal to local endeavor, self-help, sobriety, and hard work. This in itself will surely not be enough to tempt anyone away from joining a cult, fleeing the city, dropping out of school, or trying to get ahead by the use of charm. It is certainly not enough to fill that vast emptiness and that sense of disconnectedness from others that are so often a feature of the borderline adolescent.

It appears to me to be much more likely that an examination of the culture that we have with the intention of identifying some positive and available elements will be helpful. For a sense of identity we will have to return to the Eriksonian blend of private and public. The self will have to be examined and confirmed in both societal and intimate terms. In summary, then, the revulsion from the cult of the individual in society, the corrupted values of intimacy, the numbers of narcissistic and character disordered patients who appear in the clinic should not tempt one into a rapacious stance. With luck, the same processes of thesis and antitheses which resulted in the social prevalence of narcissism can produce a more positive synthesis in which the next generation will not be condemned to gazing into the mirror nor to having recourse only to despair and suicide.

REFERENCES

Erikson, E.H. 1950. *Childhood and Society*. New York: Norton.

Erikson, E.H. 1958. *Young Man Luther*. New York: Norton.

Erikson, E.H. 1969. *Ghandi's Truth*. New York: Norton.

Kohut, H. 1977. *The Restoration of the Self*. New York: International Universities Press.

Lasch, C. 1978. *The Culture of Narcissism*. New York: Norton.

Novak, M. 1971. *The Rise of the Unmeltable Ethnics*. New York: Macmillan.

Riesman, D. 1961. *The Lonely Crowd*. New Haven, Conn: Yale University Press.

Sennett, R. 1978. *The Fall of Public Man*. New York: Vintage.

Winnicott, D. 1958. *Collected Papers: Through Paediatrics to Psycho-Analysis*. New York: Basic.

Winnicott, D. 1967. The location of cultural experience. *International Journal of Psycho-Analysis* 48:371–389.

ADOLESCENCE
AND
CREATIVITY

3 CREATIVITY, ADOLESCENCE, AND INEVITABLE FAILURE

PETER L. GIOVACCHINI

The essence of the creative process is the production of something that did not heretofore exist. It may be the discovery of a realm, a new frame of reference, a better explanatory hypothesis, or a novel combination of already known factors or concepts. Our current reality is expanded by the creative product.

We can make a comparison from the psychic viewpoint. What had been previously unstructured inasmuch as it had no access to conscious or cognitive processes becomes sufficiently structured so that it can be perceived and used. Certainly the creator furthers his emotional development and attains higher levels of ego integration as a result of his creative activity. I believe that much of the appeal creativity has for many of us is based upon its potential for self-growth as the spectrum of primary to secondary process is lengthened (see Giovacchini 1971).

There are many, perhaps an inexhaustible number of perspectives by which we may explore this topic. I have investigated the relationship of the creative process to insanity (I do not believe there is any process connection between the two) and the special role of the ego ideal in the psyches of especially gifted scientists (Giovacchini 1960, 1965).

Here I will investigate the way in which the adolescent process of character development becomes intertwined with creative activity. I emphasize that I am not equating growing up emotionally with a creative act. No matter how awesome and wonderfully intricate and ingenious a fully developed human character is, we would all be geniuses if that were the case. The obvious flaw here is that we would be confusing the product with the process. I believe the word "creative" has been much misused and applied to a variety of areas and products that, at best, could be called clever and skillful but not truly creative.

During adolescence there are many internal rearrangements which have to be differentiated from creativity. Adolescence itself may supply a setting that is favorable or unfavorable to such activity. Defensive adaptations to psychopathological disequilibrium, although they may appear to involve areas that are thought of as representing creative endeavors such as artistic pursuits, in my mind, are not creative. This is a repetition of the negation that genius is equivalent to madness. Furthermore, simply because a person paints, writes, or dabbles in the laboratory does not mean that he will achieve in the sense that we would consider the psychic processes accompanying his strivings as being characteristic of the creative process. Creativity, by definition, is something special.

This does not mean that in some way accomplishment cannot have a beneficial and restorative effect on a vulnerable psyche, a vulnerability that is common among adolescents. Furthermore, the adolescent may have certain features that make him particularly receptive to the acceptance of new ideas and working them over into a useful and novel coherence. The adolescent's open character—his psychic structure is relatively unconsolidated—is a factor determining his capacity to incorporate elements within his psyche that the more structured personality could not integrate.

There are other features to the adolescent personality that facilitate innovative strivings. For example, many adolescents are typically idealistic. I cannot say whether it is true for artists, although I strongly suspect it is, but all of the highly gifted scientists I have had the opportunity to analyze were passionately idealistic (Giovacchini 1965). Within the adolescent's psyche, the intensity of the ego-ideal may be another favorable element that can be used for the promotion of creative activity.

Characterological features that are considered more or less typical of adolescence are involved in the creative process. I believe there are developmental tasks that propel a person toward the goal of being creative but which in most instances fail to achieve this aim. In some respects, failure is inevitable. The truly innovative person can convert what most often is experienced as inevitable failure into a higher level of psychic structure never being aware that his initial goal could not be achieved. He has, in effect, shifted goals as he changes his idealized objects, but before proceeding further in this discussion I will have to offer some illustrative clinical material.

Clinical Illustrations

I will first present a patient, a scientist, whom I analyzed as an adult after he had already made his mark in the world. I will focus, however, upon what I learned about his adolescence. This patient's creativity had reached fruition before entering analysis but his psychopathology interfered with his being able to continue to perform at such high levels.

When I first saw the patient, a man in his late thirties, he described his childhood and adolescence as being fairly happy. He was the second born of three children, having two sisters who adored him and, from what I gathered, still did. His father was a successful businessman who reputedly had his share of charisma. The mother, said to be a beautiful woman, apparently doted on the patient and immensely enjoyed his precociousness.

The patient was gifted and a fast learner. His father, who was somewhat scholarly, started giving his son private lessons when the patient was only two years old. He was told that he was taught arithmetic and could multiply and divide by the age of three. At four, he knew Euclidean geometry and was able to construct his own theorems. He was also taught geography and history by his father, but by the time he started school he had already outstripped his father in all of these subjects, pursuing them on his own and having developed a voracious appetite for reading books.

Contrary to being the typical bookish type, he was popular with his peers and had an outstanding number of playmates. He was also very active physically and preferred sports that stressed individual skills, such as boxing and wrestling, rather than team sports such as baseball. He played hard.

In school, he was rapidly advanced and was graduated from elementary school at the age of nine. He was able to straddle successfully different frames of reference. In the classroom he was the youngest and smallest as well as the smartest. Nevertheless, he did not threaten anyone even though he usually was the teacher's favorite. The bigger boys did not resent him because, in the physical area, he was no competition. Instead, they used him to help them; he actually did their homework for them. Since he could do it without any effort, he gladly complied. The girls thought he was "cute" and tended to mother him. He told me, with a nostalgic wistful look, how he remembered the older girls hugging him and how he loved the smell of their perfume. Apparently his female teachers were also in the habit of hugging him, something he still thought about fondly.

Outside the classroom he played with boys his size and age and he was comfortable there too. They admired his intellect, but since they had no competitive strivings in that area, they were content to just give him a nickname such as "the genius" and let it go at that. With his peers, he was accepted more as a teacher rather than as a follower and he enjoyed the position he was placed in.

At this point we might wonder why anyone with a childhood such as this, so talented and engaging and being loved by everyone, would, as an adult, be seeing a psychiatrist. Later I will briefly refer to his adult psychopathology, which at first appeared to be surprisingly severe, a schizophrenic decompensation, but which turned out to be considerably less serious.

In retrospect, the patient became aware of difficulties with his father, beginning in early childhood. He was admired by all members of his family but, he was, nevertheless, afraid of his father. At first, he viewed him as a strong, stern character who could easily lose his temper, but he had a tender loving side as well. Perhaps what disturbed the patient most was his father's emotional lability.

By the time he was five, so he reported, he had become aware that his mother hardly ever talked about her husband. From the mother's conversation, it seemed as if he did not exist. When the patient moved beyond the confines of his home and came in contact with other adults, as happens in school, he was able to make comparisons. He also noted that on the rare occasions his mother or older sister spoke about his father, they were subtly depreciating.

The patient, during the oedipal phase and early postoedipal period, had many omnipotent fantasies which continued well into adolescence, although by then they were cast in erotic tones. During childhood he would build enormous space ships in his mind and travel to and discover distant planets. He would also encounter all types of obstacles which he always successfully overcame. He would fight monsters and giants.

His dreams were especially interesting in that he had a large number of what psychologists call lucid dreams and which are said to occur particularly in creative persons. A lucid dream is one in which the dreamer is aware of the fact that he is dreaming. These are pleasant dreams in that one can do all kinds of things, satisfy diverse needs, take unusual risks, and since it is only a dream no one can get hurt. A lucid dream this patient still remembered involved his being able to fly and possess prodigious strength as evidenced by his ability to lift steamships and buildings.

As he began to idealize a teacher who had become intensely involved with him, the patient began to deidealize his father. He began to see his father's shortcomings; that underneath some superficial bluster, he was passive and submissive to his wife and older daughter. He also reported that now he feels his father could not have helped being jealous of him. Still, in spite of his superior position, one part of the patient was still afraid of the father.

He emphasized his conflicting viewpoints. On the one hand, he was clearly the victor in the oedipal triangle. On the other, he had an internalized image of his father as a powerful, strong, wise man. When the patient measured himself alongside his father, he felt inferior, a feeling he had seldom experienced.

He became passionately involved in science. Even in his prepuberty years he had a reverential awe for what he was learning and the teachers who taught him. As he advanced in school he always managed to have at least one teacher whom he idealized and who, in turn, would admire and encourage the patient to develop fully his talents. This sequence was especially interesting because some of his mentors would reveal their own personal hopes and aspirations. One particular instructor, of whom the patient was especially fond, spoke with almost religious fervor about a very famous scientist whose genius revolutionized the field he specialized in. This instructor would have liked to have studied under his tutelage, but he was not good enough to achieve this coveted position. My patient did, in fact, get his Ph.D. under this scientist and became almost equally famous.

Afterward, he continued idealizing although the objects of his idealization became increasingly more abstract. He idealized his work and the principles and goals of science, which he saw as the objective search for truth. Among the numerous books he had read, Michael Pupin's (1925) autobiography particularly impressed him since he had the same propensity for idealization of an abstraction. Pupin, for example, wrote "every American college and university could raise an invisible capital consecrated to the eternal truth and fill it with the icons of the great saints of science." He added that the "saints of science" imparted their knowledge (that is, their secrets) to their "sons," the younger, eager, sincere students of science.

Compared to his childhood, my patient's adolescence was relatively unhappy. In both high school and later at the university, he continued attracting people because of his academic brilliance as well as his personal charm. However, he was aware of a developmental lag. By the time he passed through puberty, his colleagues seemed to be well established in their sexual identity and social relationships. He was no longer satisfied being cast in the role of the young ladies' "darling." Instead, he wanted a girlfriend and a sexual partner, but he could not believe that any girl would relate to him at that level. He now suffered from feelings of inadequacy and felt defeated in an area in which he felt he did not have the endowments required for success. He thought that other young men were better looking, stronger, and more appealing.

As might be expected, he was extremely sensitive and was easily wounded by any rebuff, actual or imagined. He tried to overcome his sense of inferiority by directly confronting what he feared. During his first year at the university, he mustered his courage and started asking girls for dates. His record of success did not please him, but he managed to go out occasionally and petted fairly heavily. He also joined a fraternity, carousing a good deal with his fraternity brothers. In summary, there was some heterosexual activity, but most of his time was spent in "bull sessions" and drinking beer. He was also aware that he was covering up for his basic sense of insecurity. In the sexual area he felt very much a failure.

Academically, he continued in his usual brilliant fashion. There was no problem too difficult for him and soon he had a reputation for being able to do anything. In this regard there was an aura of omnipotence about him. He actually believed he could create at will.

His capacity for visual imagery was developed to the point that he could conjure pictures of pages he had read when he needed the information written on those pages. He did not exactly have a photographic memory, but he had the ability to produce eidetic images. He could also visualize a solution and then reproduce it and, in his mind, have a rather effortless resolution of an extremely complicated, difficult problem. Interestingly, after adolescence, his eidetic experiences disappeared although he is still able to have powerfully vivid visual experiences.

Again, the responses of his fellow students were surprising, as were the patient's response to his own talents. His peers apparently identified with his grandiosity, as evidenced by their enthusiasm and pride when they talked about his "miraculous" feats of intellect. They were proud to know him personally since he was gradually becoming a legend. Equally remarkable was that he was in no way arrogant or prepossessing. In spite of a megalomania which seemed to say, "if I can see it, that is, if I can conjure it in my mind, then it exists," he accepted this in a calm, unobtrusive fashion, and he did not threaten others.

He endeared himself to his colleagues by being interested in their interests. There was nothing that he found dull. Though deeply immersed in science, he also found his other subjects, the humanities, history, art, and music fascinating. He was a good listener as well as an eloquent speaker. Still, everything was not well.

In the sexual area he remained very insecure. The polarities were striking. Basically he considered himself a failure. He became increasingly shy around girls, and when he started graduate school, he stopped dating altogether. He became sufficiently depressed and so concerned that he contacted a psychiatrist but stopped seeing him after several months because he did not feel any better about himself. Nevertheless, he continued to do extremely well in his work, and it was this success that sustained him.

Creative persons operate within broad spectrums, a fact this patient illustrated in various ways. He demonstrated many of the qualities that have been considered characteristically associated with the creative process. He was grandiose but not arrogant, inquisitive and curious but not intrusive, and although he valued what he did to the degree of idealization, he could also appreciate the involvement and enthusiasm of others for areas in which he had little interest, such as economics and business. Roe (1953) and Stein (1953) outlined traits and qualities commonly found in the true innovator. The sense of failure, however, was not on their lists.

The clinician could rather easily focus upon elements of this patient's past history and make speculative formulations which would explain his adolescent sense of sexual inadequacy. Freud (1905) emphasized how conflicts, including guilt as well as castration anxiety, are reawakened after the latency period and during the early prepubertal period. Blos (1966) also refers to the reawakening of old conflicts during adolescence. Do feelings of inadequacy, during what many authors have considered the vulnerable period of adolescence, necessarily constitute psychopathology? Is this sense of inevitable failure perhaps part of the process of facing adult aspirations, such as sexual satisfaction, with the psychic equipment of childhood?

My patient, having sought treatment as an adult for very disturbing symptoms, indicated that his conflicts were more than just the manifestations of the insecurities inherent in a developmental phase. We can ask if his situation is a matter of degree in which ordinary occurrences become intensified to psychopathological proportions.

In the same context, we have to examine how his creative talents were related to his dilemma. Were they simply artifacts that ran parallel to his intrapsychic conflicts, thereby leading to what seemed to be enigmatic contradictions to his characterological orientation? Certainly his good feelings about his scientific proclivities and his bad feelings about his heterosexual capacities and their social extensions did not cancel each other out; this was not a neutralizing interaction (Hartmann 1955). Furthermore, the bad feelings did not "spoil" the good ones (Klein 1929). If not peacefully, they were at least able to coexist. Again, the creative factor may be implicated in that such an ego is able to keep separate these two aspects of the psyche with what we can identify as a special strength, a special ego capacity of the creative character structure.

From another perspective, we can consider whether creative talents or the infantile environment in which they developed lead to vulnerabilities which become manifest during adolescence and adulthood. I believe that focusing upon these issues will provide us with further insights about both the creative and the adolescent process and their psychopathological vicissitudes.

Another patient, an adolescent, was known to be gifted but failed to perform up to his enormous potential. He was so obviously disturbed during adolescence—in contrast to the first patient—that he and his family sought intensive treatment while he was a freshman in college.

When I first saw him, he had all the symptoms that Erikson (1959) described as constituting the "identity diffusion syndrome." Several months after having started college his personal habits broke down completely. He stopped bathing, shaving, brushing his teeth, and socially functioning altogether. He just sat in his dormitory room doing nothing. Finally, his classmates took him to see the student-health psychiatrist, who at first diagnosed him as an acute schizophrenic.

However, after his parents came to visit, the patient became less apathetic and did not have the signs and symptoms of a psychosis. He gave the appearance of a frightened, confused young man who had very little self-confidence and an amorphously constructed identity sense. The parents questioned whether analysis might be feasible, and since the patient also seemed to show some interest in intensive treatment, he was referred to me.

The patient is an only child of a wealthy, socially prominent family. Both parents are talented successful persons. From an early age, the patient showed considerable proclivity for mathematics and various branches of science—physics, chemistry, and biology. He was also interested in astronomy but dealt with it as a fascinating hobby. His parents were proud of him and doted on him. They bought him powerful telescopes, and during adolescence big motorcycles and expensive sports cars. The patient enjoyed them, but he never felt truly happy. Something was missing in that he could not experience a solid sense of gratification and fulfillment.

The father did not expect his son to succeed him in the empire he had created. He prided himself about his liberal attitudes and his respect for autonomy. I learned later that both he and his wife had been analyzed. In view of his son's interest in biology, he had hoped that he would seek a career in medicine. Ostensibly, however, he did not push him, but he did once joke when his son was only two years old that he would give him complete freedom of career choice—that he could go to any medical school he chose.

My patient quickly revealed how much he revered his parents and how he basically hated himself. The latter was based principally on his failure to live up to the expectations his parents had of him. He felt even worse because he had nothing to rebel against. These were expectations he felt they had of him, but he could not justifiably accuse anyone of having imposed anything upon him.

During treatment, it became slowly apparent that he experienced the infantile environment as oppressive to his autonomy. As an adolescent he became aware of painful feelings which he described as disruptive agitation. When he was taken to the student health clinic, he was deeply disturbed. He had withdrawn completely from the external world because he believed he could not hold himself together. He described feeling as if he would "explode," and there was nothing he could find that would calm him. The underlying sense of futility, misery, and hopelessness was most impressive. He reviled himself mercilessly for his lack of accomplishment in view of the tremendous advantages and opportunities he had had all his life. He stressed his failure.

At the same time, he was not without some grandiosity. His narcissism was not totally depleted as it might have seemed at first. In the back of his mind, he was convinced that he had the capacity to make momentous discoveries. During his treatment he often seemed megalomanic. He boasted about his brilliance, his photographic memory, and how he could conduct experiments that would prove the validity or invalidity of various controversial hypotheses. However, when he entered the area of mental development and health he was naive and sophomoric and for the most part incomprehensible, so it was difficult for me to determine whether he was being delusional about these capacities. I had no inclination to challenge him, and even if I had, the rather dismal picture he painted of himself would have forced me to remain silent.

To reinforce the assumption that I am discussing creativity when I present material about my adolescent patient, I merely need to add that some ten years later he made various discoveries that revolutionized some aspects of the industry in which he worked.

We can also profitably explore how creative ability relates to this curious clinical phenomenon.

Mental Mechanisms and Ego Developmental Processes

Both patients demonstrated a curious clinical phenomenon: contradictory ego states existing almost simultaneously. The first patient displayed the coexistence of grandiosity and a sense of failure. The second patient could feel megalomanic at the end of a session which had been dominated by bitter self-recriminations. This young man, because of the quantitative exaggeration of psychopathology, made clearer the processes and character traits illustrating certain parallelisms between elements of the creative process, adolescent character consolidation, and ego development. A mechanism, for example, which might be essential to creativity may decompensate into a pathological defense or become involved in a disintegrative, regressive current, causing it to lose adaptive and creative capacities.

I am referring specifically to dissociation, the splitting mechanisms that have been so frequently implicated in borderline psychopathology (Kernberg 1975). This mental mechanism, however, can be taken out of the context of psychopathology and viewed in terms of its adaptive capacities inasmuch as it permits the ego to continue functioning at very high levels and to reach innovative states of integration which lead to production of creative products or consolidations. Both patients used dissociation extensively, but the first patient was able to maintain self-esteem and to function efficiently and creatively.

Is dissociation a similar defense for these patients as it is for non-creative patients? Does it allow them to maintain psychic equilibrium? Ordinarily we think of defenses as reestablishing a balance, a compensation to counteract the decompensatory effects of psychopathology. At best this can be considered a psychopathological equilibrium because while the psyche expends a tremendous amount of energy to maintain a precarious balance, we would not expect there would be enough remaining for creative activity.

This was not true for the first patient. He was very productive as he maintained the split between those parts of his personality that bordered on the grandiose and megalomanic and those that caused him to feel inadequate and a failure. In fact, it seemed necessary to have the capacity to effect such a dissociation if he were able to continue functioning at such a high level. In later adulthood he temporarily lost this capacity and he was unable to continue with his creative work. The second patient could not function because he could not use dissociation well enough. He had some grandiose moments, but they were not highly cathected, as was his sense of inevitable failure.

Eissler (1958) tells of a similar situation with Goethe, who apparently had an "encapsulated" psychosis and was able to keep the creative and psychotic parts of his psyche separate. When he was unable to do so, his psychotic parts dominated and rendered him unable to function. However, it was part of his genius that he could reinstate splitting mechanisms.

Does the concept of splitting, as I use it here, correspond exactly to the dissociation we find in severe psychopathology? Inasmuch as we formulate dissociation as a mechanism in which connections within the ego are dissolved, then I believe something similar happened with my patients. This is an intraego process and involves similar levels in the psychic hierarchy; whatever splitting occurs involves the same ego subsystems. For example, in my patients we witness dissociation of the self-representation rather than of executive skills.

Norbert Wiener, the father of cybernetics, exemplifies various types of dissociation. It is reported that he was so poorly coordinated that it was necessary for his secretary to write on the blackboard for him. Yet when Wiener was doing research in a hospital in Mexico City he was a favorite among the interns. He would become involved in their two most popular pastimes, wrestling and chess. I naturally surmised that he must have been a chess master but an ineffectual, unskilled, and awkward wrestler. I was completely wrong; he was the best wrestler and the worst chess player of the group.

Regarding memory, Dr. Wiener was well known for his almost total recall for practically everything he had ever read. Still, there is an apocryphal anecdote at the Massachusetts Institute of Technology, where Dr. Wiener held his academic appointment. Around noon he was walking along and encountered a colleague. The two stopped to chat for a few minutes. Before departing, Dr. Wiener asked his friend in which direction he had been heading. After being told, he replied, "Then I haven't had lunch."

The dissociations discussed here are structurally similar to splitting mechanisms in general, but I believe there are fundamental differences. My first patient, at the time, and my second patient, later in life, had a minimum of, if any, dynamic interplay between the split-off parts of their egos. There was very little connection or continuity between the grandiose, competent self-representation and the inadequate, failing part of themselves. To maintain this separation, the first patient did not require large expenditures of psychic energy. His grandiosity and success did not constitute a compensatory defense against what he perceived as weakness and vulnerability. These were two states of mind that coexisted without intruding into each other. This isolation of structural configurations permitted him to make innovative discoveries, something the second patient could not do because he had not yet been able to achieve such a separation.

Psychopathology cannot be conceptualized on an absolute basis; it is always a matter of degree. Nevertheless, when discussing creativity, it is valuable to make as many distinctions as possible. Being able to effect a dissociation was a necessary psychic activity so that my patient could be creative. According to Eissler (1958) this was also true of Goethe. Can we then state that dissociation is a defense required for creative functioning? I cannot generalize, of course, but it is necessary for some. I would question, however, whether dissociation would be part of a defensive system if its outcome is the preservation of creativity. Here, we can distinguish an adaptation which maintains the highest level of functioning possible and a defense that protects against a psychotic breakdown.

We can question whether dissociation is fundamentally involved and intrinsically related to creativity. Both my patients emphasized how they were able to make use of splitting mechanisms since childhood. As I have stated, the patients and I concluded that their ability to not have various parts of their minds intrude into the other was a talent, a strength associated with creative capacity. Greenacre (1956) stressed that there are ego strengths, unusual discriminatory sensitivities, that are found in creative persons, but they cannot be considered etiological factors. Still, we can ask whether there are unique and special childhood environmental configurations that are particularly conducive for the development of creative ability, as Greenacre (1957) explored, or for the development of dissociative psychic mechanisms.

Environmental Factors and Psychopathology

Both patients had mothers who were unusually devoted to them. They were breast fed beyond the usual period well into the first year. The first patient actually had two mothers in that the oldest sister also doted upon him. Jones (1953) tells us about the devotion between Freud and his mother.

As their precocious talents flourished, they were increasingly idealized inasmuch as others joined the admiring throng. It would seem that they were able to incorporate life experiences, that is, to integrate them into their memory systems, since they were so gratifying. With the increased self-esteem that was produced, they proceeded to further accomplishments. This would, in a sense, constitute a positive feedback, and since there was so much harmony between the inner and outer world there would not seem to be much need for dissociative mental mechanisms.

This is where their fathers enter the picture. The first patient emphasized his disillusionment. When he viewed his father from a more realistic perspective, he was able to see that underneath the facade of competence and self-confidence his father was insecure and not successful. His mother reinforced this picture. The second patient's father, by contrast, was indeed, successful. Still, as the patient grew older he became unhappy with the materialistic attitudes that surrounded him. He wondered about his father's ethics and integrity and became less and less pleased with the gifts that his father lavished on him.

When I first saw my adolescent patient, he was, as I have described, in a state of identity diffusion. In addition to having lost, relatively

47

speaking, his sense of identity, he was in a painful quandary about his value system. He did not know what he aspired toward and what he could respect. On the one hand, he regretted the crass materialism of his father's world, but at the same time he was perceptive enough to know how pleasant and comfortable the state of lack of want could be. He enjoyed his sports cars, for example, but he felt he should not.

As treatment progressed, he relived this conflict in the transference. He reviled himself for having no integrity and for being rich and privileged. This was not the ideal image he wanted for himself. He would then attack me because of the way I lived, my high fees, and other qualities that he attributed to the materialistic, greedy Establishment. These angry attitudes are not unusual during adolescence, but what distinguished my patient was his ready propensity to internalize his feelings against himself. It became clear that he was projecting and reintrojecting his father imago.

He had been able to keep his idealization of his mentors and science dissociated from the image of the father who, during latency years, had fallen from grace. This accounted for both his self-aggrandizement and self-depreciation. The latter was the outcome of his introjected father, but as he was hating himself, he was also attacking his father.

When he first started treatment, the first patient was phenomenologically psychotic. He was an angel in God's entourage and at war with the devil and his cohorts. The split between good and evil had reached paranoid proportions, but his psychosis, if that is what it was, was colorful and even entertaining rather than grim and painful. For example, he patterned his "delusions" around the plot of Anatole France's fascinating novel, *The Revolt of the Angels,* where the forces of evil and the forces of good were not only juxtaposed but reversed. The protagonist's guardian angel rejected God and wanted him replaced by the devil.

He began treatment by challenging me to analyze him and for a long time he would not lie down on the couch. He was suspicious of me, accused me of working for the Mafia and of wanting to destroy his brain. He soon saw me as the devil but he also saw himself as behaving devilishly. At times he was the guardian angel and at other times he was the protagonist, somewhat of an amoral libertine who preaches virtue to an angel who does not believe in God. He reenacted this interplay with me, and I must confess that some of his sessions were amusing, something I seldom feel with psychotic patients. He often told me of a particular conversation between the guardian angel and the protagonist, Maurice. The angel is arguing with Maurice and trying to enlist his aid in order to raise funds so that he can organize a cadre of angels and dethrone God and replace him with the devil. As the angel argues more and more heatedly, Maurice, in an astonished voice, exclaims that it seems that the angel does not believe in God. The angel replies that, of course he believes in God, his very existence depends upon that belief but he protests that his is not a just God.

As long as he mixed his delusions with the plot of the novel, he was animated and comfortable although he was totally paralyzed as far as work was concerned. However, as he gradually internalized the feelings attached to them, he began experiencing the same coexistence of grandiosity and self-debasement and confusion my adolescent patient experienced. He also projected and reintrojected the hated parts in the transference as well as later idealizing me. Both patients carried their idealizations from my person to psychoanalysis in general.

The adolescent patient's psychopathology intensified to the point where he could not function during his teenage years, and he was not able to achieve his creative potential until late in young adulthood. It is doubtful that he would have been able to reach the heights he did without treatment. In some respects, the other patient had a difficult adolescence but he still functioned continuously at a very high level until he had his "psychotic" decompensation.

Perhaps the relationship of these patients to their fathers may have been a variable that determined whether psychopathology or creativity would gain the upper hand. The adolescent patient deidealized his father, but that did not change anything. His father continued being powerful and competent. The disillusionment concerned only one facet of his character; that which involved moral integrity. This father remained strong whereas with the other patient, the father was totally discredited. The latter patient later developed symptoms that have been associated with severe psychopathology, but he was able more easily to cling to his grandiosity and be sustained by it than was the young man. The depreciated father did not threaten his megalomania, whereas the adolescent's father's strength interfered with the patient's capacity to generate a level of self-esteem that would permit him to function and he was not able to maintain an effective dissociation between the valued and devalued parts (the paternal introject) of the psyche.

I want to mention briefly what caused these patients to decompensate and the outcome of their therapy since these are peripheral issues to the subject of creativity. The adolescent, as mentioned, could not integrate himself into his new college environment. This is a common situation with youngsters who suffer from the identity diffusion syndrome. He found himself in an environment without the usual supports. Furthermore, his adolescent sexual urges and the expectations that he be successful sexually as well as intellectually were significant stresses that caused his usual adaptations to be ineffective. The first patient's illness began after his father died. His megalomanic orientation overwhelmed him. Besides the guilt he felt at a more structured level, the omnipotence of his thoughts, or more precisely of his destructive feelings, received reality validation with his father's actual death. He had to set a massive dissociation in motion to keep his hostility from invading his ego and destroying his megalomania. He devised the colorful delusions that I have already described.

As a transference object, I was alternately assigned the role of omnipotent ally or depreciated persecutor for both patients. The latter, however, was not a grim paranoid relationship. They viewed me as someone benign but, because I valued creativity, jealous of their innovative prowess—one who would steal their ideas to become more powerful than they. They also playfully teased me about my inferiority. They had a need to feel sexually superior to me, but they were secure in the feeling that they could surpass me intellectually.

This material is not difficult to deal with analytically. They both understood that I was not threatened by either side of their ambivalence as I interpreted the transference projections. I let myself, on occasion, stray from the strictly analytic orientation by becoming interested and involved with some of the fascinating ideas they brought me. I knew they were trying to capture my interest, and they often succeeded in doing so.

The adult scientist gradually relinquished his delusional system in an unobtrusive manner. It seemed simply to disappear by blending with his creative thoughts. After several years of treatment, he terminated because he was offered an extremely attractive position in another city. From time to time, he sends me a postcard indicating that all is well and that he continues working with an almost hypomanic fervor.

The adolescent is now an adult, married, and has children. Curiously, his creativity is in the industrial realm where he has made vast sums of money for himself and his employers, including his father, a major stockholder in the company.

Omnipotence and Creativity

The truly creative product, whether it is material or an idea, constitutes something that has never previously existed. Even if its component parts are known, their combination is novel. In a sense, the creator can be thought of as producing something from nothing. Of course, the fundamental law of conservation of matter and energy does not permit a something-from-nothing sequence, but in the mind of the creator this seems to be the case and inasmuch as he has such a belief, he is being omnipotent because reputedly, only God has achieved such a feat. The sense of omnipotence and creativity are intrinsically related to each other.

The scientist patient, when he had achieved considerable integration during treatment would calmly relate how he could "will" himself to have an idea. He would describe his mind as being empty. He would then "command" himself to think of something brilliant and there, as if by magic, it would appear. We both knew it was neither that simple, effortless, or magical; that his training, experience, and knowledge were operating at levels below perceptual awareness.

As I have emphasized elsewhere (Giovacchini 1965) about the creative person, these patients did not seem at all arrogant when they talked about this feeling of omnipotence. In no way was the scientist patient offensive, and it seemed that others did not experience him in that fashion. He was casual and, although proud of his talents, not prepossessing, nor did he deprecate others who generally did not approach his level of performance. On the contrary, he respected the efforts others made and was even naively accepting of ideas that, on closer inspection, often proved to be pedantic and sophomoric.

There was an idealistic quality to his feeling of omnipotence. Ordinarily we think of idealization as consisting of the idealization of a person, an institution, or a cause. My patient idealized his own creative potential, which he considered to be a "gift from God." He had the same attitude that some very talented tenors have about their "golden" voices such as Caruso and more recently, Pavarotti, who refer to their voices as something God gave them to keep. This is an interesting combination of megalomania and modesty. The implication is that the possessors of these talents do not deserve any special credit; they were privileged in that they were bestowed these gifts by a deity for the good of mankind. They have obligations in view of this sacred trust.

Kris (1952) stressed that the creative act, in addition to the construction of something new, involves communication. The creator has to have an audience who understands what he has done. Whether or not he accomplishes this is not the point. While creating he is synthesizing and integrating in such a fashion that it is potentially understandable. My scientist patient and other scientists I have treated sought analysis because, among other reasons, they possessed a gift they could not use. They meant that they felt they could not maintain contact with the external world which heightened their sense of painful alienation.

Inevitable Failure

Adolescence, according to some authors (Blos 1966) is a stage of life in which some developmental tasks which could not be dealt with in childhood are confronted once again. Arnstein (1979) questions whether crisis is a necessary factor in the quest for identity. Sharfstein (1978) emphasizes that creative activity enhances the progression on the path toward autonomy.

Freud (1905) states that the child, as his sexual instincts develop, will experience failure which will create a breach in infantile omnipotence. This will carry over as a sense of failure in the early postpubertal age of adolescence.

According to Freud (1914), early developmental stages from auto-erotism to the secondary narcissism of beginning object relationships are characterized by a sense of omnipotence if the infantile environment has been optimally gratifying. Though there are inevitable frustrations throughout the course of development because instantaneous gratification is not possible nor, according to Freud even desirable, on the whole, the child knows that his needs can be met and that he is capable of being gratified.

In any case, when the child in early childhood faces strong oedipal urges, there is no possibility of gratification. For the child gratification would mean victory over the giant adult of the same sex. It would also mean that he has the somatic equipment by which he can achieve heterosexual satisfaction which, of course, he does not. The little boy cannot successfully pursue the goal of sexually possessing his mother. At this oedipal level, failure is inevitable. Thus, the sexual instincts become associated with failure. It might also be said that there is an asynchrony between instinctual development and the acquisition of the appropriate somatic apparatus that could be incorporated in the ego's executive apparatus which will enable a person to experience sexual fulfillment. From this viewpoint, instinctual precocity is part of normal emotional development.

It is often very difficult to distinguish what constitutes an aspect of normal development from the manifestations of cultural norms or the outcome of psychopathology. This has been an especially hard distinction to make when we study the adolescent phenomenon. Nevertheless, it is a frequent enough occurrence that the child develops feelings of vulnerability and inadequacy during the oedipal phase and that these feelings are reawakened with the biologically stimulated sexual urges of the postpubertal period. They are then felt in a pervasive fashion as a sense of inevitable failure in the anticipation of a heterosexual relationship. Establishing a sexual relationship becomes a perplexing problem.

There has been considerable cultural support for the maintenance of the sexual mystique. From a masculine viewpoint, women can never be understood by men; they are attractive but unfathomable creatures. They represent a problem that can never be solved and man will always remain inadequate in the face of its enormity.

These attitudes fit better with a mid-Victorian milieu or any society in which sexuality is to a large measure repressed. In view of the current liberal attitudes about sex this orientation would not be expected to be prevalent. Nevertheless, it is not an unusual one among a fair number of adolescents and some adults, not necessarily patients seeking treatment. However, I have seen it invariably among the creative men I have had the opportunity to analyze throughout the years.

I have discussed a scientist (Giovacchini 1971) who avidly pursued different women and who had married several times because he wanted to make their behavior predictable. Otherwise, he felt inferior and a failure. He had to master a problem and this compulsion to seek solutions carried over onto his creative work.

He illustrated an interesting conclusion first reached by Zeigarnik (1927). A completed task does not keep a person's interest. Once the problem is solved there is little further investment in it. For the creator, it loses its cathexis, or at least, its major force since he remains proud of his accomplishment. However, the act of accomplishing is much more important than what is accomplished. Zeigarnik discovered experimentally that an unfinished task, that is, an unsolved problem, retains its cathexis. If abandoned, it still vividly remains in the person's mind. Even after years have passed, an incomplete action is easily remembered in contrast to completed tasks. My patients constantly had unfinished tasks even after they gained security in the sexual area.

Creativity, Precocity, and Psychic Structure

Regardless of psychological factors, in the final breakdown, creativity is a quality found in persons with special gifts. There must be an inherent constitutional factor of which we know practically nothing. However, there are attributes of innate talent that can be understood in terms of both emotional and psychic developmental factors. I have already presented clinical material emphasizing such elements, but now I wish to derive some generalizations from data obtained from the treatment of patients.

The creative persons I have treated, read about, or known showed their proclivities early in childhood. They were destined for greatness. I know there are exceptions but, in general, the creative scientist was usually precocious and attracted attention while still very young.

Psychoanalysts have discovered that precocity may be the outcome of psychopathology, a defensive response to a traumatic assaultive infantile environment (Bergmann and Escalona 1949; Boyer 1956). The patients I have reported found that their precocity helped them maintain psychic equilibrium; whether it was primarily a defensive adaptation is difficult to determine. In view of their later creative accomplishments, it is not surprising that their talents would flourish early. Their precocity led to success.

The precociousness of the sexual instinct Freud (1905) wrote about and that of the creative person permits some interesting comparisons. Freud was referring to instinctual precocity, whereas in creative persons I am emphasizing an early unfolding, a premature appearance of talents. The ego's integrative functions and executive apparatus develop and structuralize to a degree that is further advanced that what is usual for that particular age period. In contrast to what Freud was describing, precocity here refers to overdevelopment of certain aspects of psychic structure relative to instinctual organization, the reverse of his formulation in which the instinct, the sexual instinct, is further ahead developmentally than the rest of the psyche. To repeat, these are two antithetical situations, two types of precocity: (1) psychic structure outstrips instinct and (2) instinct outstrips psychic structure.

The first type of precociousness is associated with creativity whereas the second type, according to Freud, is innate to infantile development.

In the former, precociousness can become the vehicle for a successful, creative adaptation; the latter is always doomed to failure. My patients, especially the scientists, demonstrated this peculiar combination of success and failure. Is such a combination a necessary condition to activate the creative process?

We do not know what psychological variables are involved in creativity. The psychic processes of adolescence, however, often seem to be related to creative activity. For example, as an adolescent the scientist had the capacity for eidetic imagery and a photographic memory, but these abilities diminished as an adult. He did not totally lose them but they had reached their peak during his college years.

During adolescence, there is considerable rearrangement of various psychic agencies which finally lead to character consolidation. With puberty, there is a biological heightening of sexual impulses. Unlike the child, the adolescent now has the somatic equipment to seek sexual gratification, but he does not yet have the psychic structure and orientation that would enable him to have a satisfactory experience. During adolescence, he recapitulates the oedipal failure of childhood.

The creative person can convert his failure into success. The heightened excitation induced by the hormonal accretions of puberty produces a generally higher energy level which is not restricted to sexual urges. There is an all-pervasive zest for life in the well-adjusted adolescent. For the creative or potentially creative adolescent, this energy is harnessed to serve his talent which had precociously appeared in childhood. In other words, a connection is established between precocious psychic structure and instinctual activity. Thus, sensual urges that were associated with inevitable failure during childhood become linked with successful activities and this begins during adolescence.

I do not mean that creativity is the outcome of sublimated sexual energy. I am purposely leaving the concept of psychic energy vague because I do not wish to engage in irrelevant controversy in the context of this discussion. Rather, I am stressing that to gratify needs and to function generally requires energy. This energy is used in many ways, both sexual and nonsexual. The task of adolescence is to acquire psychic structure so that a variety of needs, including sexual, can be gratified and to use the upsurge of energy that occurs with maturation in a harmonious and efficient fashion.

Instinctual forces are associated with primitive psychic levels. During the course of emotional development, there is a structural progression which establishes a hierarchy. The psyche can be thought of as a spectrum between the primitive, relatively unstructured and instinctual to well-integrated, differentiated structures that function at secondary process levels. These two ends of the spectrum are joined together by intermediary levels which are established as a smooth continuum. This continuum or bridge is poorly established in the precocious psyche of childhood and during adolescence.

During the creative act, primitive parts of the psyche governed principally by the primary process come in apposition to structured secondary-process levels. There is no bridge between the two. The continuum is temporarily relinquished. As stated, psychic structures that developed precociously become connected with instinctual elements without a modulatory bridge between the two. This lack of a bridge is characterized by what appears to be the coexistence of contradictory elements, as if the psyche were split or dissociated. The creative act culminates in a synthesis and a reestablishment of a connecting bridge which serves as a continuum.

The lack of a continuum between various levels of the psyche, as it occurs with the precocious child and during adolescence, may produce a creative person or it may lead to psychopathology or both. There are many factors which determine the final outcome as my patients demonstrated.

Conclusions

The lack of rigidity in the adolescent's character structure could provide a fertile setting for the realization of creative potential. Fluidity of character structure, however, could also be an element in the production of psychopathology and the combination of creative ability and emotional illness seems to be fairly common.

Still, comparisons and combinations do not mean that there are causal connections between what is being studied. Similarities may be only at the surface level. For example, during the creative act, the creator may seem to be using primitive psychic mechanisms such as dissociation. He may also appear to be indulging in magical thinking as evidenced by megalomania. However, on closer scrutiny, it becomes apparent that he is in control of the primitive within himself as he is simultaneously operating at higher levels of integration. The creator has a tremendous amount of energy which causes him to perceive and feel more intensely than usual.

I present two patients. The first demonstrated psychopathology in coexistence with creative capacities. His adolescence was characterized by an ego dissociation. One part of his psyche preserved his capacities for innovation, was experienced as pleasurable, and was associated with success, grandiosity, and high levels of self-esteem. The other part of his psyche contained the remnants of his childhood oedipal humiliation which he carried with him as a sense of failure and inadequacy. As long as he could maintain this dissociation he functioned well. Later as an adult he could not maintain this split and he developed symptoms that were phenomenologically psychotic but from a prognostic viewpoint not nearly so serious. The second patient decompensated into an identity diffusion syndrome during adolescence and did not realize his creative potential until after his treatment was terminated.

Various parts of the creator's psyche are hypertrophied, such as the perceptual apparatus and the ego ideal. Hypertrophied is not the most apt term because it implies constriction which is not at all the situation in creativity. I mean that these structures and functions are better developed than usual and that they become apparent earlier during the course of development. This can also be considered precocity.

I discuss two types of precocity: one characterizes the creative person and the other is an instinctual precocity which Freud (1905) postulated as typical of the sexual instinct. The former refers to ego functions and structures, such as the integrative system and the ego ideal which are advanced for the child's age, whereas the latter consists of oedipal sexual urges that are also premature in the sense that the ego does not have the apparatus to ensure their gratification. Thus, there is, on the one hand, a precocity of structure which heightens self-esteem and, on the other hand, a precocity of instinct which leads to feelings of inadequacy. Both my patients demonstrated the effects of these processes in the dissociation they experienced to a fairly intense degree during adolescence.

During the creative act the modulating bridge which forms a continuum between the primitive and the integrated structures parts of the personality is temporarily inoperative. During adolescence such a bridge is in the process of being established. The talented and secure youngster can take advantage of his relatively unstructured ego and use it for creative activity. This may be a reason why so many innovators, particularly mathematicians and physicists, have flourished during their youth.

The creative adult retains the capacity to reproduce an ego state in which connecting bridges and continuums are abolished. He is reproducing and reliving an adolescent ego state, a vibrancy and youthful zest which is the essence of the creative process.

NOTE

Presented as a plenary address on October 24, 1980, at the meetings of the Eastern Seaboard Adolescent Societies.

REFERENCES

Arnstein, R. 1979. The adolescent identity crisis revisited. *Adolescent Psychiatry* 7:71–84.

Bergmann, P., and Escalona, S. 1949. Unusual sensitivities in very young children. *Psychoanalytic Study of the Child* 3-4:333–352.

Blos, P. 1966. *On Adolescence*. New York: International Universities Press.

Boyer, L.B. 1956. On maternal overstimulation and ego defects. *Psychoanalytic Study of the Child* 11:236–256.

Eissler, K. 1958. Goethe and science. In W. Muensterberger and S. Axelrad, eds. *Psychoanalysis and the Social Sciences*. New York: International Universities Press.

Erikson, E. 1959. *Identity and the Life Cycle*. New York: International Universities Press.

Freud, S. 1905. Three essays on the theory of sexuality. *Standard Edition* 7:135–243. London: Hogarth, 1953.

Freud, S. 1914. On narcissism: an introduction. *Standard Edition* 14: 69–102. London: Hogarth, 1957.

Giovacchini, P.L. 1960. On scientific creativity. *Journal of the American Psychoanalytic Association* 8:407–426.

Giovacchini, P.L. 1965. Some aspects of the development of the ego ideal of a creative scientist. *Psychoanalytic Quarterly* 34:79–101.

Giovacchini, P.L. 1971. Creativity and character. *Journal of the American Psychoanalytic Association* 19:524–542.

Greenacre, P. 1956. Experiences of awe in childhood. *Psychoanalytic Study of the Child* 11:9–30.

Greenacre, P. 1957. The childhood of the artist. *Psychoanalytic Study of the Child* 12:47–72.

Hartmann, H. 1955. Notes on the theory of sublimation. *Psychoanalytic Study of the Child* 10:9–29.

Jones, E. 1953. *The Life and Works of Sigmund Freud.* Vol.1. New York: Basic.

Kernberg, O. 1975. *Borderline Conditions and Pathological Narcissism.* New York: Aronson.

Klein, M. 1929. Infantile anxiety situations reflected in a work of art. *International Journal of Psycho-Analysis* 10:436–444.

Kris, E. 1952. *Psychoanalytic Exploration in Art.* New York: International Universities Press.

Pupin, M. 1925. *From Immigrant to Inventor.* New York: Scribner.

Roe, A. 1953. *The Making of a Scientist.* New York: Dodd, Mead.

Sharfstein, B. 1978. Adolescents and philosophers: a word in favor of both. *Adolescent Psychiatry* 6:51–58.

Stein, M. 1953. Creativity and culture. *Journal of Psychology* 32:311–322.

Zeigarnik, B. 1927. Das behalten erledigter und unerledigter handlung. *Psychologische Forschung* 9:1–85.

4   ADOLESCENCE, MOURNING, AND CREATIVITY

JON A. SHAW

Adolescence is the phase of life in which creativity flourishes. Anna Freud (1958) has noted that the adolescent is more artistic than he will ever be again. Some authors have suggested a relationship between prolonged adolescence and creativity (Eissler 1958; Spiegel 1958). Goethe, in a conversation with Eckermann (Luke and Pick 1966), stated that "extraordinary achievements will always be found to be allied with youth . . . natural geniuses have a special peculiarity. They experience a repetition of puberty, whereas other people are young only once." The creativity of adolescence, however, ceases for most individuals with the consolidation of the psychic apparatus around the twentieth year (Spiegel 1958).

It has been noted that the "only common feature among creative people is the greater fluidity of their access to the id, or earlier ego states and the primary process" (Bak 1958). This is clearly characteristic of the adolescent process as well. The adolescent process, like the artistic endeavor, is a regression in the service of the ego. As Blos (1967) has observed, "The task of psychic restructuring by regression represents the most formidable psychic work of adolescence." With the resolution of adolescence, there will be a consolidation of the psychic apparatus, with synthesis and integration of the discontinuities of development, the polarities of active-passive, male-female, sadism-masochism, and the multiple identity fragments of one's past. The central achievement of this process will be the attainment of a self, a unitary identity confirmed by one's own experience and by others. This can only be accomplished through a process of successful disengagement from the internalized infantile objects.

Adolescence has been likened to a mourning process, in which there is a gradual decathexis of the first love objects accompanied by sad and painful feelings and the realistic awareness of the irrevocability of the childhood past (Freud 1958; Wolfenstein 1966). Anna Freud (1958) observed that adolescence and mourning share the same painful process, of having to give up a position which holds out no further hope for return of love. This process of renunciation is associated with regression as the means by which the bits and pieces of a past, loved relationship are remembered, hypercathected, and reexperienced with an awareness that it can never be again. This increasing awareness—that the reveries of the past must be left memories—leaves the adolescent acutely aware of the transience of his experiences. Every acquisition of independent functioning obtained through the adolescent process will be associated with a sense of object loss. The adolescent mourning process will be completed when the adolescent decathects the infantile object representations and moves in the direction of achieving psychological and physical intimacy with a nonincestual heterosexual object.

The interrelationship between creativity, mourning, and adolescence is evident in the adolescent poetry of many well-known poets, such as Housman, Poe, and Plath, with their themes of time, loss, and death. In an attempt to understand further the relationship between adolescent poetry and adolescent mourning, a collection of poems written by a ninth-grade English class in a public school (Kensington Junior High School 1978) and a number of poems published in a pamphlet by adolescents in a private school (Sidwell Friends School 1978, 1979) were reviewed. This review indicated that the majority were concerned with themes of time, loss, death, and the transient nature of experiences. The lack of free associations necessarily limits our understanding of the manifest themes. A few brief examples will illustrate the existence of recurrent themes associated with the mourning process.

TIME

Time is a river, with eddies and swirls,
Watching over fate, like an oyster, her pearls.
It moves so slowly, like a creek, almost dry,
Yet no one ever asks, just why?

Slowly moving it seems to you,
But only when there's nothing to do,
Moving faster, when you're in a hurry,
But only it seems, to make you worry.
People live and people die
But, time is not human and cannot cry.

[Kensington Junior High School, Grade 9]

Comment. This poem graphically portrays the capriciousness of time; like a mother, she watches over her offspring while she negligently perpetuates death and "does not cry."

Looking back one last time at the mountains
One long, last gaze at their mystifying beauty
I love these mountains
And when I am gone I will miss them

The glowing red sunsets
The view from the top
And the brilliance of the stars

But what would it have meant had you not been there?
The sunsets were a deeper red with you by my side
The view much clearer as we sat together
And seeing a shooting star gave me joy
Only because you had seen it too

You taught me the things I may never have known
You shared with me what was closest to you

Now I must leave
But what you have taught me
I will always know
And what you have given me
I will always hold dear

When I look at the mountains
They will remind me of you
And when I think of you
I will smile.

[Sidwell Friends School, Grade 10]

Comment. This untitled poem depicts the regressive looking-backward to a paradise lost of moments shared with a loved object. The poem progresses to an awareness that one must leave behind those moments of a shared union to a new independence, where the reveries will become treasured memories of a lost time, immortalized in memory but no longer the object of one's search for gratification.

IMAGES OF FEAR 1–30

umbrellas are slipping away under
my feet in reflective puddles
oily slickness of the black wet night.
oh, mother
she plucked out my eyes
and fell plunging downward
so large with child—falling, falling.
I was so frightened.
oh,
it's back at my window tonight
scratching at the pane from the outside darkness
and me inside, frightened.
oh, father,
how I miss those insane days
of the KGB and subways and late night laughter
running through those dark wet streets.
umbrellas slipping away under
our feet in reflective puddles.
we feigned foreign accents
and giggled in the elevator
whispering obscenities at rich old women.
but words had more meaning then—
they were sharp and good, and never smothered me
like they do now.
now I eat those same words
I eat this paper up
spewing discordant lines
for the sake of it.
oh, mother—
they murdered you, and father is also dead
and I am alone—the black flame
alone, silencing away all that once was life.

so self absorbed—must I die too?
oh, mother,
I am frightened
those umbrellas are slipping away from under me
and I'm falling into reflective puddles.
falling, falling, like the pregnant woman and
it's on my windowsill.
I'm falling.

[Sidwell Friends School, Grade 12]

Comment. "Images of Fear" portrays the loving memory of childhood days and the painful awareness of separation. "oh, mother— /
they murdered you, and father is also dead / and I am alone. . . ." The
fear is that separation from the omnipotent parents may bring her own
death.

A DREAM

I always liked the clinking sound of those little glass bottles
    in your bottom drawer by the sink.
I like to open the drawer (closing it wasn't quite as good)
    and look at them because they were small, but mostly
    because they were yours.
Then you read Nietzsche and said God is dead which really bothered
    me then but I believe it now because all those little
    bottles are broken to bits (someone closed the drawer too hard).
And you weren't there, so I had to clean up all the smashed glass
    and throw away my childhood in a plastic bag.

[Sidwell Friends School, Grade 12]

Comment. "A Dream" relates the lost love and dreams invested in
the parents' world, but now "God is dead." One's childhood, like
shattered, broken glass, must become a memory left behind.

GROWING UP

I know you so well, like the back of my hand
I remember the silly game we made up
    the times we laughed until morning
    the times we cried into our pillows
    the long walks in winter snow

or in the stifling summer heat
We share laughter and words
   words which tumble unceasingly between us
   words we don't even have to speak
But, we grow older
Time and responsibilities come between us
Our paths cross less often
Yet,
Each time we meet, it's as if time were
   motionless and we never really part
We are spontaneous, there is no strain
I miss the dolls and tea parties
I miss the balls we danced at, the princes, the fairy godmothers
But the bonds of friendship remain strong
Even if we are growing up.

                         [Sidwell Friends School, Grade 11]

Comment. "Growing Up" nostalgically recalls the silly games, the long walks, the shared laughter, the empathic understanding of an early loved relationship. The dolls and tea parties, the fantasies of growing up now must be left behind, for one *is* grown up. The bonds of friendship will endure, not as infantile residues, but within the context of emerging reality and responsibilities.

RAINDROPS

Like a thousand gleaming teardrops,
Rolling down the window,
The rain seems like it never stops,
But falls to the ground below.

The rain is but an ocean,
Suspended in the air,
Fleeing in panicked motion,
To get away from there.

Droplets, small and round,
Swiftly falling through the sky,
Dashed against the rock and ground
Where they splash and die.

                    [Kensington Junior High School Grade 9]

Comment. "Raindrops" is a metaphor for teardrops of sadness and farewell, of ceaseless time, and of the tragedy of an individual life.

THE DEATH OF A BROTHER

The sun will die again tonight.
The sky with his blood glow.
The stars will shudder at this sight
And bright will gleam their woe.

The time has come, the old man thought
To lay it all aside
To leave the ones for whom I've fought
So like the sun, he died.

The stars and men will join together,
To comfort one another
For this for them is their true course,
And both have lost a brother.
[Kensington Junior High School, Grade 9]

Comment. "The Death of a Brother" describes the cycle of life and death. The old man, realizing the inevitability of death, "lay[s] it all aside," for he has had his time and—"like the sun"—he dies. The image is of a loving and caring firmament that joins with those men remaining to mourn the loss of life and the inevitability of their own death.

THE HEART IS NOT A PLAYTHING

The heart is not a plaything,
   the heart is not a toy
   but if you want it broken
   just give it to a boy.

They love to mess around a lot
   with things both said and done
   but when it comes to liking girls
   they do it just for fun.

So don't fall in love my friend
   listen to what I say,
   love doesn't follow any threats,
   it happens everyday.

You wonder where he is at night
   and why he doesn't call;
   he tells you that he loves you,
   but doesn't care at all.

Each time you are together
   your heart begins to fly;
   you build your world within him,
   but he only makes you cry.

Love is fine but hurts a lot,
   the price you pay is high;
   in choosing life and choosing death
   I think I'd rather die.

So don't fall in love my friend,
   it hurts because it's true
   you see my friend you ought to know
   I fell in love with you.

              [Kensington Junior High School, Grade 9]

Comment. "The Heart Is Not a Plaything" tells of the pathos of unrequited love, the folly of building "your world within him" when "he only makes you cry." The inevitable disappointment and transience of love seem to resonate with the inevitable disappointment and transience associated with the reawakening of the oedipal conflict in adolescence.

Discussion

While there is no single meaning to any work of art, there are a number of recurrent themes which reflect the enduring existential conflicts in human life. The theme of the transience of experience in the human condition has always been reflected in art. Freud (1916) anticipated some of the recent literature on the relationship between mourning and creativity. He tells of a summer walk through the countryside with a taciturn friend, a famous young poet. The poet lamented that all beauty was fated to extinction, that summer's beauty would vanish with winter. He could find no joy but only despondency where loss was anticipated. Freud took issue with the thought that the transience of beauty should interfere with our joy in it: "A flower that blossoms only for a single night does not seem to us on that account less lovely." In fact, Freud asks, does not the very transience of beauty increase our enjoyment? His argument had no effect on the poet. He concluded that the poet was in revolt against the painful process of mourning. It is only when mourning has occurred that transience can be accepted.

Creativity seems to stand in a complex relationship to mourning. It may be a denial of transience with an underlying assertion that beauty endures forever, while in other instances it may facilitate the work of mourning. It would seem that one aspect of adolescent poetry is that it represents the work of mourning. That which is remembered and loved is expressed lyrically and painfully decathected to become a fond and loving memory, paradoxically immortalized. If the mourning of the infantile objects is successful and if the transient experience is integrated, adolescence and perhaps the creative process may both come to an end.

In recent years there has been an increasing number of studies suggesting a relationship between object loss, mourning, and creativity. While the loss itself does not account for the creative act, it seems to facilitate a creative process in some individuals. Pollock (1975) has discovered over 1,200 writers, painters, sculptors, composers, and scientists who experienced the effects of early object loss. Robbins (1969) has written that "the creative process is set in motion when painful affects related to object loss and object hunger threaten to become conscious."

The reawakening of the repressed strivings for the lost love object of one's childhood during adolescence is poignantly depicted in a poem of Sylvia Plath (1975). Plath, who lost her father in her ninth year, wrote a poem in the spring of her sixteenth year which reveals not only the sorrow of loss but the rage of abandonment. Wolfenstein (1969) has observed that rage, and not grief, is the predominant affect associated with early object loss. Interestingly, Plath titles her poem *To Ariadne (Deserted by Theseus)*. Theseus was the great Athenian hero who promised to marry Ariadne and accompany her to Athens after she shared with him the secret that enabled him to kill the Minotaur. After Theseus prevailed, and the couple put to sea, they landed on the island of Naxos where Ariadne fell asleep, whereupon Theseus sailed on without her:

TO ARIADNE
(Deserted by Theseus)

Oh, fury, equalled only by the shrieking wind
The lashing of the waves against the shore,
You rage in vain, waist deep into the sea,
Betrayed, deceived, forsaken ever more.

Your cries are lost, your curses are unheard by him
That treads his winged way above the cloud.
The honeyed words upon your lips are brine;
The bitter salt wind sings off-key and loud.

Oh, scream in vain for vengeance now, and beat your hands
In vain against the dull impassive stone.
The cold waves break and shatter at your feet;
The sky is mean and you bereft, alone.

The white-hot rage abates, and then—futility.
You lean exhausted on the rock. The sea
Begins to calm, and the retreating storm
But grumbles faintly, while the black clouds flee.

And now the small waves break the green glass, frilled with foam;
The fickle sun sends darts of light to land.
Why do you stand and listen only to
The sobbing of the wind along the sand?

[Plath 1975]

For Plath the sea was always a symbol of her father's place. Until his death, they lived in Winthrop, Massachusetts, near the sea. She would return to the sea many times, both in her life and in her poetry. The helpless rage, directed toward "him that treads his winged way above the cloud," refers to the father who had abandoned her. Her hope for a reunion, so common in those who have experienced early object loss, is doomed to disappointment: "The sky is mean and you bereft, alone." Hopeless futility and the irreversibility of loss are evident in the last stanza: "Why do you stand and listen only to / The sobbing of the wind along the sand?"

The early loss of a parent promotes a peculiar splitting of the ego which allows the individual to maintain the coexistence of contradictory ideas (Freud 1927). The death of the parent is acknowledged and the conscious attachment and relationship is given up, while simultaneously the unconscious attachment and relationship to the loved one continues. There is an idealization of the lost object which is perpetuated in fantasy. The negative side of the ambivalence is split off and directed toward the remaining parent, others, or the world at large. Instead of finding a substitute and replacement for the lost object, the child may deny the finality of the loss with conscious and unconscious fantasies of reunion and restitution, either on earth or after death.

The fantasies of reunion are beautifully and painfully described in the final lines of Poe's (1857) "Annabel Lee." Poe's mother died just before his third birthday:

> And neither the angels in heaven above,
>   Nor the demons under the sea,
> Can ever dissever my soul from the soul
>   Of the beautiful Annabel Lee;
>
> For the moon never beams, without bringing me dreams
>   Of the beautiful Annabel Lee;
> And the stars never rise, but I feel the bright eye
>   Of the beautiful Annabel Lee;
>
> And so all the night-tide, I lie down by the side
> Of my darling—my darling—my life and my bride,
>   In the sepulchre there by the sea,
>   In her tomb by the sounding sea . . .

The child interprets the world from his egocentric viewpoint. He may explain the loss of the parent by interpreting his absence as the result of the parent's abandonment, or by seeing his own evilness as driving the lost object away, or he fantasizes that the object was stolen from him.

The fantasy of the lost object being stolen is also evident in "Annabel Lee":

> The winged seraphs of heaven
>   Coveted her and me.
> And this was the reason that, long ago
>   In this Kingdom by the sea,
> A wind blew out of a cloud, chilling
>   My beautiful Annabel Lee
>
> So that her highborn Kinsman came
>   And bore her away from me,
> To shut her up in a sepulchre
>   In this kingdom by the sea.

A young individual who has experienced the loss of a primary object seems, prior to adolescence, able to put the loss out of his mind and to go about his activities without an unusual degree of sadness or depression. Once adolescence is initiated, however, there is a return of what was repressed. The hypercathexis of the internal representation of the lost object resurfaces along with a reawakening of the oedipal conflict. There may be a frantic search for an object upon which to superimpose the parental image. The internal possession of such an image seems necessary to the adolescent process, to the mourning process, and for the transfer of libidinal strivings to a nonincestual object (Freud 1958).

Children or adolescents losing an early object will be greatly impaired in their capacity to resolve the adolescent process. Instead of a decathexis and realistic appraisal of the parental objects and a gradual psychological separation and emancipation from the early objects, there is, in essence, a reversal of the task of adolescence. The infantile image of the parent is hypercathected and idealized, with a greater sense of attachment, rather than the more characteristic adolescent processes of devaluation and detachment. The idealized and glorified image of the lost parent provides a means to maintain in fantasy the image of the loved object. It is as if the individual enters adolescence and is unable to proceed further. There is often a questing or wandering motif in the lives of individuals who experienced early object loss. This is evident in the lines of Wordsworth, whose mother died when he was eight years old: ". . . roving up and down alone / Seeking I know not what" (Manley, Wordsworth, and Wordsworth 1974).

The individual who has experienced early object loss remains in a prolonged adolescent phase. The mourning process of adolescence fails to take place. There is an enhanced tolerance for ambiguity and a certain fluidity in experiencing the polarities of development (active-passive, male-female, sadism-masochism) as well as the contradictory identity fragments and the discontinuities in development. As a consequence, the adolescent process of synthesizing and integrating these disparate elements into a unitary sense of identity does not take place, and the attachment to the mental representation of the lost object is maintained with all its contradictory affective elements.

The high frequency of early object loss associated with the lives of artistic geniuses suggests that the regressive reactivation of an earlier ego state, with its splitting of the ego, is somehow facilitative to the creative process in these individuals. Two opposite views of the lost parent are maintained; the death is both acknowledged and denied. These views, although simultaneously maintained, coexist in isolation and are not mutually confronted (Wolfenstein 1969). As Wolfenstein (1973) observed in her study of two artists, a painter and a poet who experienced early object loss: "The lost parent is both dead and alive, absent but enduring, far and near. This exemplifies the ability of artists generally to dissolve the inner barriers of the mind, to combine the devices of primary and secondary processes, to subject archaic memory to the highest organizing principle. What is otherwise contradiction assumes for the artist the aspect of rich ambiguity. The boundness to an ever-living past, which prevents the neurotic from living in the present, provides the artist with the source of his work. . . ."

An earlier ego state is maintained which seems to be congruent with an ego state intrinsic to the creative process. Rothenberg (1971), in a study of the creative process, noted that one specific thought process clearly delineated in creativity is what he calls "Janusian" thinking, that is, the capacity to conceive and utilize two or more opposite or contradictory ideas, concepts, or images simultaneously—a capacity which is reactivated in adolescence.

The adolescent's phase-specific partial regression to undifferentiated object relations ushers in an ego state similar to that available to some individuals who have experienced early object loss. Greenacre (1957) has stressed the importance of the early object relationship to creativity. She notes that the potentially gifted infant responds to the primary object with an unusual sensitivity. With subsequent development and the necessary frustrations of the separation-individuation phase, af-

fects are generated which threaten to overwhelm the child. The libidinal cathexes are partially withdrawn from the primary object and re-
directed to the self and also extended out to the surround. This extension of the libidinal cathexis to the surround of inanimate objects is
determined by the infant-artist's unusual sensitivity to the sensory experience and by a need to avoid the loss of the primary object. In the
surround, objects can be selected which are not to be lost. The range of
extended experiences and affects which characterized the self-object
relationship are deflected to what Greenacre (1957) calls the "collective alternate." Various aspects and qualities of the objective reality
are interwoven with the affects of the self-object dyad and determine
the artist's love affair with the world. In the "collective alternate," the
infant creates his first artistic work, and restitution is made in the
extension of his love affair with the mother to his love affair with the
world.

In Thomas Mann's (1903) "Tonio Kröger," the adolescent Tonio
notes that it is "The fountain, the old walnut tree, his fiddle, and away
in the distance the North Sea, within sound of whose summer mur-
murings he spent his holidays—these were the things that he loved,
within these he enfolded his spirit, among these things his inner life
took its course. And they were all things whose names are effective in
verse. . . ."

In the artist, the perpetuation of the self-object relationship, with its
affective link of exhilaration, exaltation, bliss, and momentary completeness, becomes one of the self-object-affect units that make up the
repertoire of internal object relationships and that are capable of being
transposed to the external world. This enduring structure prolongs the
attachment to the primary object which interferes with the normal
progression of the infant through the libidinal phases. It is as though
there is a split in the evolution of self-representation. A firm sense of
self evolves along the normal developmental line, while the artistic self
remains attached to the primary object, continuing to reexperience the
primordial love affair vis-à-vis the "collective alternate." As a consequence, the pathway through the libidinal phases is transgressed in an
incomplete manner. There is greater fluidity and capacity to reexperience the various phases of libidinal development. The polariza-
tion of sexual differences is less complete, with the artistic individual
experiencing a higher capacity for bisexuality. The genital investment
in the oedipal object is not renounced, nor is the oedipal object completely abandoned. The artist achieves only partial resolution of the

various developmental phases, particularly the oral and oedipal phases (Greenacre 1957). The artist experiences recurrent conflict, incomplete repression, and unusual access to earlier phases of development and primary process experiences, much like the adolescent.

The adolescent is able to reexperience the early self-object relationship through a regression in the service of the ego. The adolescent experience may be characterized by transitional phenomena which provide a means of defining body boundaries and separateness from the mothering one and at the same time maintain a primal unity with the mothering one. The original primordial experience of the mother is remembered by many adolescents in the vague reverberations known as oceanic feelings. This reliving of the immortal oneness with the primal object may serve the work of mourning if there is a recognition associated with the experience of sadness that this can never be again.

Creativity may represent a synthetic attempt to complete the mourning process while, often at the same time, prolonging the psychic life of the object representation. The creative impulse in the artist springs from a need to protect himself from the transient nature of the experience. He wishes to immortalize not only himself but also the yearned-for object. This is particularly true when the artist, out of his own experience, has been traumatically sensitized to the transient experience by the early death or loss of a loved object. He takes refuge from the reality of life. The unavailability of the yearned-for object sets into motion a defensive regression in the service of the ego with a reexperiencing of earlier perceptual states which may be reproduced as art.

Creativity is the product of the synthetic function of the ego, which utilizes regression as a means of integrating multiple levels of primary and secondary experiences and seemingly contradictory elements. It is an attempt at problem solving, insofar as it serves the needs of the individual to bring into harmony the disparate parts of his intrapsychic experience. Art represents not only instinctual liberation, the expression of the pleasure principle, the recovery of a childhood experience, and making conscious what is unconscious, it also represents the elaborated product of the synthetic and integrative function of the ego. It thus gives form to feelings, compromise to conflict, and a momentary sense of closure which mitigates the conflict of coexisting contradictory elements.

If creativity is perceived as representing an aspect of the mourning process in some individuals, it should not be surprising that it is commonly found in the adolescent experience. It is the thesis of this chapter that one dimension of adolescent creativity is that it serves a Janusian function for the psychic life of the individual. On the one hand, it may be an attempt to deny transience and loss. Segal (1952) quotes Proust as noting, "The artist is compelled to create by his need to recover his lost past." She writes that: "All creation is really a recreation of a once loved and once whole but now lost and ruined object." Through the creative process, the artist may be making restitution and reparation in an attempt to recreate, restore, and retain the lost object. The aim is to achieve victory over transience (Pollock 1975). "All artists aim at immortality, their objects must not only be brought back to life, but also the life has to be eternal. And of all human activities art comes nearest to achieving immortality; a great work of art is likely to escape destruction and oblivion" (Segal 1952).

The other side of the Janusian character of creativity is that the mourning process may be served. The hypercathexis, idealization, and reliving of the early self-object relationship, expressed lyrically, may be accompanied by an increasing awareness that the idyllic and nostalgic memories of the past have to be left as memories which cannot be experienced again. The adolescent poems reveal a painful process; reality dictates an acknowledgment of transience and loss which may be opposed by a strong unwillingness to abandon the libidinal attachment to the lost object. In many of these poems, the adolescent is aware of the irrevocability of the lost relationship. We can say that mourning has been facilitated when, in the lyrical poetry of adolescents, "Each single one of the memories and expectations in which libido is bound to the object is brought up and hypercathected and detachment of the libido is accomplished in respect of it" (Freud 1917). When this occurs, the mourning process may be enhanced, creativity may slowly abate, and the adolescent experience progresses toward resolution.

Conclusions

It is my belief that the artist is an individual who, in addition to his unique talents and endowment, has failed to close off the conflicts of adolescence, to synthesize and integrate the polarities of development, and to separate fully from the primal self-object. Instead of synthesizing an integrated self and resolving his conflicts intrapsychically, he attempts to synthesize them in his creative endeavors and in the narcissistic union with the artistic product. The artist, through his creativity, reexperiences the sense of completeness that he once felt with the primal object when transience, death, and decay were absent, when his experience was one of the timeless, enduring harmony with a loved object. It is suggested that adolescent creativity, as it is manifested in the poetry presented here, represents an attempt to restore the lost childhood of the infantile objects; that the motif of transience with its themes of time, loss, and death represents the work of mourning, and that, if successful, the adolescent process will come to a close with a significant change in the dimension of creativity. In others, creativity may take the form of prolonging the affective investment in the re-experiencing of the lost past with the failure of mourning, prolonging the adolescent experience with its particular imprint on the creative process.

REFERENCES

Bak, R. 1958. Discussion: "The Family Romance of the Artist" by Phyllis Greenacre. *Psychoanalytic Study of the Child* 13:42–43.

Blos, P. 1967. The second individuation process of adolescence. *Psychoanalytic Study of the Child* 22:162–186.

Eissler, K. 1958. Psychoanalysis of adolescents. *Psychoanalytic Study of the Child* 13:223–254.

Freud, A. 1958. Adolescence. *Psychoanalytic Study of the Child* 13:255–278.

Freud, S. 1916. On transience. *Standard Edition* 14:305–307. London: Hogarth, 1957.

Freud, S. 1917. Mourning and melancholia. *Standard Edition* 14:243–258. London: Hogarth, 1957.

Freud, S. 1927. Fetishism. *Standard Edition* 21:149–157. London: Hogarth, 1961.

Greenacre, P. 1957. The childhood of the artist. *Psychoanalytic Study of the Child* 12:447–472.

Kensington Junior High School. 1978. *6th Period Poetry Booklet.* Kensington, Md.: Kensington Junior High School.

Luke, D., and Pick, R., eds. 1966. *Goethe: Conversations and Encounters.* London: Wolff.

Manley, S.; Wordsworth, D.; and Wordsworth, W. 1974. *The Heart of a Circle of Friends*. New York: Vanguard.

Mann, T. 1903. Tonio Kröger. In *The Thomas Mann Reader*. New York: Knopf, 1960.

Plath, A.S. 1975. *Letters Home by Sylvia Plath, Correspondence 1950–1963*. New York: Harper & Row.

Poe, E.A. 1857. *Poetical Works of E.A. Poe*, London: Ward, Lock & Tyler, Warick House.

Pollock, G. 1975. On mourning, immortality and Utopia. *American Journal of Psychoanalysis* 23:334–362.

Robbins, M. 1969. On the psychology of artistic creativity. *Psychoanalytic Study of the Child* 15:227–251.

Rothenberg, A. 1971. The process of Janusian thinking in creativity. *Archives of General Psychiatry* 24:195–205.

Segal, H. 1952. A psychoanalytic approach to aesthetics. *International Journal of Psycho-Analysis* 33:196–207.

Sidwell Friends School. 1978. *The Quarterly*. Vol. 77, no. 1. Washington, D.C.: American Printing.

Sidwell Friends School. 1979. *The Quarterly*. Vol. 77, no. 2. Washington, D.C.: American Printing.

Spiegel, L. 1958. Comments on the psychoanalytic psychology of adolescence. *Psychoanalytic Study of the Child* 13:296–308.

Wolfenstein, M. 1966. How is mourning possible? *Psychoanalytic Study of the Child* 21:93–126.

Wolfenstein, M. 1969. Loss, rage and repetition. *Psychoanalytic Study of the Child* 24:432–460.

Wolfenstein, M. 1973. The image of the lost parent. *Psychoanalytic Study of the Child* 28:433–455.

BERTRAM SLAFF

A small number of individuals with characters that appear to be narcissistic have the rare gift of creativity. They may suffer from difficulties derived from their narcissism and from neurotic, psychotic, or other character deformations. They may also suffer specifically from certain burdens derived from the possession of their creativity. It is essential for therapists to understand the distinction between these groups of phenomena.

Implicit in this presentation is the importance of correctly identifying the creative adolescent. Here one cannot depend upon creative achievement, since most of these youths have not lived long enough to reach that productive state. Studies of the developmental histories of creative adults can provide clues.

I have offered the following challenge to students: You are a college psychiatrist and are asked to look into a situation in which a philosophy professor is worried about the mental health of one of his students. The pupil, a seventeen-year-old sophomore, appears to be moody, seclusive, and rather odd. He participates unevenly in classroom discussions. His comments are often astonishing. They are original, disturbingly stimulating, seem to be perhaps brilliant; yet possibly psychotic. How would you proceed?

My teaching point is to stress the need for a lifetime developmental history in order to evaluate whether there is a sudden, perhaps ominous, personality change or the continuing growth of an atypical, possibly creative individual.

This challenge to students takes its origin in a referral that was made to me many years ago of a four-year-old child, then in nursery school. Warren's teachers reported that when they picked him up, it was like holding a sack of potatoes. Warren did not respond at all as an affectionate child. Concern was expressed about autism. His parents were loving, intelligent, and involved. It was brought out that in the history of the past three generations of his mother's family there were two authentic inventive geniuses and three suicides, including the maternal grandmother.

Warren was an extraordinarily "different" child. From his first meeting with me, he related as a little adult. He was formal, polite, and verbally communicative. He told me that he disliked being a child and had no intention of acting like one. Being picked up by his teachers bored him and he tried to discourage their efforts by hanging limply. He sensed that I would be likely to think he should let himself participate in being a child and informed me that he would not permit this.

For several years I saw this atypical but not autistic child in twice-weekly and later in once-weekly sessions. His parents had asked me to serve as a consultant during his growing-up years. After regularly scheduled sessions were terminated, I continued to see him periodically.

Warren's parents reacted to his atypicality with appropriate patience and understanding. They recognized that he had to be accepted as he was and could not be pressured into becoming a more typical boy of his age.

During the years I have known Warren he never evinced age-appropriate child traits. He taught himself reading, Italian, astronomy, meteorology, and aspects of neuroanatomy. At his school he felt that the other children were "childish," and he openly expressed his disapproval. When he was thirteen, he asked to go to the excellent boarding school his father had attended. In my letter to the school I reviewed Warren's development and added, "He is attracted to your school because he feels that there he will have more intellectual stimulation, his needs for privacy are more likely to be respected, and he will not be unduly pressured into 'homey' socializing activities in which he may not be interested. Atypical, rather seclusive, nonconformist, adultlike, and quite possibly brilliant, Warren would seem to merit serious consideration for acceptance at your school." He did attend that school.

Warren's story serves to illustrate the kind of challenge one faces in treating the creative or narcissistic adolescent with problems of adjustment.

During my first year of practice as a psychotherapist a young man asked permission to withhold reporting a dream until, he said, "I have finished doing my own work on it." There was an idea for a book, and he needed time and privacy to secure it. I agreed to this. Several weeks later he conscientiously described the dream in detail, associated to it, and also elaborated on the idea of the book which had been stimulated by the dream. After six months I was shown the manuscript of this work which was published the following year.

There is a specific character type, the creative personality, which in many ways resembles the narcissistic character, but with significant differences. There is considerable overlap between the commonly accepted symptoms of psychological disturbance and manifestations of the creative personality in ferment. Further complicating the picture is the capacity of the creative person to develop neurosis, psychosis, or character disorder as any person might. In the treatment of these individuals, efforts to relieve the stress of psychopathology are entirely appropriate. Stress as a function of the creative process cannot be avoided. The creative individual can be helped to cope satisfactorily with his creativity and the difficulties associated with it.

Most of us live multilevel existences. Freud (1915) contrasted the primary process thinking of infancy and dreaming with secondary process thinking, the logical thinking of which the more mature personality is capable. Flavell (1963) summarized Piaget's work in exploring and describing elaborately the transformations of thinking throughout the child and adolescent phases of the life cycle. Piaget delineated the sensorimotor phase from birth to one and one-half to two, the preoperational or egocentric stage until six or seven, the period of concrete operational thought until about eleven, and the potential for abstract operational thinking beginning in early adolescence. In both the Freudian and Piagetian approaches there is a hierarchy of values among the thinking capacities in which secondary process and abstract operations are accorded the highest position.

I believe that concurrent with these capacities there are aspects of earlier developmental levels of thinking and feeling which contribute to the totality, to the final common path of mental life. These may exist within consciousness, in the preconscious, or in the unconscious. For example, dreams have been described as a royal road to the unconscious reaches of the mind (Brenner 1955). Expressions of primary-process thinking, they are related to aspects of sensorimotor and preoperational thought mechanisms.

Let us review some of the generally accepted qualities of primary-process thinking: symbolization; condensation and its opposite, dispersion; displacement; distortion; denial; reversal; association; splitting; exaggeration and its opposite, minimizing; identification; internalization; externalization; incorporation; and projection. Additionally there may be secondary elaboration, reaction formation, irony, alliteration, punning, and metaphor. It is at once apparent that many of the qualities of primary-process thinking are also the qualities of poetry, however, very few of us are vouchsafed to become poets. The question is posed: From an ubiquitous potential for creativity, what factors propel particular individuals toward actual creative achievement?

I conceive of the term "creative" as embodying the qualities of invention, discovery, and originality, all ultimately to be submitted to judgment and critical review, but not necessarily at once. It is my impression that the psychodynamics of creativity are similar for those in the arts and those in the sciences.

The creative individual is someone who is less likely to respect uncritically the hierarchy of values among the thinking capacities, in which secondary process and abstract operations are accorded the highest position. He or she is not afraid to dream, to imagine, to "fool around with," to play, to experiment, to try new combinations, juxtapositions, relations, to "defamiliarize," to "waste time." He is likely to be extraordinarily curious and perceptive; what many others will take for granted, he challenges. He often is neither conformist nor anticonformist, but rather is nonconformist. He is usually very talented and highly intelligent, but may disconcert his teachers by asking original questions about the material being studied that challenge the teacher's perceptions and understanding.

An atypical personality, he may reject the tried and true paths of scholastic advancement by which organized and devoted mastering of academic requirements is rewarded. He may be considered troublesome. The creative individual has an unusual capacity to bounce, so to speak, within the levels of unconscious, preconscious, and conscious mental functioning. Similarly he can be said to be able to bounce within the various time levels of his experience, actual or imagined, past, present, or future. He is likely to be open intellectually and affectively.

Kris (1952) describes in such individuals "the capacity of gaining easy access to id material without being overwhelmed by it, of retaining control over the primary process, and perhaps specifically, the capability of making rapid or at least appropriately rapid shifts in levels of psychic function."

It is my impression that creative people have a less effective stimulus barrier than do most individuals. They are extraordinarily responsive to perceptions from without and from within. This sensitivity greatly expands their areas of awareness, which can be a most enriching factor.

Greenacre (1957) suggests four characteristics of creative talent: a greater sensitivity to sensory stimulation, an unusual capacity for awareness of relations between various stimuli, a predisposition to an empathy of wider range and deeper vibration than usual, and an intactness of sufficient sensorimotor equipment to allow the building up of projective motor discharges for expressive functions. She postulates that this unusual capacity for awareness of relations between various stimuli must "involve sensibility of subtle similarities and differences, an earlier and greater reactivity to form and rhythm—thus a greater sense of actual or potential organization, perhaps a greater sense of the gestalt."

Greenacre provides a hypothetical example of a potentially gifted infant's reaction to mother's breast. She described the intensity of the impression of warmth, smell, moisture, the feel of the texture of the skin, and the vision of the roundness of form—according to the time and situation of the experience—as greater than might be true in the less potentially gifted infant. She conceives that for the more gifted infant the primary object which stimulates certain sensory responses is invested with a greater field of related experiences than would be true for the infant of lesser endowment. There would inevitably be a greater harmonizing of "inner object relationships (as the perception of the object reacts on and combines with other body sensations) and the world of sensory impingement."

Greenacre uses the term "collective alternates" to describe the range of extended experience which may surround or become attached to the main focus of object relationships. She then states, "In this connection it seems to me that this may be the beginning of the love affair with the world which seems to me an obligatory condition in the development of great talent or genius."

Glynn (1977), discussing Greenacre, notes that the love affair with the world grows out of and alongside of the original intense relationship to the mother, but it comes to assume greater importance. Competing with growing success with that and subsequent personal relationships, the gifted gratifies wishes and needs through the collective alternates, keeping them active and potent: ". . . the adult artist will have a 'porous' personality structure, one of polymorphous energies, where the primitive and infantile will have ready routes toward consciousness."

Clinical Issues and Creativity

Important questions are raised for clinicians dealing with the creative personality. If there is clear evidence of psychopathology, what may be the relationships, if any, between it and creativity? Is creativity likely to be a help or a hindrance in overcoming neurotic, psychotic, or character problems? What is the risk of diminishment or loss of the creative drive if psychological stresses are successfully alleviated?

Let me address the last question first. I have been privileged to work in analytic psychotherapy with a number of creative individuals. Drawing from these experiences I believe that *creative achievement is an ego-syntonic gratification of the highest order for the creator. It is indeed a blessing.* Creativity can be further liberated through psychotherapy; it cannot be opposed. I agree with Kubie's (1958) view: "No one need ever fear that getting well will cause an atrophy of his creative drive."

Creative individuals have at least the same likelihood as others for having a difficult childhood and conflicted human relationships, with the potentiality for developing psychopathology. There are additionally certain psychological burdens which are related to the creative capacity. The creative individual is restless. No matter what he has achieved, or what recognition he has been given, he is not able to interrupt the constant questioning, searching, and striving. There is a driving quality which forces the scientist, the artist, the inventor to pursue further his quest, competing often with himself, to go beyond frontiers into the unknown. A young physicist, who was later to receive the Nobel Prize, told me of the terror which accompanied his discovery that a particular "law" which had been taught to him by his great teachers was flawed and that they were all in error. He felt desperately alone.

I have alluded to the ability to bounce among various levels of consciousness and among various time periods. It is not difficult to conceive that the venturing into the unknown creatively might stimulate the reliving of childhood experiences involving various unknowns. Fear of the dark, separation anxiety, primal scene experience or fantasy may all be tapped. These may be extraordinarily painful to the creative individual.

Despair is another emotion intimately connected with the creative experience. One is dissatisfied with the present understanding of a situation; one stews, ruminates, broods, obsesses; there seems to be no answer. One despairs, feels that the gift of creativity is gone. Without creativity, what is there? Bleak depression may ensue, with suicide a temptation and risk.

Here I would like to propose a revision of Greenacre's (1957) concept of the artist's "love affair with the world." It is, I believe, rather a love affair with one's own creations, with the original self-object or fantasied original self-object transformed into an intense commitment to the collective alternates, perhaps to be considered as a transitional object, resulting ultimately in artistic or scientific achievement.

The creative struggle is a wrestling with unknowns, a working through at all levels of the process of discovery. Subjectively this period is often experienced as a block, a blind alley, a loss of creative capacity, with a resulting feeling of exhaustion and perhaps annihilation. Such an individual may present clinically as a person in a depression.

At some point there is likely to be a breakthrough, and a resolution of the creative challenge becomes apparent. When it erupts into consciousness there is an extraordinary sense of rescue, relief, and happiness. If the new synthesis satisfies the critical judgment of the originator, despair is gone, depression is relieved, and there is likely to be the high of a great challenge, successfully mastered.

What I have just described is almost a paradigm of manic-depressive illness, the often sudden reversal from severe depression to elation. And of course creative persons can be manic-depressive and manifest a history of bipolar affective disorder. Nevertheless, in most instances, I aver the despair followed by happiness at the successful confrontation with a creative challenge is a function of the creative process at work. It is not a psychopathological experience. Lithium is not indicated.

I have used the terms "nonconformist" and "atypical" to describe the creative personality. Many of these individuals can further be characterized as loners, as eccentric and withdrawn, "marching to the beat of a different drummer," self-involved, perhaps fantasy ridden, preoccupied, as "internal émigrés." These qualities often define what is known as the schizoid personality. Although the behavioral similarities of creative individuals and schizoid persons may be remarkable, psychodynamically I believe there are major differences.

The creative person has retreated from conventional reality to free himself from its restrictions so that new advances can be essayed. Kris (1952) has called this "regression in the service of the ego." Wertheimer (1959) considers creative thinking "the process of destroying one gestalt in favor of a better one." Koestler (1964) used the phrase *"reculer pour mieux sauter,"* to take a step backward in order to make a leap forward. The schizoid individual is thought to have developed these qualities as defenses and coping techniques. These frequently serve restrictive rather than expressive or inventive purposes. There is likely to be rigidity instead of fluidity; a fixed, sometimes stereotyped quality of behavior.

Adolescence and Creativity

The contemporary teenager is in a developmental phase characterized by intense peer pressure to conform. The creative youth, generally unable to do this, is prone to be ridiculed as a "bookworm," a "crazy," or "not one of us." He may suffer acutely from social isolatedness and the absence of group support for his endeavors. If he lacks the gratifications that come with creative achievement, which probably still lies ahead of him, this may lead to a split in his sense of identity, with the creative self at war with the social self. Of course this conflict between the creative self and the social self may continue throughout life, since loneliness is one of the burdens of the creative individual.

Atypicality in sexual and interpersonal relationships is often observed in creative individuals. Passionate involvement in one's creative strivings may reduce the psychic energies available to the social self, in the pursuit of sexual and affectional goals. The solitary nature of the creative function can easily be experienced as coldness and withdrawal by the intimates of the creative person.

Let me summarize: there is an entity, the creative personality. There is a magnificent reward for this individual, the creative achievement, the blessing mentioned in the title of this chapter. Major burdens may accompany this gift: loneliness, terror, never-ending restlessness and searching, frustration, depression, suicidal risk, sexual difficulties, and interpersonal disharmonies. It should be clear that I consider creativity

85

to be a most important aspect of the health of the individual with that rare gift. Yet the burdens associated with it can be overwhelming. It is incumbent on the therapist to seek to help the creative person to cope successfully with his creativity and whatever burdens are associated with it and with any other problems he may have.

Earlier I raised the question: Is creativity likely to be a help or a hindrance in overcoming neurotic, psychotic, or character problems? Because inventiveness, daring, and openness to new ideas are qualities associated with creativity, individuals with this resource are more likely than others to discover newer, less rigid, more adaptive techniques in living. Storr (1962) states, "What is distinctive is the creative person's superior ability to synthesize and make new wholes out of opposing aspects, not the presence of opposition within."

Now to the question, what is the relation, if any, between creativity and psychopathology? It is abundantly clear that psychopathology most commonly exists not associated with creativity. Developmental studies of creative persons and the experiences of creative individuals in psychotherapy make clear that there frequently is psychopathology.

Conclusions

The gifted individual, extraordinarily endowed with those special capacities described by Greenacre, develops on a different track from most people. His gratifications come from his love affair with the products of his creative drive. Achievement of his goals may provide ecstasy at times. Frustration in gaining achievement may make him seem worthless to himself. If his identifications are with himself as creator, interference with creativity may be experienced as annihilation. Growing up differently from most people, he is likely not to have developed successfully the kinds of support systems more generally available, such as stable and predictable family and career anchorages. He is likely to be unique and alone, sometimes gloriously so, sometimes devastatingly so.

REFERENCES

Brenner, C. 1955. *An Elementary Textbook of Psychoanalysis*. New York: International Universities Press.
Flavell, J.H 1963. *The Developmental Psychology of Jean Piaget*. Princeton, N.J.: Van Nostrand.

Freud, S. 1915. The unconscious. *Standard Edition* 14:159–215. London: Hogarth, 1957.

Glynn, E. 1977. Desperate necessity: art and creativity in recent psychoanalytic theory. *Print Collector's Newsletter* 8(2):29–36.

Greenacre, P. 1957. The childhood of the artist. *Psychoanalytic Study of the Child* 12:47–62.

Koestler, A. 1964. *The Act of Creation*. New York: Macmillan.

Kris, E. 1952. *Psychoanalytic Explorations in Art*. New York: International Universities Press.

Kubie, L. 1958. *Neurotic Distortion of the Creative Process*. Lawrence, Kan.: University of Kansas Press.

Storr, A. 1962. *The Dynamics of Creation*. New York: Atheneum.

Wertheimer, M. 1959. *Productive Thinking*. New York: Harper.

6 THE NEEDLE OF CARING, THE THREAD OF LOVE: CREATIVE WRITING ON AN ADOLESCENT MEDICAL WARD

ADELE D. HOFMANN AND NANCY R. LEWIS

I was like an old piece of clothin' and the doctors were my tailors. I was old, beat up, torn at the seams, ready to be discarded. But they saw the silver lining and decided to remake me into something useful and fashionable. They took the needle of caring and the thread of love and sewed me back together. Now I'm ready for use once again.

["Handsewn," Wendy, age seventeen:
heart surgery]

Adolescent medicine is the primary care of young people between twelve and twenty-one years. It is committed to a comprehensive approach, integrating biological, emotional, and social factors into a holistic set of concerns. It also recognizes the unique developmental issues of these years (Erikson 1950; Tanner 1962) and their critical significance for the implementation of any health-care plan. This approach is derived from both a comprehensive definition of primary care as well as necessity. The intense interplay between biological and psychological factors so characteristic of adolescence cannot be ignored if care delivery is to be effective. Adolescent medicine not only attends to specific organic issues but also incorporates a strong element of preventive mental health through guidance in effective decision making, support for the assumption of self-responsibility, as well as brief (and, sometimes, not so brief) interventive psychotherapy—all under the rubric of "counseling."

The delivery of adolescent health care often requires a team approach. The needs of this age group cannot be met, in many instances, without the alliance of a variety of professionals: physicians, psychiatrists, psychologists, nurses, social workers, educators, and recreation workers. The adolescent-life worker is a relatively new and important addition to this team, particularly on the adolescent medical ward, bringing developmental training, professional discipline, and therapeutic purpose into the formerly superficial and limited role of "play lady" and recreational volunteer. It is the purpose of this chapter to demonstrate the function of this new professional in exploring one facet of the adolescent-life program at Bellevue Hospital—creative writing.

But before proceeding, we will outline the developmental dilemmas facing hospitalized adolescents and summarize responsive therapeutic principles as defined by Hofmann, Becker, and Gabriel (1976). We also will examine theoretical concepts underlying creative writing and its significance as a support system for physically ill and injured youth. Our analysis of the writing itself is predicated upon these fundamentals.

Hospitalized Adolescents: Developmental and Therapeutic Considerations

To recapitulate briefly the two major developmental task areas of identity formation and emancipation (Erikson 1950), adolescents are heavily invested, first, in attractiveness, physical prowess, and other determinants of masculinity or femininity and, second, in mastery, control, and independence. Being ill, disabled, and hospitalized directly challenges each of these tasks.

Emancipation drives are thwarted both by enforced dependency consequent to being ill and by administrative regulations prohibiting customary mobility. Perceived loss of control is further escalated by the need for others to assist in the performance of formerly autonomous functions, particularly in such intimate matters as bathing and toileting. To make matters worse, biologically disruptive, invasive, and painful therapeutic procedures must be tolerated passively, accepted as beneficial, even with appreciation of staff efforts to help; and this a staff of strangers legitimately endowed with the power to examine and treat even the most heavily invested anatomical part.

Excepting those for whom long-standing chronic illness has brought familiarity, hospitalization usually is an unprecedented event for the adolescent. It requires adjustment to a host of threatening circumstances in terms of both present and future implications. There also are frequent life-death undercurrents that cannot wholly be denied. Such unique confrontations require the mounting of new systems of defense and adaptation. The impact on body image and emerging concepts of adult sexuality is a significant one. Conditions that interfere with physical attractiveness, limit athletic ability, delay puberty, cause wasting and debility, or otherwise preclude full normalcy according to peer-group standards inevitably bear a potential for serious psychological consequences.

Older adolescents may be less stressed by independence issues or concepts of sexuality—if these have already been secured at this stage. But young people will be challenged by possible compromise of educational and vocational goals, prospects for marriage, and a family or life style—all concerns of the incipient young adult in establishing his or her functional identity.

Increasing competence in abstract thought (Piaget 1969) introduces another set of considerations. On the positive side, the ability to abstract permits adolescents to understand better their situation and its implications. In turn, this facilitates compliance with therapeutic requirements and effective adaptation. On the negative side, the enhanced potential for unbridled fantasy may well lead to misinterpretation and magnification of justified and unjustified fears. In any event, it is important to recognize that maturing intellectual capacity remains the only dimension of the young person that is not compromised de facto by illness or injury (excluding organic brain syndromes). Intellectual functioning is a major resource in any preventive or therapeutic plan, enabling the disabled or disfigured adolescent to define effective coping mechanisms in adaptation and secure compensatory self-esteem.

The psychological management of the hospitalized adolescent responds to all these issues through an approach which encourages continued normal psychosocial development and counters specific threats thereto. Young people should not be dealt with as if they were dependent children. Adolescents are no longer passive recipients of parent-physician decisions made unilaterally on their behalf—to be coaxed, cajoled, or coerced into compliance. Rather, adolescents are served better when treated as active, collaborative partners in the health-care process. Mastery and control needs are recognized, given credence, and supported by proffering adolescents as much knowledge about their condition as they are ready to assimilate and an opportunity to direct their own health affairs with physician guidance to the degree that is realistically possible. Teenagers who know their diagnosis, understand its implications, and perceive that they have been active participants in establishing the management plan feel far less helpless and are far less likely to maladapt than when kept in passive and protective ignorance.

The failure to take developmental issues into account at best risks poor compliance and acting out; at worst it can provoke persistent regression or developmental arrest. Optimally, a comprehensive management plan not only results in constructive adjustment to the immediate situation and an ultimate return to the normal business of growing up, but also provides opportunity for the discovery of new and heretofore untapped inner strengths.

> I thought I was NEVER going to live through being in the hospital. But I did! Here I am! One week before I go home. I feel brave! Good old me! Now I can go through ANYTHING if I've gone through all this!　　　　　　　　　　[Dorothy, age thirteen: orthopedic surgery]

Creative Writing: Theory and Implications

Creativity is the questioning and challenging of reality and life through reflection and recreation; the eternal unquenchable dissatisfaction with the merely existing (Hacker 1965). The creative process involves the channeling of energy and the act of a personal statement into an art medium such as paper, canvas, or clay. This requires a reaching into the inner parts of oneself with a new level of awareness and manifesting these freshly discovered insights outwardly. Creative work inherently offers the expansion of horizons, an enriched perspective of oneself in relation to the external world, and opportunities for gravitating from isolation toward connectedness with others. "The artistic process in general may be said to consist of two processes: the immediate and essential one which has always been known as inspirational and which psychologically we describe as an access to the deeper layers of the unconscious; a secondary process of elaboration, in which the essential perceptions and intuitions of the artist are woven into a fabric which can take its place in the organized life of conscious reality'' (Read 1966). Read (1945) also contends that all expression and all perception is inherently artistic and seeks an esthetically satisfying configuration. Imagination is the common factor in all subjective aspects of art and is that which reconciles their modal diversity through invariable laws of objective beauty and order.

> I was very awake up there. More, I think, than the doctors knew. . . . They were sculpting my face. The chiselling, hammering and molding made me feel like a piece of clay. The only reason that the thing didn't horrify me more is that I could relate to what they were doing because I work with clay. Working with clay gives me the supreme sense of control. Doctors must feel that way too. It must be a real power trip. They are controlling the way I look just as I control the clay. It's really a form of creation, assuming the surgeon takes some pride in his art.
>
> ["Pain as a Work of Art," Trina, age seventeen: surgical repair of a fractured nose]

During adolescence there is a discrepancy between paintbrush and pen as expressive modes. Kramer (1971) observed that children's art work, generally expressive and original in nature, undergoes constriction with increasing age. She contends that a certain rigidity in attitude toward art work is introduced with adolescence owing to anxiety concerning the production of photographic representations. We ourselves hypothesize that young people do not wish to risk criticism and devaluation of "incompetent" art. They resort, instead, to safer, more easily rendered and stereotyped themes: hearts, graffiti and stick, stylized, or cartooned figures. Creative writing offers the adolescent greater accessibility to the imagination and self-expression; a word is, after all, only a word, while art equals performance.

WRITING BY HOSPITALIZED ADOLESCENTS

A great deal has been written about the content and benefits of art therapies for patients in mental institutional settings—dance, drama, poetry, painting (Jennings 1974; Kramer 1971; Leedy 1969; Nordoff and Robbins 1971; Way 1967). Considerably less has been published about the creative arts, and creative writing in particular, on childrens' or adolescents' medical wards. Bergman and Freud (1965) secondarily illustrate their analysis of emotional problems encountered by chronically ill children and adolescents with a few examples. Schowalter and Lord (1972) are, to our knowledge, the only authors who have taken creative writing by adolescents on a medical ward as the primary subject. While we view Schowalter and Lord's discussion of the implications of such writing in analytic understanding of the hospital experience as a signal contribution, the works themselves do not demonstrate the full potential of this medium. Writing in this report was not introduced as part of a definitive therapeutic support system nor as a structured experience by a creative-writing specialist. Rather, it was introduced as a simple, open-ended, self-directed exercise in making a contribution to the ward newspaper. From our perspective, this methodology does not reflect the therapeutic potential: ventilation and sublimation.

Creative Writing on the Adolescent Medical Ward

Creativity requires an inner drive, an inner tension, a generative force—inevitable accompaniments to the hospital experience. Also tension is inherent in the need to submit, to be passive, to restrain the self in the face of aggressive attacks in the name of therapy: needles, painful procedures, immobilization, anesthesia, various bodily invasions. It may be quite legitimate to express one's outrage at a rapist by combative force but not at a gynecologist about to perform an examination for possible pelvic inflammatory disease. The need to displace these tensions is further compounded by the need to deal with the companion issues of mortality, frailty, and vulnerability. The hospital situation, in all its parameters, uniquely provides precisely that milieu in which the creative process can occur if fostered.

> It's so long
>> that it looks like a skinny man
>> that's so mad
>> that he could go through my body.
> Inside me it fights the bones
>> like a snake throwing his poison.
> The needle is like an animal fighting another animal

93

It scratches my bones and it's not nice to me.
It's too mean for me.

["The Needle Is Like an Animal,"
Jimmy, age thirteen:
acute appendicitis and appendectomy]

For many adolescents, hospitalization can be the first occasion where the confluence of circumstances, time, and opportunity force inward reflection about the current state of affairs. Further, hospital life depersonalizes and diminishes individuality through the uniformity of plastic name bracelets, hospital pyjamas, identical beds, and professional "whites" (Lewis 1978). Creative writing offers opportunities for putting these concerns into some sort of order, for promoting greater insight about past and immediate experiences, and for maintaining self-awareness. The patient thus continues to listen to himself or herself and be heard by others as an individual.

I am society's child; who am I?
I am your lack of understanding.
I am all of your fears.
I am the "what if " of your thoughts.
I am the dislike to your eyes.

You are my prison and jailer.
You are the law of my happiness.
I must look like you
To have a full life in your world.
You have yet to learn that
I am human like you.

I give you my forgiveness gladly,
For you are normal in our social structure,
And that is your handicap.
I give my pity,
For it is no more your fault
That you were born normal
Than I was born abnormal.
I pity you that you may
Never have the chance to

> Feel my pain or know my feelings
> About being "Society's Child."
> ["I Am Society's Child," Alison, age seventeen:
> craniofacial reconstruction]

Hospitalization poses certain threats and hurdles for inner-city adolescents in particular. Ghetto health care is frequently crisis oriented and episodic rather than anticipatory or planned. The underlying perception of hospitals is likely to be one of helplessness, intimidation, and alienation rather than benevolent aid and humane concern. Further, due to impoverished environmental and educational factors, inner-city adolescents seldom have been encouraged to speak of their experiences in a personal, expressive, or imaginative way. The deprived young person emerges from a background where the average individual is not concerned with self-expression and where the locus of control tends to be perceived as external. Creative writing for these adolescents has an additional meaning in the opportunity to discover new tools and skills to be put to the service of mastery, control, and self-determination.

> When you're a doctor and you see people like raised up in the ghettos, you have to think, "Let me find a way to speak to patients so that they can understand me better." Some doctors come out with these words you hardly understand and some talk to you in a way you understand—a street talking way. . . . And there's always some who talk in a way that you think, "God! this dude's been reading a lot of medical books!" [Jose, age fifteen: cellulitis and abcess of buttocks]

Methodology

The adolescent medical ward of Bellevue Hospital cares for young people from thirteen through seventeen years of age; the daily patient census varies from eight to fifteen. Most patients are inner-city youths of Hispanic ethnicity. But a significant number are black, oriental, or white. All adolescents presenting to the hospital and requiring admission are placed on the ward regardless of diagnosis or assigned service with the exception of pregnancy, concomitant emotional disorders re-

95

quiring a locked ward, and youths under police detention. The types of conditions seen are those which would be encountered in any adolescent population and are reflected in the diagnoses of our young writers.

An extensive support system is provided each youth. In addition to pertinent medical and surgical staff, each patient is seen and evaluated by a member of the adolescent medical unit core team; this includes the unit director, fellow in adolescent medicine, nurse coordinator, social worker, adolescent-life therapist, and liaison psychiatrist. The patient's developmental and social status, implications of the health problem at hand, and actual or potential adjustment problems are reviewed in team conference and a prescriptive plan drawn up and implemented.

The creative-writing specialist, a member of the child and adolescent life staff, as well as adjunct to the unit core team, frequently is requested to work with a patient in motivating him (or her) to express feelings about hospitalization. This is done by placing creative modalities at the patient's command in whatever manner is appropriate in helping him realize his potential. Aware of the particular adolescent's special needs, the specialist goes to the bedside and engages the patient in dialogue. Any comment or remark, however inconsequential, can serve as catalyst for developing these thoughts further on paper. Alternatively, the specialist may show the work of other patients which seems pertinent to the situation, prompting the individual's own response. The actual writing may be done either by the patient directly or by dictation. The latter is appropriate when a patient is physically incapable, or when it is apparent that the act of writing will impede the creative process due to self-consciousness about the lack of writing skills.

Patients' writings, with their permission, are made public in various ways. They may simply be typed up, copied, and passed around, published in a ward periodical, or posted on one of several corridor bulletin boards. To see one's creativity so valued as to be formalized in type and distributed or posted makes a definitive statement as to its worth.

While the writings presented in this chapter were not obtained under controlled circumstances, the opportunity was consistently offered to all patients capable of participating in this experience and physically well enough to do so. All works were voluntary and of spontaneous, undirected content. Selections from 250 pieces collected over a two-year-period (1976–1978) comprise the foundation of this study. Obviously, not every piece could be included and we admit to some bias in our choices. On the other hand, for each one we do present there were many others of similar and equally insightful nature.

In many respects, it is tempting simply to present the poetry and prose of our young writers without commentary. Each piece speaks eloquently for itself. No deep analysis is necessary to hear these adolescents loud and clear. Indeed, the true authors of this paper are our patients, not ourselves.

Creative Writing: Analysis and Implications

An analysis of the writing reveals certain recurrent themes. They speak to the fears, frustrations, angers, fantasies, stresses, adaptations, and appreciations of the ill and injured youth. They provide unique insight, permitting us to gain greater understanding of the experience of hospitalization through the adolescent's own mind's eye.

ATTITUDES TOWARD STAFF

Adolescents' views about the hospital staff are particularly common topics. These include both negative observations and positive expressions of identification and appreciation.

> You know how there is a wall-to-wall carpet?
> Well, there is wall-to-wall doctors too.
> Right in this hospital!
> And when you are surrounded by wall-to-wall doctors
> You can't even breathe!
>
> [Dorrie, age fourteen:
> fever of unknown origin]

I find my doctor special. He took time out to be with me when he could have been doing other things. . . . He took time out every day. Even if we are talking about nothing, he would take time out and talk about nothing . . . [W]hen he wasn't able to make it and had other things to do, he would come and tell me. . . . Most doctors, if they . . . have a lot of things to do, they're not gonna stop to tell you. . . . They're gonna keep right on going. In a way I felt special, not to be selfish or anything, but I felt special!

[Denise, age eighteen:
pelvic inflammatory disease]

A theme variant consists of idealized concepts of what staff members should be like.

> What makes a good doctor and a nurse? Their personality and the way they treat patients. They should be nice to us and not come off cute. They can tell us the truth, nice and straight, as long as they tell us with kindness and love.
>
> [Eunice, age fifteen, and Eva, age fifteen:
> diabetic acidosis and repair of burn scars]

It is of interest that writings in this category invariably are limited to doctors and nurses, those who are most immediately and intimately involved in the care of the medical or surgical condition and its outcome. Few pieces speak of other professionals even when uncommonly involved.

PAIN

Drawing blood, injections, and intravenous fluid administration regularly provoke statements of resentment and anger. The intensity of these feelings frequently goes well beyond the actual intensity of the pain involved, appearing to be exaggerated by the associated requirement of voluntary submissiveness to an invasive procedure and the misinterpretation of staff professionalism as insensitivity.

> It blows my mind and makes me sad
> Of the evil feeling that I've had.
> Doctors really don't understand.
> Their feeling is different than the one in my hand.
> Oh God, it hurts! What can I do?
> The feeling travels down to my shoe.
> I have a suggestion. Before graduation
> Doctors should learn their bedside mannerization.
> Then doctors would understand
> About the feeling in our hand. . . .
>
> [Charles, age sixteen:
> diabetes]

Postoperative or traumatic pain also are regular topics, but more from the perspective of bearing it and surviving it. Rarely is there the same degree of underlying rage or the element of conscious submission.

> I pick up this pencil
> (I know that I am in pain)
> To get my mind off my leg.
> It's only a game. . . .
>
> I look at my leg
> And think of the time.
> All these things are
> Hurting my mind.
>
> I want it finished.
> I want it to end.
> I don't want to lie back
> And just pretend.
>
> One of the famous questions
> In life is, "What do you want to be
> When you grow up?"
> Who ever said, "A cripple"?
>
> > [Mickey, age seventeen:
> > leg injury with
> > potential permanent damage]

It is also of interest here to note the virtual absence of comment about the loss of blood despite the frequent vituperations about the act of drawing blood. Yet the meaning of blood as a life force, at a time when life-death issues are inevitable confrontations at some level, would suggest that this would be at least a sometime theme.

CHRONIC ILLNESS

Adolescents with long-standing health problems characteristically speak of the implications for their lives. Young people with congenital orthopedic disabilities tend to do better than those who acquired their disease later in life. Contrast the first piece by an adolescent with cerebral palsy with that of another with chronic asthma.

I am a girl with cerebral palsy. I have different problems I have to cope with. The way I do it is very easy. I look at things with a different outlook than some other people do. . . . I've always been in a wheelchair so I don't really miss being well. It doesn't mean I wouldn't like to walk. It means I've already decided how I'm going to live my life; as best I can, as fully as possible.

> [Donna, age fourteen:
> surgical stabilization of scoliosis
> secondary to cerebral palsy]

Sometimes I wish I was dead. My asthma started when I was six. Now I'm fifteen years old. I suffered alot way back in those years. I went to hospitals many times and I had a lot of shots and needles. Now I still go to hospitals. When I get asthma I feel like I'm going to die. It feels like I am catching a heart attack.

> [Michael, age fifteen:
> chronic asthma and
> suicidal preoccupation]

The totality of the adolescent experience with chronic illness from the developmental perspective is insightfully expressed by this seventeen-year-old, also with chronic asthma.

Nine out of ten cases of asthma are results of growing pains; . . . how to grow out of it. I feel I have been exploited because of my asthma. You come into the hospital and the attitude is: "What brought it on this time?"; "Oh, you're back again!; Mommy didn't give you allowance?" You can get a very mixed attitude.

You have to find something else to replace asthma; find something else in your life that's bigger. . . . There are three steps really. The first is facing reality and realizing you are screwing up somehow. . . . You have to deal with your weaknesses . . . that are going to remain there. You may find out that . . . you've dealt with it so that it's not a major factor in your life. It still might reoccur once in a while, but when it does you have to learn to say, "Big deal; shots, medicine, and it's over with."

Your attitude might change, but the problem is that others, such as doctors and social workers, don't necessarily. You have to learn how to read other people; not let them frustrate you. . . . Just because someone says something doesn't mean it's true. . . . [K]eep your own principles.

Ice skating, painting, drawing, martial arts; the more physical it is the better. . . .

I do have one friend who also has asthma and found a way out of the pit. He's someone I can look up to—a big brother. . . . He tells me, ". . . What's really important is to have someone behind you saying not to give up." I know now not to look for it to be your parents or sibs. They see you in a different perspective. They're on a guilt trip. They failed. Someone outside the family can see you differently. . . .

Advice for a mother of an asthmatic would be, first, not to feel guilty; it's not her fault. Second, her kid is probably a lot stronger than she thinks he is. And, third, give him room to find himself. Don't give him too much slack. Stay behind him. Monitor him but don't possess him.   [Chang, age seventeen:
chronic asthma]

FATAL ILLNESS

Our adolescents with potentially fatal disease have not shied away from writing about this in a poignant manner. The invitation to write validates staff recognition of their deepest fears and gives them opportunity to speak of the unspeakable. Writing also proffers assurance of immortality in some small measure, leaving something of themselves behind, not to be forgotten. Several writers in this group wished to be assured that their particular piece would be made public and that friends and family would receive a copy.

When I heard the truth about my disease I wanted to cry at first, but I didn't 'cause my family was in the room. They weren't supposed to know yet that I knew that I had leukemia. I really didn't know what the disease was all about, so it didn't bother me too much. When the doctors told me all about the disease, I didn't take their word for it. So I looked it up. I found out that what they were telling me was the truth. I felt I shouldn't let it bother me. Like if I had a short time to live that I should enjoy my life—the time I had got left—instead of just thinking about it in misery. It ain't gonna do no good.

I have a little altar at home, with a couple of saints. . . . I always keep a candle lit . . . and I will never lose my faith. . . . I find myself kind of lucky 'cause there are people worse than I am. I probably

won't have all the luxuries in the world, but I have the main
thing—and that's love. [Martha, age seventeen:
acute myelogenous leukemia
(died ten months later)]

A further refinement of the life-death theme (and virtually the only
symbolic writing) was the use of either flowers or trees to express
feelings of vulnerability, frailty, and transience on the one hand, while
affirming immortality in the eternal process of the flower's life cycle on
the other hand. After looking at a picture of a bud, one patient wrote
these words:

Once the bud knows that it is a flower, it would open up and
become a flower. Maybe at times of it's life something would give
it a burst ahead toward finding out what it is. . . . When it knew
that danger was coming, it would leave seedlings behind so that
the life of the flower would continue on into the seedlings. When
the flower would just about find that it's a flower, someone would
come along and destroy it. But it's main wish was that it's memory
of life would carry on to the seedlings to help the seedlings find out
who they are. [John, age sixteen:
hemophilia]

BODY IMAGE

Concepts of the physical self are paramount in adolescence and are
particularly apt to be at the forefront of thought in ill and injured
youths. It is to be expected that body image issues are frequent themes.
Most of our patients express their distress about impaired function or
appearance in negative terms; how they perceive others to see them.
The intent appears to be both ventilatory and communicative, bringing
feelings into the open for both the patient and others to deal with in
direct terms.

I wish regular kids could see more children like us to see what we
have to go through. Maybe then they wouldn't be as uptight about
meeting us. We're really just the same. We just have special
needs. [Sylvia, age fourteen:
spina bifida and paraplegia]

Everybody has something wrong with them. . . . It could show; like with me it shows. With other people it doesn't show. I imagine it's easier when it doesn't show. . . . People are reluctant to come near me on the street.
[Frank, age fifteen:
severe eczema]

THE ILLNESS EXPERIENCE

The experiences and associated feelings surrounding illness, injury, or hospitalization comprise a particularly common theme. By putting down these events, often with great humor, adolescents appear to gain mastery and control over their situation and affirm, in the process, that they are coping to the best of their abilities.

You want to know what my breakfast was like? NASTY! Raw eggs are nasty! The bacon is as hard as a rock! You could hit somebody over the head with it. The toast is cold and real rubbery. It really means up my mind. Now I feel MEAN!
[Juan, age fifteen:
appendectomy]

Isolation is a lonely place to be in because when you have visitors you feel strange. They have to wear gowns and masks and you feel that you're different than they are. . . . I, myself, get depressed and cry because I am so lonely. I wish I didn't have to stay in isolation. I hope for the doctors to tell me I can leave the room soon and be with the other kids on the ward. . . . The only sound I hear is people walking back and forth and I wish I was out of here.
[Diane, age sixteen:
cavitary tuberculosis]

Inherent in many of these narratives is the subissue of the need to know what is happening, what to expect in detail, and to feel that he or she has been party to the evolution of therapeutic plans, again speaking to mastery, control, and autonomy.

"Is this gonna hurt Doc?
Will I have to cry?"
"No, you won't feel a thing.
Would your doctor lie?"

Now I won't have to prepare myself to receive any pain.
I'll just sit back and relax and count the links on that chain.
All of a sudden my hopes are let down.
I was in so much pain
I wish I was six feet underground.
"Why did you lie, Doc?"
I said with tears in my eyes.
But the doctor didn't answer me.
I guess he is not too wise.
Doctors should always tell the patient
Exactly what they ask.
They should try to be more human.
Doc, come out from behind that mask.

> [Daniel, age seventeen:
> recent quadriplegic from a sniper's bullet
> undergoing wound debridement]

OTHER PATIENTS

Peer relationships continue to be important, not only to the normal peer group process but also for peer support in a time of crisis. Sometimes peer support is perceived as even more meaningful than that of the staff. Friendships and appreciation of the help offered by other patients on the ward are frequent themes.

> I had a special friend while I was in the hospital. Her name was Carmen. She was so nice to me. She pushed my stretcher wherever she went. We played together and laughed together. She was so nice to me. When she left I was really sad. But I got over it. Me and Carmen was just like sisters.   [Anna, age thirteen:
> slipped femoral epiphysis]

A singular omission, however, is reference to patients of the opposite sex, although keen interest is readily evident to any observer of ward behavior. It is hypothesized that this is such a sensitive issue, and particularly so in the face of the hospital setting, that denial or repression precludes writing about matters with obvious sexual implications.

Another aspect of interpatient relationships is the concern of adolescents for those who are younger. (A number of six- to twelve-year-olds are on the same ward for bed utilization reasons.) In part, this clearly reflects displacement, but it also speaks of the personal rewards, enhanced self-esteem, and sense of mastery gained by helping others who are perceived as more vulnerable.

> Marianne [age six, congenital heart disease] was crying. She was awake. I opened her drawer and looked for a doll for her, and then I gave it to her. At first she didn't want it. So I put it back, started to close the drawer. And then Marianne opened it back up again and she takes the doll. Then she was holding the doll next to her and I asked her to give me her hand. . . . Then she put her hand back in her bed and fell asleep. [Lourdes, age thirteen: fracture of arm]

Last, the death of another patient poses particular challenge to the youth's own perceptions of invincibility. This may well be the first time that death has been encountered in such direct terms, forcing previously unadmitted concerns to the surface. Several of our adolescents used the writing mode to mourn the loss of a fellow patient and the loss of their own innocence about mortality. The following lines are about a dying twelve-year-old:

> She hardly never talked.
> She was always very quiet.
> She was feeling a lot of things though.
> I guess she knew partly everything that was going on.
> She would feel scared but she would also feel there
>   has to come a time when
> She just wouldn't be able to keep on living.
> She tried to be calm 'cause she knew it would be coming.
> She wouldn't be crying or screaming,
> She'd be calm. . . .
>
> Everyone knew it was the end when they put on her
>   pints of blood and I.V.'s and oxygen mask so
>   she could breathe.
> Everything came together like a bundle.
> It felt to me like I was losing a sister.
> Like she was part of me.

We were together so long. . . .
And, like, when I heard it, I felt they had broken or
  taken a part away from me.
It's like losing a part of me and I need that part.
I guess I'm gonna have to pretend I have that part
  there with me.

      ["The Girl Who Died Quietly," Maria, age fourteen:
      acute appendicitis]

FAMILY

Properly, this topic should not be listed as a recurrent theme. To the contrary, parents and home are rarely addressed in writing. Although most of our patients appropriately look forward to going home, this does not appear to be high on the agenda of stressful concerns, in contrast to the primacy of the separation issue for the younger child. We conjecture that the normal developmental distancing process attendant to emancipation relieves the adolescent of this burden.

Two exceptions are evident. First is the particularly immature adolescent who resorts to regression as a major coping mechanism, reverting to much earlier parent-dependency ties.

When I'm near my mother it's like a warmness that's coming into your chest. Like it's telling you that it's your real mother without your needing proof. It's like your food and water; You can never leave it. . . .

      [Diane, age fourteen:
      idiopathic abdominal pain]

Second is the seriously ill adolescent of any developmental age who looks to his or her family as a vital support system.

When you go through what I've gone through, it makes you want to live more. If you have your mind set on living you can go through anything. When I had my operation I knew I was on my way out.

My color went out of me, my kidneys stopped and my heart for a little while. All I knew was that I had to get better, set my mind on living. For a while I felt I was in another world, a peaceful world though. And when my family came to see me, we would hug each other in a way we only usually do after we haven't seen each other in a long time. And everybody that came to see me, I'd grab their hand real hard.   [Ginny, age eighteen: congenital heart disease]

Our patients' writings clearly validate our theoretical considerations of the impact of illness and hospitalization on development. Pervading most of the writing are concerns for loss of control, impaired identity, and diminished self-esteem. In an incomparable manner they let us into the world of the hospitalized adolescent and increase our awareness of and sensitivity to the inner conflicts, fears, confrontations, and challenges facing these young people. The writing also points to the depth and richness of adolescents' intellectual capacity, even those of the inner city, and provides convincing evidence that teenagers are capable of far greater insight than generally believed.

In the individual case, creative writing also gives us vision of the true genesis of maladaptive behavior in compassionate and empathic rather than alienating terms. Reciprocally, we are given a glimpse of the vulnerabilities of those who outwardly appear to be unperturbed and doing well.

As a Medium of Communication

Adolescents believe it is risky to tell doctors or nurses directly their negative or positive feelings. Expressions of anger and resentment bear the distinct possibility of precipitating counteranger or even abandonment by precisely those individuals whom the adolescent must rely upon. The adolescent's own experience has found this to be frequently true in other settings (e.g., the punitive response of a teacher or the abandonment by a peer). The adolescent has no basis on which to believe that a health professional might behave differently (and reality dictates that sometimes they do not behave differently). Many of our young patients' writings were specifically intended for posting on the bulletin board or publishing in the ward magazine with the intent of telling a staff member just how the author feels, but in a manner that does not risk rejection.

My doctor, he's gotten so important that he has forgotten all about his patients. He used to be a very nice and considerate person.

107

When I got my first operation, he was the one who put my I.V. in and put me to sleep. When I woke up he was by my side. He used to come every day to see me. But when the years kept passing, he got more and more important. He's still nice, but he's changed in a lot of ways. He hardly ever comes to see me when I'm in the hospital. . . . I'm not saying that he has to be every day by my side, but he should come and see me at least and say how I'm doing or what he's going to do. I think that people shouldn't change just because they are a little important. They should think that people are human and they have feelings.   [Anonymous]

Conversely, to speak too warmly of appreciation also is difficult for adolescents whose transference and feelings of affection for their physician are not entirely divorced from sexual and seductive fantasies. Face-to-face expression of gratitude bares the possibility of saying more than is intended, risking emotional embarrassment. Writing permits the stating of exactly what one wishes to say without a compromising excess.

> He's nice.
> I like everything about him.
> He's patient.
> You can play with him.
> He's just like someone you've known a long time.
> He comes here every morning.
> No matter where he is, he comes here every morning.
> He always remembers us.
>
> [Isobel, age sixteen:
> Hodgkin's disease]

Writing is also a way for patients to convey what they feel to busy staff members who may not take the time to listen; or to express what one would like to say, but cannot out of feeling inhibited in the presence of adults seen as overwhelmingly omnipotent.

> Nurses and doctors are sometimes nice.
> They are sometimes good in advice.
> But after a while they can become a pain,
> And then it's best to keep cool and refrain.

Play along with what they say,
And then it won't be so hard to obey.

Let the doctors have their fun
When they come with blood guns.
And then, after a while, they will be done.
So then you can get up and run.

Let the nurses have their fun too,
Because they go along with the rules.
They will help you in every way
To make you have a pleasant stay.
But remember, some can be a pain too.
Like tell you things that are not true.

But we put up with the mess
Just not to become a pest.
For you will see, when they are through with you,
That you are a different person and feel different in
   a certain way.
That they have done what they did
To make you feel this way. . . .

                [Daisy, age seventeen:
                  lupus erythematosus]

Last, writing also is a way of countering the depersonalizing experiences commonly met in an institutional setting—a way the patient can be seen for himself or herself, not just simply a disease.

As I sit here and . . . look at these strange faces and cold hands, I feel like I'm a football and the doctors and medical students are football players. Every time I see a crowd of doctors and medical students coming to look at me, I start to get the feeling I'm on display. The doctors look at my leg and say words I don't understand . . . it makes me feel scared like I never did before. Every day when I see the doctors coming, I wonder when or if they will tell me I can't walk again.   [Gino, age thirteen:
            severe fracture of leg and in traction]

PEERS

Our patients' writing often has the intent of establishing ties with known and unknown peers—ward mates and those yet to come. Many have expressed their pleasure in knowing that their work will be made available to others and may be helpful to those who must someday go through the same course; an altruistic theme encountered with some regularity. Writing in many instances is specifically meant to both give and receive peer support in validation of continued esteem, even in the face of significant loss.

When I saw Marilyn, she was really scared and every time I tried to talk with her she never answered back. I knew right away she was scared. I felt so sorry for her that she had to go through everything I had already gone through. . . . They tell you so many things. It hits you all at once; needles, blood, the traction. . . . I felt like crying when they told me all those things I'd have to go through. Peter . . . really saved my life. He told me that traction wasn't so bad. He softened me up. Right after talking to him I knew what was coming. Since Peter told me, I wanted to tell someone else who was just as nervous as I was.

[Wanda, age thirteen: scoliosis repair]

As a Therapeutic Tool

The act of writing and the setting down of thoughts, feelings, and experiences into tangible form has a number of specific benefits which, collectively, support the more adaptive of coping modes. We do not wish to imply, however, that creative writing is sufficient unto itself. Obviously, much more is needed and support is best provided in a multi-faceted manner. But the analysis of a single element of the support system is illustrative and prototypical of the management approach in toto.

VENTILATION AND SUBLIMATION

Patients on a medical ward are not always given opportunity to express themselves in emotional terms. Expectations of intellectualization and a "stiff upper lip" philosophy more often prevail. Yet ventilation of pent up anger or simply a personal review of current events and associated fears is an important first step in adaptation. Fostering ventilation through writing diminishes the possibility of acting out taking place through more behaviorally unacceptable terms. The act of writing also serves to sublimate anxieties by the very process in an approved, even humorous manner.

> There are nurses,
> Then there are nurses,
> And then there is THE nurses.
> This third set wish you would leave in hearses.
> The same ones want to make you sit and suffer.
> If you show them your discomfort, they show you their
>   laughter.
> People wonder of the experience in a hospital.
> The news is somewhat confidential.
> Yet frequently patients scream of pain.
> But the third set of nurses hope you get it from
>   your toes to your brain.
> So if by some misfortune, you get the third set of nurses,
> Remember—
> Do as you please, but don't expect results or something.
> If by luck it comes, it's better than anything.
>
> > [Tina, age sixteen:
> > comminuted fracture of leg]

MASTERY AND CONTROL

Writing is an effective way in which the patient can be given tangible evidence that he (or she) is at least master of his thoughts and in control of his words, if nothing else. Setting down one's thoughts to be read by others provides a sense of accomplishment and self-determination. Additionally, the act of putting feelings into written words gives structure and form to diffuse anxiety. In turn, this aids putting anxiety into manageable proportions, decreasing the risk of escalating anxiety and impulsive maladaptation.

> My mother said, "Don't worry. Don't worry. Everything is going to be alright." But it's like you don't know what's going to happen, how it's going to feel. Like you have to find out for your own

self. You can't really say that you're scared, but you'd be imagining in your head all different kinds of things than they tell you. Tomorrow is a big day because I never gone through nothing like this before. It's something new to me. I'll just bear with it and let it heal.

> [Nicole, age fifteen:
> sickle cell anemia with cholelithiasis
> before surgery]

Control also may be afforded through the impact of a patient's writing on staff response. It is not unusual for a distributed poem or piece of prose to modify the negative view and defensive posture of ward personnel toward an adolescent perceived as "difficult," coming instead to see him or her in undefended terms. On the youth's part, he comes to perceive that he is not entirely helpless in the face of authoritarian adults and, in some measure, can promote a more supportive, kindly, and tolerant demeanor toward him by his own constructive act.

> . . . They gave me four spinal taps. Now they want to operate and I'm really scared for an operation because the way the doctor told me. It was frightening. He opened his eyes wide when he told me and he had a strong voice and was real big. I didn't like the surgeon who told me that. And my heart started pounding real fast.
>
> [David, age fourteen:
> old unhealed skull fracture]

IMMORTALITY

Writing offers the possibility of continuity, even immortality, for those who are seriously ill. This, in turn, helps counter feelings of impending isolation and abandonment through a sense of connectedness and permanence. This is not always implicit in the writing itself, but it is often quite clear in the context, with the patients requesting that the piece be given to his or her family and posted in the hall.

> You know this forest. . . . There was green and yellow from little flowers—dandelions. They sat and they just blew, gentle and softly, staying in one spot. It wasn't on my block; my block was too small. . . . One day my uncle and I saw a lot of men cut down

trees. They were left there in long logs and the tops of them were
thrown out. The logs were strong-looking and brown. Full strength
it dies. And there are a lot of flowers around the log that makes it
look even better. They were dandelions. The log was surrounded
by all these flowers.   [Barbara, age seventeen:
                          cerebellar astrocytoma, terminally ill]

INTELLECTUAL STRENGTHS

The invocation of intellectual strengths in substitution for that which
has been lost often can help to counter diminished self-esteem and loss
of independence, invariable accompaniments of hospitalization. Writing not only offers channels for constructive coping through intellectualization, but also through compensation when the creative
product is endowed with credibility and value by others and the young
person himself.

The more science there is, the more pain it is for the person to get
cured. Now-a-days it's like more complicated and more painful. . . . It can make people well, but they should also understand
how much pain is inflicted on the other person. They should find
out always what the potential of the pain is for the benefit of the
creator and the participant. That's really the heart of success.
                                    [Liz, age fifteen:
                          regional ileitis (Crohn's disease)]

DEVELOPMENTAL ALTRUISM

In a number of instances, writing has served to support the adolescent's growing sense of idealistic altruism by intending his work to be
put to the help of others who may benefit from reading it, sharing a
common set of concerns. The validity of this perception has been repeatedly confirmed by the expressed reassurance and relief of other
patients who later read such pieces and came to know they were not
alone or unique in their fears.

Let's say the doctor tells you about an operation and he explains
why you need it and why they feel it's best. You should think
about it and then come to the best decision that you can. Tell your

parents what you've decided, but it's got to be the best decision.
Don't get too worried because they've got things that will cool the
pain down. Of course one of the things will be a needle. Always
ask the nurse to help you, you know; hold your hand or whatever
it is. After that, the needle will help you get to sleep. If you don't
like a couple of nurses and doctors, try your best not to ask for
their help too much. But if they're the only ones there, you'll have
to accept it. When you're really sad, the best advice is to pray; that
really calms your nerves down—or to talk to someone you
trust. . . .

[Meg, age thirteen:
spina bifida with paraplegia]

INNER-CITY YOUTH

Creative writing has unique implications for ghetto adolescents on
the ward. Few adults have been responsive to the needs of these young
people or have taken time to listen to them unless they act out. Ghetto
adolescents have particularly deep-rooted feelings of helplessness and
hopelessness; validation of the self often only coming through street
survival techniques. Further, they commonly have received little encouragement to express themselves in a creative manner, much less
discover this potential. Encouragement in the supportive milieu of the
adolescent medical ward can open doors heretofore unknown, both for
more effective coping with hospitalization and enhancing the quality of
life in broader dimension. A borderline delinquent and dropout wrote
thus:

"Don't worry Mr. Mendoz, you're going to be fine." I wish I
could tell you what's really on their minds. "Lie back Mendoz,
please relax. After the tests we'll know some facts."
"Yeah, but what seems to be the problem? What could be
wrong?"
"Please, Mr. Mendoz, this won't be long."
"I'm a little worried. What's that machine?"
"Calm down Mendoz! It's not as bad as it seems. Take off your
pants. Take off your socks."
You tell me not to worry and you're going to plug me into that box!

[Raphael, age sixteen:
traumatic injury to the peroneal nerve]

Conclusions

The hospitalized adolescent is singularly vulnerable, unguarded, and potentially open to new methods of coping with stress. Former denying concepts of magical invulnerability are no longer valid or effective. The creative-writing experience brings unconscious concerns to the surface, but in measurable and manageable terms. It can help the young patient look at life-death, despair, damaged body image, threats to identity and self-esteem, frustrated emancipation, or anger and rage. These thoughts are brought out into the open where they can be dealt with in direct, honest, and supportive terms rather than through denial.

We further suggest that this may be a unique opportunity in an adolescent's life. Capitalizing on an unavoidable, stressful, and, often, pivotal life-event by raising fundamental issues to a conscious level frequently initiates a process of continued insightful reflection about the self. Vague feelings and thoughts become crystallized to be put in the service of rational consideration of the present and future, contributing to self-directed and thoughtful acts rather than impulsive behavior.

The discovery of the creative seed can be a new resource in health as well as illness. Discovering that he (or she) can perceive and express thoughts in ways and depths not previously experienced, the adolescent gains a new set of skills to the enhancement of self-awareness and promotion of understanding others.

> I feel like this whole experience changed me. I'm not the person I used to be. I feel that since I took so much pain that I'm now more of an adult. . . . If this accident had not happened, life would have been as usual. But this has happened and now I have a totally different attitude about a lot of things, like life. I was looking at life with a negative attitude; seeing people fight, be violent, and racial conflict. The positive attitude toward life is nature. To stroll through the park again; to look at the sun, the blue sky and to be content. . . .

> I saw myself in a mirror before the operation. I just gazed and gazed and gazed. "Take it out" I said, "I don't want to look that way any more." The eye was destroyed. I thought this decision through on my own. . . . The night before the operation to take out

my eye, I was thinking not only about my eye and the accident but the expression on my mother's face. Tremendously sad, I used my eye for the last time. I cried. And cried. Let the eye cry for me because it's the last time that it will accompany me in my crying, sorrow.
[Robert, age seventeen:
traumatic rupture of eye]

REFERENCES

Bergman, T., and Freud, A. 1965. *Children in the Hospital.* New York: International Universities Press.

Erikson, E. H. 1950. *Childhood and Society.* New York: Norton.

Hacker, F. J. 1965. *Creativity in Childhood and Adolescence.* Stanford, Calif.: Science & Behavior.

Hofmann, A. D.; Becker, R. D.; and Gabriel, H. P. 1976. *The Hospitalized Adolescent.* New York: Free Press.

Jennings, S. 1974. *Remedial Drama.* New York: Theatre Art.

Kramer, E. 1971. *Art as Therapy with Children.* New York: Schocken.

Leedy, J. J. 1969. *Poetry Therapy.* Philadelphia: Lippincott.

Lewis, N. R. 1978. The needle is like an animal. *Children Today* 7(1):5–8.

Nordoff, P., and Robbins, C. 1971. *Music Therapy in Special Education.* New York: Day.

Piaget, J. 1969. The intellectual development of the adolescent. In G. Caplan and S. Lebovici, eds. *Adolescence: Psychosocial Perspectives.* New York: Basic.

Read, H. 1945. *Education through Art.* New York: Schocken.

Read, H. 1966. *Art and Society.* New York: Schocken.

Schowalter, J. E., and Lord R. D. 1972. On the writings of adolescents in a general hospital ward. *Psychoanalytic Study of the Child* 27:181–200.

Tanner, J. M. 1962. *Growth at Adolescence.* 2d ed. Oxford: Blackwell.

Way, B. 1967. *Development through Drama.* London: Longmans.

ADOLESCENCE
AND
DIVORCE

7 DIVORCE AND CHILDREN AND ADOLESCENTS: AN OVERVIEW

ALLAN Z. SCHWARTZBERG

During the past decade, the incidence of divorce has been accelerating at an alarming rate. In 1976, 1977, and 1978 there were approximately, on an annual basis, 1.1 million divorces in the United States and 2.2 million marriages. For every two marriage licences issued during the year, one divorce was granted (U.S. Dept. of Commerce 1979). Three times as many children experienced divorce of their parents in 1976 as was the case twenty years earlier. While two out of every five couples who divorce have no children, divorces where there are children usually leave the custodial parent with two or more children to care for. Approximately 19 percent of households with children under eighteen years of age are one-parent families, 17 percent are maintained by the mother alone, and only 2 percent by the father. Thus, the most frequently found family situation in the immediate separation and post-divorce period is one in which the children live with a single mother and have intermittent or no contact with the father.

While a number of excellent statistical and demographic reports exist concerning marriage and divorce, there is much less information available on the characteristics of psychopathology in children whose parents are divorced. Few studies of psychopathology controlled for such variables as sex, age, socioeconomic status, time lapse since parental separation, as well as the quality of the parent-child relationship before, during, and after divorce have been reported. Similarly, there have been few direct behavioral observations of nonclinical populations of children and adolescents at the time of parental divorce (Hetherington 1972; McDermott 1968).

119

This chapter will review some of the relevant literature on the divorce process and its effects on children and adolescents. The chapter will focus on the effects of divorce at various developmental stages and the implications for appropriate therapeutic interventions.

The Divorce Process

Divorce may be viewed as a process in which the family system is altered but not terminated. A family perspective on divorce emphasizes continuity and mutuality with reciprocal obligations and responsibilities extending well beyond the legal act of divorce. The process of divorce can be divided into three phases: an initial predivorce phase; a phase of separation; and the postdivorce phase.

A variety of types of marriages and motivations precede the final decision to divorce. In many marriages parents have stayed together "for the sake of the children," attempting to present a united front until heightened stress, communication breakdown, and increasing distance, often precipitated by an extramarital affair, present the final impetus to the decision to divorce. Anthony (1974) describes how the nature of the marital conflict prior to divorce influences the type of psychological reactions manifested. He noted that in one study a majority of grown-up children (80 percent) recalled the predivorce period as one in which the families were closely united and free from overt conflict, with only a minority (20 percent) reporting constant open warfare between the parents. Anthony stated that a hostile parental relationship results in children with increased irritability and aggressiveness, while children from devitalized marriages generally react with flatness and lack of zest. In intense marital relationships with overt hostility, children often serve as pawns, scapegoats, manipulators, and allies of the conflicting parents.

Despert (1962) noted that "emotional divorce" begins a long time prior to the actual divorce. She postulated that it was not divorce per se but a bad marital relationship with or without divorce which determined the child's adjustment. She noted that a child would be disturbed when the relationship between the parents was disturbed. While emotional divorce usually precedes legal divorce, it is not always followed by legal divorce.

Anthony (1974) observed that child and adolescent reactions to divorce depend on the age, stage of development, sex, quality of the early environment, the amount of stress previously experienced, and the ability of the parents to provide security. Additional reactions depend on the nature and extent of family disharmony prior to divorce, the parents' and adolescents' personality structures, and the parents' relationship during the separation and divorce period.

Initially, nearly all children and many adolescents experience divorce as painful and traumatic. Wallerstein and Kelly (1974, 1975, 1976a, 1976b) note that anxiety is related to a heightened sense of vulnerability, sadness at the loss of the noncustodial parent and the protective and supportive family structure, guilt over fantasized misdeeds, worry over distressed parents, anger at the parent or parents who have disrupted their world, often shame at the parental behavior, and a deep sense of aloneness. There is a concern with being different from peers.

Wallerstein and Kelly noted in their studies of normal preschool children in families of divorce that the youngest children, ages one to three, experienced regression, bewilderment, irritability, separation anxieties, sleep problems, and a state of neediness. The disturbance was strongest where parental discord continued following the divorce and when the custodial parent was seriously impaired in family functions. The best adaptation was made by those children where there was consistent parenting and affection by both parents.

In the middle preschool group there was an increase in aggressive behavior coupled with a fear of regression. The children of this age group experienced unpredictability and undependability in relationships and a good deal of insecurity. There was evidence of self-blame and reduced self-esteem. The children displayed increased inhibition, constriction in play and fantasy, diminished self-esteem, and continuing sadness. The older preschool children showed evidence of anxiety, irritability, and aggression. Vulnerable children in this group have particular difficulty in resolving oedipal conflicts; five- and six-year-old girls were noted to continue to cling to fantasies of the father's return. However, others in this group were able to place distance between themselves and the parents without impairing their development. Latency-age children were noted to be depressed and vulnerable to regression. There was a strong sense of loss felt by younger boys, especially in regard to the departing father.

At a one-year follow-up, Wallerstein and Kelly noted that many normal preschool and latency-age children were significantly worse psychologically. In the later latency-age group they gave evidence of consolidation into troubled and conflicted depressive behavior patterns. There was evidence of chronic maladjustment with continuing depression, low self-esteem, and frequent school and peer difficulties. Deterioration one year after parental separation was correlated most significantly with continuing family disorganization, unremitting anger, and/or the psychological elements of the custodial parent (i.e., impaired coping). For relatively intact children, the resumption of developmental growth seemed primarily related to the availability of support systems and the relationship between the custodial and noncustodial parents.

Wallerstein and Kelly (1974), in their study of twenty-one adolescents from divorced families, noted that the family disruption "poses a very specific hazard to the normal adolescent process of emancipation from primary love objects. If the disruption does not come prior to normal detachment, independence and maturation may even be facilitated. The adolescent may be able to 'transform' feelings of helplessness into a sense of control by active mastery."

In adolescents, some of the prominent effects related to considerable sadness and a sense of loss and betrayal by the parents. There was evidence of recurrent themes of anxiety about future marriage, worry about money, abrupt deidealization of parents, heightened awareness of parents as sexual objects, and often intense loyalty conflicts. Adolescents who coped best were able to make a strategic withdrawal from the parental conflict, allowing for a more objective assessment of parental behavior, enabling them to proceed with normal adolescent developmental tasks. Wallerstein and Kelly noted three major psychopathological formations: prolonged interference with entry into adolescence, temporary interference with entry into adolescence, and pseudo-adolescence. Schwartzberg (1980) in a study of thirty adolescents from divorced families noted similar psychopathology. Subsequently Wallerstein and Kelly (1980) found a close connection between continued contact with the noncustodial parent and the adolescent's self-esteem. This connection was especially strong among older teenagers, particularly boys. There was a significant link between depression and children at the five-year mark and disrupted or impoverished contact with the noncustodial parent.

The Stress of Divorce

It is difficult to generalize about the psychological effects of divorce on children and adolescents. The immediate reactions depend on the cumulative stresses from the predivorce period and vary with the particular circumstances triggering the divorce, whether alcoholism, mental illness, adultery, desertion, or cruelty. If the predivorce marital relationship has been reasonably amicable, the children will often react with transient situational adjustment reactions. The major task relates to the need to work through the losses that the child sustains. These losses generate a wide range of affective reactions including anger, guilt, hurt, anxiety, mood fluctuations, and impaired functioning. While there is a similarity between divorce and the loss of a parent through death, there are also significant differences. In death, the absent parent is usually idealized; in divorce, the absent parent is usually devalued. While it is essential to work through the loss of the departing parent, frequently powerful resistances of repression, denial, and acting out develop to interfere with the mourning process. Some authors have noted that the child's tendency, in reacting to the death of the parent, is to avoid acceptance of the reality of the emotional meaning of death and to await the return of the deceased parent (Deutsch 1937; Fleming and Altschul 1963; Wolfenstein 1966). Similarly, in divorce, reconciliation fantasies are typically present, especially in preschool and latency-age children, and persist for prolonged periods of time, even after a subsequent remarriage of one or both parents.

Problems in the Single-Parent Family

A number of authors (Hetherington 1972; Hetherington, Cox, and Cox 1977b; Ilgenfritz 1961; Weiss 1975) have described the stresses present in the single-parent family. These stresses operate on the custodial parent, usually the mother, and affect competence and coping ability. Task overload includes the multiple daily tasks of homemaking functions, holding a full or part-time job finding adequate child care, along with the provision of emotional support, financial security, as well as the enhancement of self-esteem and promotion of an effective parental role model.

All too often mothers in single-parent families are isolated socially and lack social and emotional supports. This is especially true in a mobile society. Hetherington (1972) noted that social isolation is often associated with acute depression. Single mothers are likely to have fewer friends, belong to fewer organizations, and participate in fewer recreational activities than do married women (Pearlin and Johnson 1977). A social network in the formation of friendships and intimate attachments seems crucial to alleviating intense loneliness and social isolation.

Hetherington, Cox, and Cox (1976, 1977a) have examined the complex emotional reactions precipitated by marital dysfunction. They noted that divorced parents felt more anxious, depressed, angry, rejected, and incompetent than married persons. Divorced men and women both experience these changes in self-concept. Fathers felt a lack of identity, rootlessness, and complained of a lack of structure, whereas women complained of feeling unattractive, helpless, and of having lost their identity as married women. Weiss (1976), in a study of 150 separated men and women, noted that even when love and other positive feelings between the separated couple faded there was a persistent strong attachment which remained even when alternative relationships had been established. Weiss compared this marital bond to the attachment of children to parents described by Bowlby (1960, 1978). Separated spouses and children separated from parents both had reactions that included rage, anxiety, maintenance of strong fantasy relationships with the lost person, and persistent efforts at reunion.

There is evidence that the stress on the single parent has reciprocal effects on the children, who in turn trigger stress in parents. In short, the effects of divorce represent a process and a dynamic interaction through time and involving different phases. Hetherington et al. (1976, 1977a) conducted a two-year project on the effects of divorce on family interaction functioning by intensively studying families of forty-eight nursery school–age boys and girls from divorced families with a control group of children from intact families. The results showed that divorced persons have difficulty parenting, particularly mothers with sons, and that they did not communicate very well with their children, were not very affectionate, and were inconsistent in disciplining their children in contrast to the parents of intact families. They suggested that disruptive behavior, especially in boys, can cause emotional responses in mothers such as anxiety, feelings of helplessness, incompetence, and depression. Under such pressure the mother often becomes an ineffective parent and provokes further negative behavior in the children.

Coping with Emotional Reactions to Divorce

Attachment theory provides a theoretical framework in which to view divorce as both a process extending over time as well as involving specific tasks related to the task of working through the experience of loss. Bowlby (1960) has described the occurrence of four phases of reaction to separation: denial, protest, despair, and detachment. Reactions to loss may be temporary or prolonged and are dependent upon the child's and parent's age, coping capacity, support systems, degree of stress experienced, and the extent to which previous losses have been mastered and worked through. The pattern occurring not infrequently is where a departed parent, usually the father, has left because of an extramarital affair. The custodial parent is confronted with the need to work through feelings of shock, hurt, anger, guilt, depression, despair, and the wish for revenge. Often this period occurs at times of greatest stress with the immediate crisis period both before and after separation. Thus, the crisis of separation can be characterized as a time of great stress, increased needs of both parent and child, often with decreased support systems, regression, and temporarily impaired coping and parenting ability.

The child, too, needs to work through the stages described by Bowlby. Additionally, the child usually experiences intense and continuing loyalty conflicts. The intensity of the conflict depends not only on the child's relationship with each parent and the coping capacity of each parent, but also on the degrees to which the parents have been able to negotiate their differences. It is possible, with the current trend toward development of joint custody, that the intensity of loyalty conflicts will be lessened. Many children experience sympathy and support for the departed parent as somehow being disloyal to the custodial parent.

After-Effects of Divorce on Children

Anthony (1974) has written about the postdivorce period which he characterizes as a "neurosis of abandonment." This period is marked by alternations between inner depression and outer aggressiveness, a grieving for the lost family unit, and feelings of being small, weak, and intensely vulnerable. McDermott (1970) in a study of nearly 1,500 children from divorced families up to age fourteen noted several symptom clusters. These included depression of moderate to severe intensity in approximately one-third of the children, running away episodes, delinquency, and very poor home and school behavior.

A number of studies (McDermott 1970; Wylie and Delgado 1959) demonstrate a direct association between divorce and delinquency.

Delinquent children have been noted frequently to come from homes broken by separation and divorce. McDermott speculated that running away had to do with attempts at reunion with the absent parent. In some cases there is a reaction to a submerged depression which can no longer be tolerated. McDermott also noted special problems with identification and superego development. There appeared to be a definite relationship between the presenting symptoms of delinquency and acting-out behavior and the image of the devalued father. Some children seemed to be reenacting the father's role when the mother referred to the father as no good, promiscuous, unfaithful. McDermott observed that frequently an unconscious conspiracy of both mother and child occurred to recreate the lost father through the child's identification with his traits. This process seemed to provide a mechanism through which the mother could continue to express anger, guilt, and punish the father through the child.

Superego development appears to be affected by divorce in view of the frequent experience of parental regression, poor impulse control, distortions, and inconsistencies, both in their relationship with each other as well as with the children during the separation period. McDermott concluded that there was a high correlation between the child's presenting symptoms and the description of the absent parent, suggesting identification with a part or a fantasied part of that parent as a way of dealing with the loss and the conflicts surrounding it for both mother and child. The largest group of children consisted of those whose symptoms erupted during a subclinical depression period after the divorce experience with the symptoms classified as predelinquent, eventuating in a part of their character formation.

Hazards of Divorce for Adolescents

Sorosky (1977) noted special psychological vulnerabilities that may occur in adolescents: a fear of abandonment, rejection, or loss of love; interference with the resolution of typical adolescent conflicts; and an intense fear of personal marital failure. In addition to these vulnerabilities, the child is often confronted by conflicting loyalties as described by Wallerstein and Kelly (1974). They noted that the conscious or unconscious expectation that the child align with one parent against the other in a continuing struggle resulted in frequent feelings of despair, guilt, and depression. In their case series, more than half the adolescents were profoundly conflicted with issues of allegiance and loyalty. They angrily protested the role they felt was being forced upon them, but at the end of one year, virtually all were able to disengage themselves from active loyalty conflicts. This is in marked contrast to latency age children, many of whom were unable to detach themselves from this destructive process due to their age and dependence on their parents for continued support. Additional issues involved blurring of generational boundaries, role reversal, and exploitation and manipulation of one or both parents by the child.

The loss of the marital partner tends to lessen the defined roles and generational boundaries between parent and child. It was much harder for the parent to maintain authority and control, especially in mother-son relationships. It was much easier for the father than for the mother to assume the culturally defined role as disciplinarian, especially with boys. The need of the custodial parent, usually the mother, to have a confidante leads to blurring of generational boundaries, greater difficulty with discipline, and often heightened anxiety, especially in boys, over reawakened oedipal conflicts and guilt. In order to defend against the anxiety created by blurred generational boundaries, many children will resort to acting-out behavior and adopting an aggressive and masterful stance (Tooley 1976).

Role reversal occurred not infrequently and depended on the severity of parental regression. With severe regression, there was often a need and wish for the parent to be parented by the child, causing potential interference with developmental tasks. This interference, if prolonged, can lead to a pseudoadult stance denying dependency needs which are age appropriate.

If divorced parents continue to relate with intense anger and conflict, a child may exploit the situation and play one parent against the other for his own advantage.

Therapeutic Implications of Research Studies

Clinical experience indicates that the separation and divorce process for many children and adolescents is highly stressful. In general, the earlier a child is deprived of a healthy relationship with each parent, the greater the vulnerability to developing psychological reactions to the loss.

It is important to view divorce as a process involving different phases over an extended period of time, often two to three years or more. The greatest stress appears to occur at the time of separation.

127

Parents need to be adequately educated about the divorce process in order to provide effective guidance and support while working through their own emotional reactions of anger, anxiety, guilt, hurt, and the sense of loss and abandonment. Recognition of the different phases of divorce will allow for greater therapeutic effectiveness through intervention before, during, and after divorce. A psychoanalytic developmental perspective combined with a family systems approach is particularly useful. Parents need to communicate to children that the decision to terminate their relationship with each other does not terminate their relationship as parents. Children also need to understand that they are not responsible for the parental decision to divorce and should in no way feel guilt or blame. The alleviation of guilt and the reassurance of parental commitment, loyalty, and affection require reinforcement.

All too often children and adolescents and their families receive too little education, support, counseling, and therapeutic intervention. Often, therapeutic intervention, when it does occur, comes long after the predivorce and separation phases, when depression and behavioral problems have become entrenched. The studies cited in this chapter highlight the importance of early intervention at the time of crisis. The best coping responses to divorce occurred in children and adolescents who demonstrated good predivorce ego strength and good relationships with both custodial and noncustodial parents. Positive responses were also associated with effective coping responses of the custodial parent, the ability of parents to communicate in a reasonable fashion, the availability of a supportive network, and the absence of continuing anger and depression (Wallerstein and Kelly 1980).

It is important to identify children and adolescents at high risk for the development of psychopathology. High risk is clearly dependent not only on the child's premorbid ego functioning, but also on the emotional stability of the custodial parent. Wallerstein and Kelly (1980) noted in a five-year follow-up study that "good father-child relationships appeared linked to high self-esteem and the absence of depression in children of both sexes and at all ages." This important finding gives impetus to the need for the child's access to both parents on a continuing basis. The data raise basic questions about the thesis advanced by Goldstein, Freud, and Solnit (1973) stressing the importance of the "single psychological parent who has sole legal custody and decision-making power, including visitation rights of the noncustodial parent." In the Wallerstein and Kelly study, approximately one-third of the children and adolescents were significantly depressed and 39 percent felt rejected by the father.

It is clear that the current adversary process of divorce can delay and intensify the working through of losses. New and promising trends to mitigate the effects of litigation and costly court and custody fights involve the advent of a new professional, that is, the family mediator-therapist, as well as the development of joint custody arrangements.

Preventive efforts to minimize the effects of divorce are still in a nascent state. Prevention is especially important so that the child can work through and integrate losses and change with as little interference as possible with negotiating successive developmental tasks. More preventive efforts are needed through special programs in schools, domestic courts, social agencies, churches, and synagogues. Similarly, not only do mental health professionals need further education, but so do all those professionals who work with troubled children and families, including attorneys, physicians, educators, and the clergy.

For the young child, work with parents through education and support often provides successful intervention. For the latency-age child, a combination of individual psychotherapy and parent-focused intervention is recommended (Derdeyn 1980). The major obstacles to the successful resolution of loss for the child are denial with maintenance of the fantasy of reconciliation.

Therapeutic work with adolescents should not only be ego supportive and assist with ventilation and working through anger, loss, and grieving for the lost family unit, but should also provide an opportunity to work through age-appropriate adolescent developmental issues. The therapist needs to understand the adolescent's particular anxiety about future marriage as well as concerns about developing potential ego and sexual identity impairment in the wake of parental divorce. The therapist can facilitate resolution of loss through the role of a transient ego ideal. Encouragement of a supportive network of relationships and specialized groups can be helpful. Family therapeutic intervention is often necessary with participation of both parents encouraged wherever possible. Family therapy requires appropriate neutrality, flexibility, empathy, and sensitivity.

Conclusions

Relevant literature on the divorce process and its effects on children and adolescents at different developmental stages has been reviewed.

Divorce has been stressed as a process occurring in different phases, altering but not terminating the family system and network of relationships. Factors favoring successful resolution of loss relate to good premorbid ego functioning, good coping and adaptive capacity of each parent, a positive relationship with both the custodial and non-custodial parent, and a reasonable communication pattern between the parents. The special stresses operating on the single-parent family have been noted. The effects of divorce on superego development and resolution of oedipal conflicts have been stressed, particularly with boys and mainly with the custodial mother.

The importance of early and effective intervention during the crisis of separation was particularly noted to prevent the development of severe and chronic psychopathology. It is clear that controlled studies of children and adolescents are needed at different stages of the divorce process to further increase our knowledge and understanding. It is essential that children and adolescents be able to integrate their losses and to express feelings of anger, sadness, abandonment, and anxiety in order to negotiate age-appropriate developmental tasks. When the work of mourning occurs successfully, often aided by effective family intervention, the crisis of divorce can develop into an opportunity for continued growth and development.

REFERENCES

Anthony, E.J. 1974. Children at risk from divorce: a review. In E.J. Anthony, and C. Koupernik, eds. *The Child and His Family: Children at Psychiatric Risk.* New York: Wiley.

Bowlby, J. 1960. Grief and mourning in infancy and early childhood. *Psychoanalytic Study of the Child* 15:9–52.

Bowlby, J. 1978. Attachment theory and its therapeutic implications. *Adolescent Psychiatry* 6:5–33.

Derdeyn, A.P. 1980. Divorce and children: clinical intervention. *Psychiatric Annals* 10(4):22–47.

Despert, J.L. 1962. *Children of Divorce.* Garden City, N.Y.: Doubleday.

Deutsch, H. 1937. Absence of grief. *Psychoanalytic Quarterly* 6:12–22.

Fleming, J. and Altschul, S. 1963. Activation of mourning and growth by psychoanalysis. *International Journal of Psycho-Analysis* 44:419–432.

Goldstein, J.; Freud, A.; and Solnit, A. 1973. *Beyond the Best Interest of the Child*. New York: Free Press.

Hetherington, E.M. 1972. The effects of paternal absence on personality development in adolescent daughters. *Developmental Psychology* 7:313–326.

Hetherington, E.M.; Cox, M.; and Cox, R. 1976. Divorced fathers. *Family Coordinator* 25:417–428.

Hetherington, E.M.; Cox, M.; and Cox, R. 1977a. The aftermath of divorce. In J.H. Stevens, Jr., and M. Mathews, eds. *Mother-Child, Father-Child Relations*. Washington, D.C.: National Association for the Education of Young Children.

Hetherington, E.M.; Cox, M.; and Cox, R. 1977b. Beyond father absence: conceptualization of the effects of divorce. In E.M. Hetherington, and R. Parke, eds. *Contemporary Readings in Child Psychology*. New York: McGraw-Hill.

Ilgenfritz, M.P. 1961. Mothers on their own: widows and divorcees. *Marriage and Family Living* 23:38–41.

McDermott, J.F. 1968. Parental divorce in early childhood. *American Journal of Psychiatry* 124(10):424–432.

McDermott, J.F. 1970. Divorce and its psychiatric sequelae in children. *Archives of General Psychiatry* 23:421–427.

Pearlin, L.I., and Johnson, J.S. 1977. Marital status, life strains, and depression. *American Sociological Review* 42:704–715.

Schwartzberg, A.Z. 1980. Adolescent reactions to divorce. *Adolescent Psychiatry* 8:379–392.

Sorosky, A. 1977. The psychological effects of divorce on adolescents. *Adolescence* 12:123–136.

Tooley, K. 1976. Antisocial behavior and social alienation postdivorce: the "man of the house" and his mother. *American Journal of Orthopsychiatry* 46:33–42.

U.S. Department of Commerce. 1979. *Divorce, Child Custody, and Support*. Current Population Reports. Special Study Series, P-23, No. 84. Washington, D.C.: Government Printing Office.

Wallerstein, J., and Kelly, J. 1974. The effects of parental divorce: the adolescent experience. In E.J. Anthony, and C. Koupernik, eds. *The Child and His Family: Children at Psychiatric Risk*. New York: Wiley.

Wallerstein, J., and Kelly, J. 1975. The effects of parental divorce:

experiences of the preschool child. *Journal of Child Psychiatry* 14(4):600–616.

Wallerstein, J., and Kelly, J. 1976a. The effects of parental divorce: experiences of the child in early latency. *American Journal of Orthopsychiatry* 46(1):20–32.

Wallerstein, J., and Kelly, J. 1976b. The effects of parental divorce: experiences of the child in later latency. *American Journal of Orthopsychiatry* 46(2):256–269.

Wallerstein, J., and Kelly, J. 1980. *Surviving the Breakup: How Children and Parents Cope with Divorce*. New York: Basic.

Weiss, R.S. 1975. *Marital Separation*. New York: Basic.

Weiss, R.S. 1976. The emotional impact of marital separation. *Journal of Social Issues* 32:135–145.

Wolfenstein, R.S. 1966. How is mourning possible? *Psychoanalytic Study of the Child* 21:93–123.

Wylie, H.L., and Delgado, R.A. 1959. A pattern of mother-son relationships involving the absence of the father. *American Journal of Orthopsychiatry* 29:644–649.

8 OBSERVATIONS ON ADOLESCENT RELATIONSHIPS FIVE YEARS AFTER DIVORCE

JOAN B. KELLY

The dramatic increase in the rate of divorce in the past two decades in the United States has generated new interest in understanding the overall effects of divorce on the ongoing development of children and adolescents. A large population has been touched—1 million children and adolescents each successive year since 1972—and estimates are that more than 30 percent of all youngsters born in the 1970s will experience at least one parental divorce before their eighteenth birthday (Bane 1979).

Research investigating the adult experience of divorce has been prolific (Levinger and Moles 1979; Sell 1977), and data from longitudinal studies of divorced adults have recently begun to emerge. But within the same time period, surprisingly little attention was devoted to studying the longer-range impact of divorce on children and adolescents in either the general nonclinical population, or among those receiving psychotherapeutic intervention.

One aspect of normal adolescent development that has generated considerable interest in relation to the potential disruptive influence of divorce has been the course of adolescent object relationships subsequent to parental divorce. Mental health professionals and lay persons alike have expressed curiosity about the future dating and marital relationships of those youngsters who were adolescents when their parents divorced. Some have expressed cautious optimism that once freed of the pathogenic parental marriage, these youngsters would gravitate toward healthier interpersonal relationships. Others have doubted the youngsters' capacity to overcome the destructive or unsatisfactory models of marital interaction internalized during their earlier years.

Because of the importance of object relationships in a successful negotiation of the adolescent developmental process, this chapter will present selected observations of the postdivorce heterosexual relationships of a small group of adolescents, as seen five years after their parents divorced. Of particular interest are those patterns, attitudes, and views of interpersonal relationships, including marriage, which emerged within the longitudinal context, and which seemed to be divorce engendered.

The Adolescent Group

Eighteen adolescents ranging in age from thirteen to eighteen were part of a larger five-year investigation of the impact of divorce on 131 children and adolescents from sixty families. They were first seen soon after the parents' separation, within the context of a brief preventive intervention (Kelly and Wallerstein 1977; Wallerstein and Kelly 1977), and then returned again for clinical research interviews at eighteen months and five years postseparation. Because of an interest in exploring the normative responses of children and adolescents to divorce, youngsters were excluded that had a prior history of psychological difficulties as identified by parents or the school.

The initial responses of this small group of adolescents to their parents' separation and divorce have been described in considerable detail elsewhere as have those various factors, both predivorce and postdivorce, found to be significantly related to eventual outcome or adjustment (Wallerstein and Kelly 1980). The separation and divorce was a major crisis for almost all of these youngsters, and ushered in a prolonged transition period of family instability, change, and personal turmoil. The divorce was seen to cogwheel with the normal adolescent developmental process as described by Blos (1962) and others in a painful way. Among those normal phase-specific tasks affected were the progressive decathexis of the parents and the subsequent move toward other significant heterosexual objects, the gradual deidealization of the parents accompanying this process, and the slow achievement and consolidation of greater autonomy and moral integrity. The divorce itself, and in particular the many psychological changes in the parents and in their functioning in the parental role engendered by the divorce, was seen to burden, although not necessarily overwhelm, the adolescent ego. These adolescents experienced an acceleration and intensification of those developmental processes crucial to a normal adolescence. Parents, for example, became precipitously devalued objects. The normally slow deidealization process was telescoped into a painfully shortened period of time, resulting in anger, disenchantment, sadness, and bewilderment. Adolescents once dependent upon parental advice and guidance were suddenly themselves called upon to be sources of strength and support. Some were exploited in new and unaccustomed ways, or tempted to form alignments which had a bitter rejection of the other parent as its core dynamic. Whereas the adolescent normally moves outward in progressive steps toward independence, alternating with regressive retreats to the safety and acceptance of the family, these youngsters suddenly felt called upon to be adults, watching out for disorganized and hurting parents in striking reversals of role that simultaneously enhanced their sense of being valued and needed and that potentially hampered their ability to attend to their own adolescent development. Many became wary of marriage, shaken as they were by the undependability of human relationships they previously thought permanent.

By the first follow-up, the adolescents were, for the most part, less acutely distressed by the divorce; the initial crisis period had come to an end. But two identifiable groups had emerged. The first group of youngsters had been able in the intervening year to resume their developmental agendas and were proceeding slowly in the direction of young adulthood. The second group were disrupted, delayed, or fixated in their development. These latter vulnerable youngsters had entered adolescence with some troublesome but largely unidentified psychological problems which were then exacerbated by the many changes precipitated by the divorce. Parental regressions and prolonged diminished capacity to parent left these youngsters confused and floundering without adequate guidance and support. Overwhelming bitterness between some parents, which continuously drew the youngsters into the cross fire, left them feeling conflicted and abandoned. For these adolescents, the divorce seemed to have overburdened their fragile capacities to cope with work, friends, and the tasks of growing up. Yet, as with the better-adjusted group, things were still very much in flux, and a more final verdict on the divorce impact was not yet clearly in sight.

Five Years after Separation

At the second follow-up, this same group of adolescents ranged in age from seventeen to twenty-three. Two had married, and the parents of two adolescent siblings had remarried each other again. Five of the original group of eighteen were assessed as being in good or excellent psychological condition, three were functioning at an average or adequate level with a mixture of successes and failures in school or relationships, and the remaining ten had significant psychological difficulties. This psychologically dysfunctional group were all in need of extensive psychological intervention yet none had sought help. Among the ten youngsters in trouble was one young man who sustained permanent brain injury in an accident and whose deterioration was only in small part related to the divorce.

HETEROSEXUAL RELATIONSHIPS

An examination of the adolescents' heterosexual relationships nearly five years postseparation revealed interesting and consistent configurations associated with the quality of their psychological adjustment.

Among those adolescents assessed as being quite well adjusted, none had yet developed an appropriate or enduring relationship with someone of the opposite sex. These youngsters had all dated and continued to be engaging in the normal adolescent process of heterosexual object finding and object relinquishment. Yet, they seemed to bring to the dating situation scars and reservations which they (and we) felt were engendered by the divorce. For the most part, their relationships were short lived and more often terminated by them rather than by their partners. Fears of involvement appeared to figure prominently in this pattern. These well-adjusted, competent, and articulate adolescents recognized, more clearly it seemed than adolescents from intact families, that a meaningful relationship involved commitment, but were afraid to venture. Clearly, the pain of rejection and the intrapsychic chaos observed in their parents after separation had left a strong impression.

Ann, now almost eighteen, was characteristic of these youngsters. A senior in high school with plans for college, Ann had been elected to several leadership positions at school and had a small group of carefully selected female friends. In sharing information about her dating activities, Ann asked if she could discuss some reactions that had been troubling her. When she started to like somebody socially and sexually, Ann had noticed that once back in the privacy of her bedroom she would review all the negative or less attractive aspects of her beau and, within a short period of time, found herself not liking him anymore. Asked what she thought was happening, Ann replied that she had given it some thought and wondered if she was afraid to be involved with someone of the opposite sex. She found it hard to be trusting and felt the divorce had made its mark in this way. Ann's need to defend against sexual and loving feelings partly derived from her self-identifications as a good and responsible adolescent. Indeed, she had taken on the role postseparation as an "example setter" for her younger siblings. And the oedipal anxiety and anger stimulated by her father's social and sexual activities with younger women soon after the separation may as well have encumbered the integration of a more mature capacity for heterosexual and tender love.

Two of this small group of competent adolescents had earlier been involved in relationships which lasted several years. In each case, the relationship had captured an essential aspect of their parents' unsatisfactory marital relationship.

Tom had an exclusive relationship for two years with a younger girl who, in his words, "always ordered me around." Initially, Tom was not discomforted by her demanding, bossy behavior although his friends often questioned his judgment. When Tom terminated the relationship, he had come to recognize some unhealthy parallels to the prior relationship of his parents. By the five-year follow-up, Tom found himself unwilling to be involved and, like the other well-functioning adolescents described, seemed doubtful of the value of an enduring relationship.

The remaining group of adolescents, those functioning at a barely adequate level and those with serious, chronic psychological difficulties, demonstrated a different configuration in their heterosexual relationships. Instead of a fear of involvement, these adolescents clung tenaciously to heterosexual relationships which were uniformly impoverished, immature, and ungratifying. They had rushed into heterosexual activity at the expense of personality differentiation and were incapable of making judgments about the adequacy of their relationships or of being discriminate in their heterosexual object choices. Characteristic of these young men and women were low self-esteem, depression, and an intervening history of minimal performance or failure in school. They defended against their emptiness by passively accepting and clinging to whatever came along. The relationships were long term, had a high level of sexual activity from their inception, and were most often terminated by the other partner. As might be expected, these relationships replicated important fragments of the parental marital interaction in the conscious or unconscious identifications with one or both parents.

Sandy was nearing her high school graduation when seen for the second follow-up. A shy, awkward, childlike adolescent, Sandy was naive and vague about her future and seemed content to float along without creativity, planning, or energy. She had a core group of female friends whom she described as fellow "misfits." Her boyfriend, ten years her senior, was in jail on a robbery conviction. While he had amply demonstrated his incapacity for commitment, either to rehabilitation or to their relationship, she wrote to him sporadically and planned to live with him when he was released. The impoverishment in the relationship was stark. There were none of the hallmarks of mature heterosexual love, no evidence of concern, respect, or reciprocity, only a feeling on Sandy's part that "I get along with him." Sandy's parents had lived in a loveless, barren marriage in which the father, a brutal unpleasant man, would disappear for periods of time without explanation. When he did return, the only communication was via cursory notes left on the mantelpiece, a condition the mother tolerated for a number of years. After separation, Sandy's father totally disappeared from her life. Just as she had no expectation of nurturance or even a physical presence from her father, so she made no demands upon or expected anything for herself from her boyfriend.

Nicole, now nineteen, had dropped out of high school and was working as a restaurant busgirl. Soon after the separation, when Nicole learned the details of her father's affair, she entered a period of frenetic sexual activity. She acquired a boyfriend who moved into an apartment built for Nicole by her father in the basement of the family home. Nicole's mother was totally unable to provide any limits or guidance, saying helplessly, "After all, she did just lose a father." Mother and daughter recreated a bizarre variant of the intact family with Nicole's new boyfriend. When that relationship was terminated by her boyfriend, a replacement was found. At the second follow-up, having decided that she could no longer depend on her parents, Nicole lived in an apartment with her third consecutive long-term boyfriend. But at work and within this stormy heterosexual relationship, Nicole's efforts to re-create a sense of family were pathetically evident. Now more obviously needy, easily frustrated, angered, and depressed, Nicole entered each new job situation with high hopes for a "family atmosphere." When she was treated as an employee and the longed for nurturance was not forthcoming, Nicole became quickly disappointed, felt exploited and angry, and moved on to another job. Her need to be cared for and protected and her inability to achieve an autonomy more characteristic of her age were equally evident in her relationship with her boyfriend. She wanted only pleasurable experiences, felt she deserved, and had earned, instant gratification without perseverance, and resented the demands of housework and the worries of bills.

The two marriages that occurred among this group of poorly adjusted adolescents were disastrous. One male, now twenty-three, had married eighteen months earlier, when his partner's pregnancy was discovered. In an identification with his father, this young man was cruel and abusive to his fragile and dependent wife, who required psychiatric hospitalization soon after the birth of their son. He then abandoned his family, as had his father years earlier, and moved in with another woman. An abuser of alcohol and drugs with a felony and jail record, his increasingly destructive behavior was alarming.

ATTITUDES TOWARD MARRIAGE

One of the striking findings five years after separation among the clear majority of the entire adolescent group was the very negative view of marriage which remained. When initially seen, soon after separation, adolescents were overwhelmingly skeptical of marriage and proclaimed their intent to chose partners more carefully than their parents. By the first follow-up, there had been some apparent softening of that attitude. Yet, five years postseparation, at an age when many young adults either marry or give considerable thought to it, marriage was not seen as a desirable objective or outcome for two-thirds of these adolescents.

The persisting doubts about marriage were found among the entire group, regardless of psychological adjustment status, but personal opposition to marriage was particularly pervasive in the average and well-adjusted groups where seven of the eight adolescents and young adults expressed their negative attitudes and perceptions firmly and articulately.

Ken, now a junior in college, strongly doubted that he would ever marry and related his feelings specifically to the impact of his parents' divorce. He felt that divorce "wrecks a lot of lives" and seemed to anticipate that his own marriage would inevitably lead to divorce. If he ever married, Ken reflected, he would live with the intended spouse for at least a year, and she would have to be economically independent with her own career (in contrast to his dependent, psychologically unstable mother).

Ann also told us that she would only marry after living with someone but quickly added that she saw no particular reason for marrying. Speculating that if she had a child she would probably have to marry, Ann's lack of enthusiasm conveyed the conviction that marriage had little to offer that was nourishing or valuable and betrayed as well a fear of the undependability of human relationships.

Even among those poorly adjusted adolescents who had been involved in long-term pathological relationships, there was little investment in the concept of marriage. Sandy wanted to live with her boyfriend when he was released from prison, but had no marriage plans. She most definitely wanted to avoid divorce, and felt she would wait at least ten to fifteen years before marrying.

What emerged from the interviews with all these doubtful youngsters was a sense that the divorce profoundly affected their ability to believe in the goodness and potential for love and commitment in a marital relationship. They seemed to have no visions of the intimacy, companionship, and nurturance that can exist and develop in a marriage. Indeed, they had lived for the major portion of their lives in families where the marital relationship lacked intimacy and love, and some lived in families where hostility and violence punctuated the marital existence. But equally important seemed to be the searing impressions of the divorce itself, its impact on their parents and particularly on them. Even if they felt that in the long run the divorce had benefited the lives of their parents, and for a few, themselves, these adolescents had witnessed turmoil, pain, rage, and humiliation in the unfolding of the separation period, and they remained unwilling to subject themselves to that experience. They seemed not only cautious but haunted by the potential ravages of their own anticipated divorces.

Conclusions

We have described two distinctive configurations in the heterosexual relationships of adolescents that emerged in the five years postseparation. The outcome for those well-adjusted adolescents fearing and avoiding intimacy and involvement in mature heterosexual love is unknown. While they gave evidence of a successful and consolidating move into late adolescence in their purposeful action, their constancy in emotion, their stabilizing self-esteem, and the integrations of their impulses and defenses, there seemed to be a postponement of that capacity to love and be loved in the mature heterosexual sense. Only a further longitudinal study would determine whether this represented a delay in their otherwise normal developmental process or a more permanent developmental arrest which will have longer lasting detrimental effect on their adult lives.

For those poorly adjusted adolescents who clung indiscriminately to immature heterosexual relationships, the future seemed bleak. In their failure to negotiate the often difficult but essential course of normal object relationships during adolescence, they seemed destined to lead lives of emptiness and disappointment.

REFERENCES

Bane, N.J. 1979. Marital disruption and lives of children. In G. Levinger and O. Moles, eds. *Divorce and Separation: Context, Causes and Consequences*. New York: Basic.

Blos, P. 1962. *On Adolescence*. New York: Free Press.

Kelly, J., and Wallerstein, J. 1977. Brief interventions with children in divorcing families. *American Journal of Orthopsychiatry* 47:23–39.

Levinger, G., and Moles, O., eds. 1979. *Divorce and Separation: Context, Causes and Consequences*. New York: Basic.

Sell, K. 1977. Divorce in the 1970's: a subject guide to books, article, dissertations, government documents, and film on divorce in the United States. Salisbury, N.C.: Catawba College, Department of Sociology.

Wallerstein, J., and Kelly, J. 1977. Divorce counseling: a community service for families in the midst of divorce. *American Journal of Orthopsychiatry* 47:4–22.

Wallerstein, J., and Kelly, J. 1980. *Surviving the Breakup: How Children and Parents Cope with Divorce*. New York: Basic.

LEE H. HALLER

How often will someone have to decide with whom a child will live when his or her parents divorce? The following statistics provide us with the unfortunate answer. In 1976, one of every two marriages ended in divorce (Wallerstein and Kelly 1979). For that same year, 1.1 million children were affected, a figure which is typical for the 1973–1976 time period. Even assuming a slower rate of divorce in the 1980s from the 1970s, this translates into the projection that in 1990, one-third of all children under age eighteen will have lived with a divorced parent at some time. For black children, the problem is even worse. A full 45 percent of those born in 1977 will live with a divorced parent before they reach the age of eighteen (Glick 1979).

Having examined the statistics of divorce, one can easily see the enormity of the problem for children and adolescents. Unfortunately, although the problem is perceived easily enough, it becomes a difficult task for the psychiatrist to have a significantly positive impact in alleviating the acute difficulties at the time of divorce and subsequently. One of the most difficult areas for the mental health expert to tackle successfully is child-custody evaluation. This task not only challenges the clinician's clinical acumen in terms of gathering and interpreting data but also demands that one deal with the potential pitfalls of the legal system. It is hardly surprising that many mental health experts choose to avoid this task, given the fact that to involve oneself means having to work with attorneys, to write detailed reports, to submit oneself to examination and cross-examination, and to spend time in a courtroom waiting for a case to be called. Yet, somehow, judges must arrive at a decision when parties oppose each other for child custody. The help that a psychiatrist can provide via his recommendations as to a custody and visitation plan can go a long way towards setting the stage for maximum growth of a child or adolescent in the future. No one else can provide the same degree of expertise. Therefore, since we have something significant to say, and since the courts are often willing to listen, it behooves us to consider involving ourself in this, "the ugliest litigation" (San Diego County Bar Association 1976).

Strategies of Custody Evaluation

This chapter is designed to familiarize the clinician with what he is likely to encounter in performing a custody evaluation and how to do it as successfully and as expertly as possible. There are other situations that demand a similar kind of evaluation such as abuse and neglect hearings, termination of parental rights, and adoption proceedings. The specific difficulties involved in those evaluations will not be addressed here. However, many of the principles stated herein are applicable. This discussion will be limited to the situation where two parties are competing for custody of a child, whether it be two natural parents, or a natural parent and a third party.

At this point you are concerned with what you have just read; you hear your phone ringing. On answering it, you find a person who, in a friendly yet professional way, describes how he has heard of your expertise in the field of psychiatry and is desirous of your help. He goes on to indicate that he has a client in the process of divorce and is seeking custody of the children. He gives a few details about the problems of the marriage, adds a few facts about the children, and finishes by requesting that you examine his client and the children and then send him a report as to whether his client would be the better of the two parties to have custody. Immediately, you are confronted with a decision as to whether to accept involvement. Assuming you decide you are willing to participate in this type of case, you will want to do so not as an advocate for either parent, but rather as an advocate for the child. Therefore, it is generally accepted that it is not in the best interest of the children to participate in a case without seeing all the parties involved. Your response to the attorney's request should reflect your position.

There is a rationale for involving yourself in a custody case only when you, as the examiner, are allowed to see all the parties involved.

Without having seen both parents (or both competing parties if the litigation is not between the two natural parents) and the child, and without being able to contact other relevant personnel (such as pediatricians, previously involved mental health personnel, or school teachers), the end product of your evaluation will necessarily be incomplete. Although you might be tempted to draw some tentative conclusions about the mental health of the party not seen, based on the history from the party you do see, avoid doing so. The historian you see may be too negatively biased for you to rely on the accuracy of that person's perceptions. Therefore your conclusion from having seen only one of the competing parties and the child or children involved must be limited to whether or not that parent is a fit and proper custodian for the child. This response will be of little help to the court in deciding who is the preferred parent to raise the child, especially since the other side may well have its own psychiatrist to testify to the fitness of that party.

There is another potential pitfall to doing an evaluation of only one of the competing parties and the children involved. That difficulty arises should you conclude on the basis of your examination that the party you have examined should not have custody of the child or children. In this instance, since your report is going only to that party's attorney, your report will never get in front of the court. This is because the attorney is an advocate for his client, the parent. Since your report is unfavorable to his client, it would not be ethical for him to bring that information to the court.

For these reasons it is generally accepted that a custody evaluation should be done only when the mental health expert is free to see everyone involved in order to determine the "psychological parent" (Goldstein, Freud, and Solnit 1973). There are a few exceptions to this. The first involves a situation wherein the attorney is not asking about the best interests of the child, but is interested in rebutting an allegation that his client should not have custody because of mental illness. In that case, your evaluation of only one of the parties and the children can be appropriate. You are in a position to answer the referral question. Even in this situation, however, it is necessary to see the children involved. This is because mental illness or mental retardation on the part of a parent, even if present, is not necessarily a bar to that parent having custody except as it affects the children. (These issues usually arise in a proceeding to terminate parental rights.[1])

The second exception occurs when one of the competing parties is currently residing and working out of state, such that it is extremely inconvenient, or even impossible, for him or her to get sufficient time off work to come to your office. This obstacle can often be overcome by arranging appointments on Saturday, when that parent comes for visitation. If the party refuses this option, then there is likely to be some other reason for the resistance.

This brings up the third exception, which arises when the other party refuses to become involved in a psychiatric evaluation. In this instance, one course of action could be for you to contact that party and the attorney in order to convince them of the benefits of an independent psychiatric examination. Should either refuse, you can let that person know that the refusal will be noted in your final report. This may change his or her mind. A word of caution. Do not contact the other side without first getting clearance to do so from the attorney who called you.

In each of these last two exceptions, you might wind up seeing only one side. However, there is another route to explore before doing so. Ask the attorney who called you to file a motion with the court requesting an evaluation of all parties by a single examiner. Often a court order will achieve the desired result.

Returning now to the attorney who is waiting on the phone for your answer, it is appropriate to inform him of your prerequisites for entering the case. This can be followed up by the suggestion that he contact the other attorney to see if the two of them can agree on retaining you as the independent expert. You will want the permission of both attorneys, as well as their clients, to submit your report to both sides and, possibly, to the judge.

The attorney on the phone may agree to do this and then suggest that you start your evaluation so as to avoid any further delay. Although avoiding delay is certainly something you want to encourage for the welfare of the child, this is not the time to go along with the recommendation. The basis for this initial delay is that you may wind up seeing the parent for the initial interview before the attorney you have spoken with has gotten an affirmative reply from the other side. The process of agreement involves one attorney contacting the other, who must then discuss this with his client, and then relay the answer to the first attorney. This process may take several days at least, and perhaps weeks. In addition, if the attorney you spoke with was not entirely convinced about the benefit of doing the evaluation in the manner you suggested, he may delay contacting the other side in order to consider your proposal. Needless to say, this adds another delay in all parties reaching agreement that you function as an independent expert.

If, during this process of communication between the attorneys and the client, you have already started your evaluation, counsel for the other side is less likely to see you as a truly independent expert. Therefore, he may either decline the offer entirely and get his own expert or, alternatively, may agree to the proposal of an independent expert, but decide against you being that person and suggest that someone else perform the evaluation. Thus, any time that you have already invested seeing any of the parties involved may not be productive either for you or for the parties seen. It may, indeed, prove a hindrance to any further evaluation. This is more likely to be true if you have already seen an adolescent involved in the case. He may have decided to share his concerns with you. Then, when he finds that you will not be involved, he may decide not to open up again, or at least not as readily, to the next examiner.

Therefore, in responding to the attorney who is still waiting for your answer on the phone, it is prudent to decline his offer to start on the case until he has reached some sort of agreement with the opposing attorney. However, you certainly will want to offer your assistance to him in describing your plan of action to the opposing counsel and to answer any questions he may have directly. You will want to convey this information to the parents as well, but this move can be delayed until your first session with each of them. It is extremely important that you do share with the parents and the child(ren) why you are doing what you are doing. More will be said about this later.

The method of entry into the system just described (as a result of having been contacted by an attorney representing one of the competing parties) is only one of the ways mental health experts can enter. Sometimes the request may come directly from the court (Derdeyn 1975, 1976). In this instance you will be responsive to the court and should have free access to all parties and to all information. Additionally, a report will go directly to the court, as well as to the attorneys involved. Another method of entry into the process occurs when you are contacted by a guardian *ad litem* for the child or by an attorney for the child (Derdeyn 1976). Here again, you are in a position of being able to function independently; your report will go not only to the parents' attorneys, but also to the guardian or child's attorney.

There is yet another situation wherein you may be asked to participate in a child-custody dispute. This occurs when a patient whom you currently have in treatment, or have had in treatment, becomes involved in the process of a divorce. This becomes a very difficult situation, regardless of whether your patient is one of the parents or one of the children whose parents are divorcing (Benedek and Benedek 1980). In general, the wisest course to take in this instance is to maintain your role as therapist and decline the offer to do the custody evaluation. The logic of this is obvious if it is the parent that you have in treatment. Clearly, you cannot continue to see one parent in a therapeutic role while, at the same time, evaluating the other parent and the children. To do so would interfere with the therapeutic alliance. You would not be in a position of being free to recommend custody to the parent who was not in therapy with you since to do so would jeopardize the therapeutic alliance to such an extent that the patient would flee treatment. It is reasonable, however, for you to provide information to the evaluator about your patient, should the patient so desire.

If it is the child you have in treatment, the decision to avoid serving as the evaluator for determining custody is not as obvious. Indeed, in at least one case the therapist did choose to become involved, and the outcome was positive (Miller 1976). The biggest potential problem, should you decide to involve yourself, is if the court should disagree with your recommendation and award custody to the other party. Then there would be a clear danger that the party who did get custody would pull the child out of treatment. Even if that parent left the child in treatment, your ability to do any sort of parent-guidance work might be impaired by negative feelings on the parent's part toward you, thus leaving the child caught in a loyalty conflict.

If you are no longer treating any of the parties involved, but have done so in the past, it still is advisable to abstain from doing the evaluation, at least if your patient was one of the parents. Given the therapeutic relationship, it would be extremely difficult to see the other competing party and maintain true objectivity. Even assuming that you were able to do so, your previous relationship with the parent would certainly give the appearance to any outsider of a bias. If the child was the patient, the treatment was successful, and both parents were involved, then consideration might be given to agreeing to the evaluation. However, as in the other case, before doing so, the evaluator must make absolutely certain that there are no remaining countertransference issues interfering with objectivity.

Preparation

Before actually embarking upon the custody evaluation, there are several things you need to take care of in the way of preparation. First, you need to be certain of the purpose of the evaluation. Check to see that what you anticipate doing is what the attorneys expect of you. This can most easily be done via a brief letter to both attorneys. Obviously, the major question will be which of the competing parties should have custody of the child(ren). However, your evaluation should go beyond answering this question. You may well wish to address yourself also to the question of visitation. If you do not comment on this, there is a fair likelihood that the judge will grant "reasonable rights of visitation" to the noncustodial parent in the custody decree. As a result of your interviews with the parents, you may arrive at some pertinent conclusions as to what visitation should be like. For example, you may want to recommend frequent and liberal visitation, restriction of overnight visitation, or, perhaps, even total denial of visitation by the other parent. (For divergent views on this see Benedek and Benedek 1977 and Goldstein et al. 1973.) Therefore, before beginning the evaluation, keep in mind that you have the option of making recommendations as to visitation. This should be clarified with both attorneys. The third task of the evaluation is to assess the nature and extent of psychological disturbance in the child and the parents, at least in so far as it affects their parenting abilities. Numerous authors have noted the adverse effects of the divorce process on children (e.g., Anthony 1974; Despert 1962; Wallerstein and Kelly 1974, 1975, 1976a, 1976b, 1979). So some type of stress response will likely be observed. Look, as well, for evidence of longer standing psychopathology in the child so that a recommendation for periodic psychiatric follow-up or even psychotherapy can be made, if indicated, both to the parents and the attorneys. On the other hand, your task with the parents is to identify psychopathology only as it is relevant to the child. This is not to say that mental illness not falling within this realm should be ignored. If noted, it can be discussed with that parent during the interpretive interview but need not be unduly emphasized to the other parties in the litigation.

Not only must you know what questions you will be answering in the course of your evaluation, but also what the legal criteria are for arriving at a determination. In order for your report to be effective and helpful to the judge, it must be phrased in terminology that fits the state statute. Thus, you will want to know what the criteria are for determining custody in your state. Is the test still the "tender years" presumption or is there a "best interest of the child" standard (Freed 1980)? Some states have very specific factors which are listed and must be addressed in arriving at a determination of custody (e.g., Michigan).[2] Be sure to check the statute before you begin so you know if there are any specific questions you need to ask in order to conform to the state code. Furthermore, you will want to know if the child's opinion has any legal standing in court. There are some states where a child over a certain age is entitled to express an opinion which must be given a certain amount of weight (Freed 1980). Additionally, you will want to know about any specific rulings in the state court as to how certain issues do or do not bear on the ability of an individual to have custody or be allowed visitation. For example, formerly a homosexual would not be allowed custody and perhaps would even be denied visitation unless away from his or her sexual partner. Recently, more courts are recognizing that there are few absolute bars preventing any particular class of people from having custody or visitation rights. This includes homosexuals[3] and adulterers.[4] The test seems to be not whether any of these circumstances exist, but rather what effect they have on the child or children. Thus, if a parent is homosexual, but this life-style does not adversely affect the child, then there should be no legal bar to the child having the opportunity to visit or live with that parent. Should you discover such a situation, you need not feel constrained from recommending custody to the homosexual parent, should you find it appropriate. Caution should be used in making this recommendation, however, since the data as to the effects on children being raised in a household where homosexuality is practiced is not yet clear (Javaid 1980). Likewise, there are some jurisdictions where custody can be awarded to a parent who has a "live-in lover" of the opposite sex, provided that the effect of this is not adverse to the child.[5] On the other hand, some jurisdictions still treat this situation as a bar to custody of minor children.[6] Although you, as the evaluator, may not know of all these specific decisions and need not necessarily be aware of them, one does need to be attuned to the fact that there may be statutes or case law relating to these unusual types of settings. Thus, should one encounter this type of problem during the course of an evaluation, you will be aware of the fact that you need to check with an attorney as to what the status is in your jurisdiction.

Another issue that must be dealt with before embarking on the evaluation is that of payment of the fee. This is best handled before starting the evaluation, since it is frequently a source of disagreement between the competing parties. Settling the issue with one party is not sufficient because, as with several other issues in the divorce and custody litigation, there may well be disagreement as to who is responsible for what. If the issue of payment of the professional fee is not settled before the evaluation is begun, should a disagreement arise in the midst of the evaluation, it is possible that one party will refuse to cooperate. Not only will this leave some portion of the bill unpaid, but more importantly, may prove unsettling to the child involved, especially if the diagnostic sessions with him or her are incomplete.

It is reasonable to expect payment at the time of each visit. If you wait until the completion of your evaluation to submit a bill, you may find that the party who was seeking custody and did not get it will not want to pay for the services rendered. Also, it is acceptable in this setting to bill for any significant period of time spent on the phone with attorneys, teachers, and any other people with whom you had to speak. Custody evaluations sometimes require substantial time on the phone. You should be reimbursed for this, as well as clinical time spent. However, if it is not your standard practice to bill for time on the telephone, this additional fee should be explained to both of the competing parties prior to or at the start of the evaluation and some agreement should be reached as to who will pay that portion of the bill. Likewise, it is reasonable to submit a bill for time spent writing your final report, since this will involve a substantial investment of time. As with the billing for telephone conversations, this issue should be addressed prior to or during the first interview with each of the competing parties. Finally, should you be asked to go to court to testify, it is admissible to inquire as to how much time will likely be involved and to ask for payment in advance for that service (Goldzband 1976). Since fees for time spent in court can be rather substantial, you may be asked by the party who calls you to accept payment at a later date. Should you decide to do so, it is recommended that you work out some kind of payment schedule.

There is another issue that can be addressed prior to actually starting the evaluation. This relates to having the parties provide you with relevant reports from other individuals who have seen the child, such as pediatricians, school personnel, psychologists, or other mental health workers. You will also want reports from other mental health personnel who have seen either of the competing parties. Unlike the other issues which should be handled prior to starting the evaluation, obtaining reports is optional. This must be done at some time during the course of the evaluation but not necessarily before the evaluation begins. However, to ask that reports be provided to you before you start is expedient since it often may take several weeks for the requests to be honored and for the reports to reach your hands. To get the ball rolling before the evaluation starts will speed up the entire process. On occasion, you may find one of the competing parties hesitant to provide you with information. This may have to do with a number of concerns, although one of the most frequent is that the party may not want the school system to know that the child is seeing a psychiatrist. If you meet with any resistance, the judicious tactic is to defer this issue until it can be discussed during one of the initial interviews.

Performing the Examination

Having taken care of the preliminaries, you are now ready to begin the evaluation itself. In order to get a thorough picture of the situation, each of the parents (or competing parties) should be seen on at least two occasions. Each of the children should be seen a least once individually and with each of the competing parties. You may also want to see both of the competing parties together. Some evaluators find this helpful (Rogers 1976), but it is not generally accepted as being an essential part of the evaluation process. In scheduling the appointments, it is often best not to schedule back-to-back individual appointments with the two parents. This only serves to put the parent who is seeing you second on edge and may add an unnecessary interference to conducting the interview itself. Occasionally, one parent may express a strong preference for being seen first so you are not "biased" by the other side. It is probably best to accommodate this request, provided there is no objection from the other side, and also to take into account the clinical data that accompanies this sort of request.

In the first interview, the ground rules for the evaluation should be briefly reviewed with each of the parents. The parents' waiver of privileged communication should be obtained both verbally and in writing. The release of information form they sign should give permission for you to release information to the opposing attorney and court not only about the parents, but also about the child. (Failure to obtain such releases may leave you vulnerable to a successful suit for breach of the physician-patient privilege. A recent suit, however, was unsuccessful, holding that the privilege belonged to the child.[7]) In addition, if any releases of information are needed for other outside personnel, these should be obtained during the initial interview as well.

In doing the parental interviews, one obviously wants to get a sense of them as both individuals and parents. Thus, time should be spent evaluating the psychological status of each of the parents and the presence or absence of psychopathology. One wants to look at their track record as parents—that is, their involvement with the child in the past in such areas as discipline, amount of time spent with the child, ability to share activities, and overall sense of the child as an individual. In looking at the parents' past behavior, be sure to ask about the distant past and not just the recent past, since frequently parents will try harder at being a good parent when they file for the divorce and are seeking custody. Sometimes this is for the benefit of the psychiatrist or a court; sometimes it is in an attempt to buy the affection of the child through gifts or special trips. Therefore, it is important to assess their involvement over the period of several years. Also, you will want to inquire about future plans should custody of the child be awarded to them. Do they intend to stay in the area or move far away? What plans if any do they have in mind for care of the child while they are at work (assuming that this will occur)? Who else, if anyone, will be living in the house? If they anticipate having someone else living in the home who will be involved in the care of the child, it will be important to see this person as part of your evaluation. Furthermore, it is important to ask why the parent seeks custody. In evaluating their answers to all these questions, it is necessary, just as with any other information obtained in a clinical evaluation, to listen to not only what is said about the child, but how it is said.

While discussing the child with the parent, it is important to get some sense of how the parent may interact with the child and his or her perceptions of the child as an individual. In looking at the issue of custody of an adolescent in particular, you will want to assess whether this particular parent has the ability to tolerate the normal growth of an adolescent with the concomitant movement away from the parent as primary love object or whether the parent seems to have a need to keep the adolescent excessively close and in a dependent position. You will need to assess whether there is any indication that the parent needs the adolescent for his own support and whether there is any tendency evident towards viewing the adolescent as a peer and companion rather than a child. If custody involves a child of the opposite sex from that parent, look for indications of seductiveness on the part of the parent.

Also, listen to see if there is any covert sense that the parent wishes custody in order to get revenge at the child, whether he or she blames the child for the breakup of the marriage, and whether there is any projection onto the child of qualities he or she has previously attributed to the spouse.

In evaluating all these areas, it will be important not only to listen to what the parents say, but also to assess them during a joint interview between the parent and the child. However, before doing any joint interview, it is generally advisable to see the child or adolescent alone first. As with any psychiatric evaluation, the child should be prepared for an evaluation by whichever parent currently has custody. In interviewing the adolescent, the initial part of the first interview, at least, should be a rather standard unstructured interview designed to allow you to learn about the adolescent's personality, developmental phase, and reaction to the divorce. As with any interview, you will want to elicit the adolescent's thoughts as to the purpose of the session. In this particular setting, it is important to do this at the beginning of the interview. Allow the adolescent to express any thoughts and feelings about the evaluation and the contest over his custody. It is important to let him know that the confidentiality normally attached to a psychiatric interview does not exist in this evaluation, since you are under an obligation to help the court or judge decide with whom he should live. Therefore, it will be necessary for you to divulge some of the information that is discussed between you. At some point later in one of the interviews with the adolescent, you will want to elicit his wishes about custody. It is important to do this in as nonthreatening a manner as possible. This is one place where you really do need to know the statute in regard to custody, since, in some states, the wishes of an adolescent over a certain age regarding custody are controlling or at least must be given strong weight by the judge (Freed 1980). Thus, you may not be able to give adolescents the reassurance that you can give to younger children that their decisions about custody are not the controlling factor. On the other hand, if the particular statute in your state does not address the issue of the adolescent's expressed preference, then some reassurance may be given to free him to more openly discuss his feelings about his parents.

In eliciting and assessing information from the adolescent about both parents it is important to keep in mind some of the frequent responses seen by Wallerstein and Kelly (1974) in their research on divorce. In this study, the authors describe some of the common responses of adolescents on divorce. Among other reactions, there was "precipitous deidealization of the parent." They also noted that the adolescent "feels personally betrayed by this parent's divorce and often vigorously defends against such feelings of loss by expressing considerable rage. In the process, he overzealously undervalues and derrogates at least one of these fallen parents." Another frequent response they note is loyalty conflict: ". . . One or both parents consciously or unconsciously require that the child align with him in the continuing struggle. This demand on the adolescent frequently resulted in feelings of despair, anger, guilt, and depression. At the time of the initial conflict, early in the divorce proceedings, more than half of our adolescents were profoundly conflicted by issues of allegiance, loyalty, and angrily protested the role they felt was being forced upon them." In addition, the authors note that the adolescents had a "heightened awareness of parents as sexual objects." Thus, the task of evaluating who should be given custody of an adolescent becomes an extremely difficult task due to the fact that one must sort out prior allegiances and psychological ties from the defensive reactions of the adolescents to the divorce process.

Another important area to evaluate (sometimes given less emphasis in a standard psychiatric examination) is the adolescent's ties with his siblings. This is particularly important because, perhaps more so than other developmental phases, there might be a tendency to award custody of adolescents to the same-sex parent. This would separate the siblings if both an adolescent male and female were involved. Generally, splitting of siblings is not recommended. When the parents are fighting with each other, siblings tend to rely more on each other for a support system. Investigation might disclose, for example, that although a young adolescent male might seem to prefer the father as custodian over the mother, he might be inclined in the opposite direction if given the data that his sister is likely to wind up in the mother's custody. This particular aspect of custody evaluation may become important enough that you will want to see the siblings, even if their custody is not being contested.

Not only is it important to elicit the adolescent's feelings about custody, it is also important to discuss feelings about visitation. This becomes even more important than in doing the evaluation of the younger child since an adolescent is old enough to refuse visitation and make his refusal effective by leaving home at the time when the noncustodial parent arrives. Should this happen, there is a fair likelihood that the

154

noncustodial parent will accuse the custodial parent of sabotaging the visitation which will lead to further litigation. Whatever you can do during the initial custody evaluation to forestall this event will be beneficial to all parties.

Arriving at a Decision

Having completed the evaluation, the task is to answer the question or questions posed by the attorneys. Obviously, the first and foremost question is who should receive custody of the child or children. The possible options are several. Obviously, custody of all the children may be awarded to one parent or the other. Or, it may seem most advisable to split custody of the children between the parents. More recently, there has been a tendency on the part of some courts or state legislatures to encourage joint custody (Benedek and Benedek 1979; Foster and Freed 1979, 1980). This tendency toward encouraging a decision of joint custody exists in spite of the fact that there is a paucity of good research that supports this as being a viable solution to the problem. Given the lack of research, the most prudent course is to assess this option on a case by case basis. As indicated by Benedek and Benedek (1979) there are both potential benefits as well as risks involved in this type of arrangement. One of the possible benefits they detail is that this solution, more than the others, keeps both parents involved with the children. This means that the feelings of loss which attend a divorce are minimized. On the negative side, they comment on the shuffling back and forth which is entailed for the children and the confusing differences between two home atmospheres. Instability and inconsistency might create such problems in a particular child that the benefits are outweighed. Generally it seems reasonable to expect that the solution works best when the parents live in relatively close proximity to each other and can communicate with each other about the children without becoming embroiled in old marital disagreements. One author has even suggested that joint custody can work when there is animosity between parents, provided that there is some method of transferring the children between homes without the parents coming into contact with each other and starting an argument. An arrangement can generally be accomplished under which one parent takes the child to school in the morning and the other picks up the child in the afternoon (Grief 1980).

There is yet another option in the matter of the custody dispute. That option is to recommend that neither parent be given custody of the child or children. There may be occasions when you conclude that neither of the competing parties is a fit parent. Should such a problem arise, it will be helpful to both attorneys and the court if you make some recommendation as to another caretaker. This might mean interviewing grandparents or aunts or uncles (Angell and Angell 1980). Another possibility is that the offspring be placed with relatives or in temporary foster care, with court-ordered treatment for the parents (Laybourne 1979). One must make this recommendation only with the greatest caution since there are numerous difficulties with the foster care system (Schetky and Slader 1980). If there seems to be no hope for rehabilitation of either of the potential caretakers, a recommendation might even be made for termination of parental rights (Frankel 1978; Haller, Dubin, and Buxton 1979; Shetky and Slader 1980). Quite possibly when one considers this alternative, it will be because abuse is involved. Thus, there will be a need to involve the Department of Protective Services.

Having made the decision as to who will be the more fit parent to have custody of the children, the next question is that of visitation by the noncustodial parent. It will not always be necessary for you to make a recommendation as to visitation, especially if you think that the parents can work this out between themselves. However, you may have some thoughts as to how involved the noncustodial parent should be with each particular child involved. If you have suggestions, they should be included in your discussion with the attorneys and parents, as well as in your report. For example, you may feel that visitation with the noncustodial parent should be curtailed on a temporary basis due to psychopathology of that parent which will adversely affect the development of the child. If you believe this is the case, it is important for you to so state. In addition, if you have any hypotheses about whether psychotherapy might be of help, this can be included in the report as well. On the other side of the coin, you may feel that the noncustodial parent plays a particularly significant role in the child's development, in which case you would want to recommend frequent visitation.

The presence of any special needs of the child or children you evaluated is another area that needs your attention. Examples of this would be the child who needs psychotherapy, or the child who is mentally retarded to such a degree that he or she will not be able to function independently, even when he or she is chronologically an adult. The reason for commenting on these special needs is that they require special funding and your comment allows the attorneys and parents to be aware of this so that the property settlement, including child support, will take these needs into account.

Communicating Your Findings

An important part of successfully finishing the evaluation is the timing of your meetings with the attorneys, the parents, and children, if appropriate. In order to be fair to all parties involved, the information should ideally reach all of them simultaneously. This would mean meeting with the attorneys, who can be seen together, followed immediately by separate meetings with each of the parents. Following this, the children can be seen, if appropriate, based on your clinical evaluation.

Usually, it is helpful to sit down and meet with the attorneys to go over your findings with the two of them together. There will be several questions that each of them has which need to be answered in detail. Communication should be made with both attorneys prior to the meeting to see if they are willing to meet with you before having a chance to review a written report, or whether their preference is to see a written report first. Sometimes, the parties will be able to work out an agreement as to the issues at hand without there being any need for the extra expenditure of time to write a formal report. However, even if a formal report is not written, the organizational work necessary to write a report must be done. It is necessary because the presentation of your findings to the attorneys must be done in a logical and coherent fashion. Review the history you have obtained, state your clinical findings, and then pull the two areas together in conclusion. It is extremely important that you use evidence from the history and examinations to document your findings. This will mean explaining the psychological significance of much of the interview material. Although this can be a tedious task, it is necessary since the attorneys must have at least a basic understanding of the rationale of your recommendations and the feeling that you have done a competent job. Moreover, in stating your conclusions it is important that you rely upon the statutory language. You might decide, for example, that the child should go with one parent because it is in the "best interest" of the child, but should this recommendation not adhere to the legal test for custody in the state, your conclusions are open to challenge, and, in that way, less helpful.

When meeting with the parents, it is again important that you go through your findings in an orderly progression to support your conclusions in regard to custody and visitation. As with the attorneys, it is important to allow sufficient time for questions. If your presentation is well prepared and you are able to answer all the questions the parents have, especially those of the parent who is not getting custody, then it becomes less likely that the matter will go to court. However, it is important to remember that it is the right of either party to challenge your findings by going to court. You should never presume to take on the role of the judge. To do so is an omnipotent stance that can only interfere with your effectiveness in fulfilling your role as a psychiatric expert who has been called to render an opinion.

When seeing the party to whom you are not recommending custody be given, you may feel threatened and respond by becoming overbearing since this party will likely see himself or herself as the loser in the battle and thus may well react by becoming hostile toward you. It is important that you allow this party time to ventilate his or her feelings and that you maintain an empathic stance. Eventually, during the course of the interview, you will want to explain why you decided as you did, giving the individual specific indications of what problems you have seen with him or her as a parent. If psychotherapy is indicated, recommendations should be made. The positive aspects of the individual's personality should be emphasized and some time should be spent focusing on what role he or she can play in the child's life through visitation. (This is assuming that you are recommending visitation. Various experts have disagreed on what role the noncustodial parent should play.) In this regard, it is important to stress that the noncustodial parent may still play an important role in the child's life (Friedman 1980) and that visitation rights are a responsibility, not a consolation prize.

The interview with the parent to whom you are recommending custody will obviously go more smoothly. There is likely to be a sense of relief and gratification on the part of that parent. There may also be other feelings, such as concern for whether he or she can handle the responsibility of being the single parent. As in the interview with the noncustodial parent, it is important to allow time for ventilation. Just as with the party to whom you are not recommending custody, it is also important to focus on any problems that you see and to recommend psychotherapy, if indicated. Also, if you are recommending visitation by the other parent, it will be important to discuss your rationale. Emphasis needs to be given to the importance of visitation so that this parent will work to ensure that the visitation does occur. In discussing visitation with both parents, the necessity of predictability in visitation should be emphasized. The child should be ready to go for the visitation at the appointed time and the noncustodial parent should be on time to pick the child up as well as return him on time.

Finally, in doing the interpretive interview with the parents, it will be important to point out any difficulties you have noticed the child to be experiencing. To the extent possible, a true interpretive interview should be done, indicating strengths, weaknesses, and any needs the child may have from a psychiatric standpoint. If it is clear that the child needs psychotherapy, this should be recommended. It should be kept in mind, however, that children and adolescents frequently show signs of emotional distress during the acute phase of a divorce. This is not necessarily indicative of their general level of functioning. Therefore, great caution should be used in recommending psychotherapy at the time of custody evaluation. Generally, a better course is to indicate what problems the child is having currently and that if these symptoms continue unabated, psychotherapy might be indicated. A reasonable recommendation is to suggest a follow-up visit in three months for reevaluation of functioning at that point.

After the Interpretive Interview

The next step after the interpretive interview will often be writing a report. In some cases, this is not necessary. In other cases, one or both of the lawyers may have wished to have the report before your conference with them. In still other cases, the request will come after the joint meeting. When a report is required, it becomes a tremendously important document and should be treated as such while you plan and write it. Just as with your oral presentation to the attorneys, the report needs to be thorough and orderly, with a detailed history, examination, and conclusions that are supported by the data. The recommendations with regard to custody, visitation, psychotherapy, and special needs of the child must be specific and unequivocal. Be absolutely certain that you answer all the questions that were asked in the initial consultation.

A well-written report serves not only to explain your conclusions, but can be a source of education as well to those who read it. Another, and equally important, function the report can serve is to refresh your memory as to why you recommended what you did should the case go

159

to trial. In fact, the report becomes an extremely helpful aid should several months lapse before you are called upon to testify.

If you are called on to go to court, do not panic. Going to court need not be a painful experience. In fact, it can be most rewarding if you know what you are doing. Although a comprehensive review of handling yourself in court is beyond the scope of this chapter, there are several authoritative articles on the subject (e.g., Benedek 1980b; Roberts 1975). A few brief comments here, however, might be helpful. Most important, remember that you are required to give an opinion designed to assist the judge in making a decision. You are not on trial. Therefore, your role should be to present your opinion in as professional a manner as possible and not allow yourself to become defensive under cross-examination. Do not be surprised if the attorney from the opposing side treats you harshly, in contrast to your congenial contacts with him outside the courtroom. He is merely doing his job, and, once the trial is over, you may find him amiable again. During cross-examination, he will attempt to discredit your opinion in any way that he can. In order to do so, he will use any number of tactics. As long as you confine your testimony to facts and opinions you are sure of, you should be on safe ground. But you will run into possible trouble if drawn into making speculations based on inadaquate information. You should avoid this at all costs since going beyond the bounds of your knowledge can ruin your position. Thus, if you are asked a question that you cannot answer, do not be afraid to state that you do not have enough information to answer or do not know how to answer the question. In this way, you maintain the credibility of those statements you are sure of. Be well prepared before you go into the courtroom. This entails reviewing your notes and having a pretrial conference with the attorney who has called you to testify.

One final note needs to be added to this discussion of custody. The focus of this chapter has been on the original determination of custody. However, a large percentage of the cases that go to court regarding custody are requests for change of custody based on a change in circumstances. Should you be called upon to do an evaluation of this sort, the process is the same, with one exception. In doing the evaluation, it is important for you to examine the nature and extent of the alleged change in circumstances. Once made, a custody decision should ideally be a final determination (Goldstein et al. 1973). This is important because for a child's or adolescent's emotional growth to continue, they have to be able to count on stability and continuity. If the child is repeatedly subjected to suits for a change of custody, his stability will be adversely affected by fears that the parental support system will be undone. It is incumbent upon you as the evaluator in this type of situation to look very closely at the circumstances. A change of custody should not be recommended lightly. Rather, the evidence should be extremely convincing before you make such a recommendation.

Conclusions

Performing an examination to answer questions about custody and visitation can be a challenging experience. However, owing to the enormity of the problem of divorce and the vast number of children affected, it is a challenge we must accept. Although initially one might be hesitant to become involved, the examination itself is much like any other psychiatric examination, but with some added facets. The keys to success lie in adequately attending to the preparation, doing a thorough evaluation, and adroitly conveying your findings. Application of the principles as stated here should render any difficulties manageable and, hopefully, leave you with a sense that you have helped the family members with this aspect of the divorce process.

NOTES

1. Helvey v. Radnour, 408 NE2d 17 (Ill. Appt. Ct., 1980); State of Utah in the Interest of E. and B. v. J. T. 2 Ment. Disabil. Law Rptr. 707 (Utah Supreme Ct., 1978); In Interest of M.M.C. 227 NW2d 281; 5 FLR 1885 (N.D. Supreme Ct. 1979); Matter of Welfare of Kidd 261 NW2d 833 (Minn. 1978), especially at 834.

2. M.C.L.A. sec 722.21 et seq. (P.A. 1970, No. 91, Eff. Apr. 1, 1971).

3. Nadler v. Superior Court, 255 Cal. App. 2d 523, 63 Cal. Rept. 352 (Calif. Superior Ct. 1967); Miller v. Miller 5 FLR 2032 (Mich. Supreme Ct., 1979); Belmont v. Belmont, 6 FLR 2075 (N.J. Superior Ct., 1980).

4. Hackley v. Hackley, 380 S2d 466 (Fla. App. Ct., 1979); Davis v. Davis, 280 Md. 119 (Md. Ct. of App., 1977); U.S. cert. denied, 434 U.S. 939; reh. denied, 434 U.S. 1025.

5. Davis v. Davis, 280 Md. 119 (Md. Ct. of App., 1977); U.S. cert. denied, 434 U.S.; reh. denied, 434 U.S. 1025.

6. Jarrett v. Jarrett, 382 NE2d 12 (Ill. 1978); reversed 400 NE2d 421

(Ill. Supreme Ct. 1979); cert. denied U.S. Supreme Ct.; Washington Post Oct. 21, 1980.

7. Last v. Franzblau—New York Supreme Court, August 1979 as reported in *Clinical Psychiatric News* vol. 8, no. 2 (February 1980).

REFERENCES

Angell, R.H., and Angell, K.S. 1980. Grandparents, grandchildren, and the law. Presentation at the annual meeting of the American Academy of Child Psychiatry, Chicago, October 1980.

Anthony, E.J. 1974. Children at risk from divorce: a review. In E.J. Anthony, ed. *The Child in His Family.* Vol. 3. New York: Wiley.

Benedek, E.P. 1980. The expert witness. In D.H. Schetky and E.P. Benedek, eds. *Child Psychiatry and the Law.* New York: Brunner/Mazel.

Benedek, R.S., and Benedek, E.P. 1977. Postdivorce visitation. *Journal of the American Academy of Child Psychiatry* 16(2):256–271.

Benedek, E.P., and Benedek, R.S. 1979. Joint custody: solution or illusion? *American Journal of Psychiatry* 136(12):1540–1544.

Benedek, R.S., and Benedek, E.P. 1980a. Participating in child custody cases. In D.H. Schetky and E.P. Benedek, eds. *Child Custody and the Law.* New York: Brunner/Mazel.

Derdeyn, A.P. 1975. Child custody consultation. *American Journal of Orthopsychiatry* 45(5):791–801.

Derdeyn, A.P. 1976. A consideration of legal issues in child custody contests. *Archives of General Psychiatry* 33:165–171.

Despert, J.L. 1962. *Children of Divorce.* Garden City, N.Y.: Doubleday.

Foster, H.H., and Freed, D.J. 1979. Joint custody: a viable alternative? *Trial* 15(5):26–31.

Foster, H.H., and Freed, D.J. 1980. Joint custody: legislative reform. *Trial* 16(6):22–27.

Frankel, S.A. 1978. Intervention with overtly rejecting parents: a suggestion for a collaborative legal and psychiatric approach. *Journal of the American Academy of Child Psychiatry* 17(3):498–504.

Freed, D.J. 1980. Divorce in the fifty states: an overview as of August 1, 1980. *Family Law Reporter* 6(42):4043–4066.

Friedman, H.J. 1980. The father's parenting experience in divorce. *American Journal of Psychiatry* 137(10):1177–1182.

Glick, P.C. 1979. Children of divorce in demographic perspective. *Journal of Social Issues* 35(4):170–182.

Goldstein, J.; Freud, A.; and Solnit, A.J. 1973. *Beyond the Best Interests of the Child.* New York: Free Press.

Goldzband, M.G. 1976. A friendly word of welcome—"go to hell." In Child Custody: The Ugliest Litigation. Symposium by San Diego County Bar Association, San Diego, California, January 17.

Grief, J.B. 1980. Joint custody: a sociological study. *Trial* 15(5):32–33.

Haller, L.H.; Dubin, L.A.; and Buxton, M. 1979. The use of the legal system as a mental health service for children. *Journal of Psychiatry and Law* 7(1):7–48.

Javaid, G. 1980. Children raised by lesbians develop bisexual identity, behavior. *Clinical Psychiatry News,* vol. 8, no. 7, reporting on paper presented at the annual meeting of the American Psychiatric Association.

Laybourne, P.C., and Krueger, J.M. 1979. Is the psychological parent immutable? Ramifications regarding custody decisions. Presentation at the annual meeting of the American Academy of Child Psychiatry, Atlanta, October.

Miller, E. 1976. Psychotherapy of a child in a custody dispute. *Journal of the American Academy of Child Psychiatry* 15(3):441–452.

Roberts, L.M. 1975. Some observations on the problems of the forensic psychiatrist. In R.C. Allen, E.Z. Ferster, and J.G. Rubin, eds., *Readings in Law and Psychiatry.* Baltimore: Johns Hopkins University Press.

Rogers, T.A. 1976. The crisis of custody: how a psychiatrist can help. In Child Custody: The Ugliest Litigation. Symposium by San Diego County Bar Association, San Diego, California, January 17.

San Diego County Bar Association, San Diego Psychiatric Society, and Department of Psychiatry, School of Medicine, University of California, San Diego (sponsors). 1976. Child Custody: The Ugliest Litigation, a symposium for attorneys and psychiatrists, January 17.

Schetky, D.H., and Slader, J.D. 1980. Termination of parental rights. In D.H. Schetky and E.P. Benedek, eds. *Child Psychiatry and the Law.* New York: Brunner/Mazel.

Wallerstein, J.S., and Kelly, J.B. 1974. The effects of parental divorce: the adolescent experience. In E.J. Anthony, ed. *The Child in His Family.* Vol. 3. New York: Wiley.

Wallerstein, J.S., and Kelly, J.B. 1975. The effects of parental divorce:

experiences of the preschool child. *Journal of the American Academy of Child Psychiatry* 14(4):600–616.

Wallerstein, J.S., and Kelly, J.B. 1976a. The effects of parental divorce: experiences of the child in early latency. *American Journal of Orthopsychiatry* 46(1):20–32.

Wallerstein, J.S., and Kelly, J.B. 1976b. The effects of parental divorce: experiences of the child in later latency. *American Journal of Orthopsychiatry* 46(2):256–269.

Wallerstein, J.S., and Kelly, J.B. 1979. Divorce and children. In J.D. Noshpitz, ed. *Basic Handbook of Child Psychiatry*. Vol. 4. New York: Basic.

PART II

DEVELOPMENTAL ISSUES AND ADOLESCENT PROCESS

EDITORS' INTRODUCTION

The chapters in this part range from the theoretical and conceptual aspects of life-cycle theory to the more pragmatic issues of parental styles of communication, to the importance of transitional objects in the developmental process, with a final focus on effects of adolescent pregnancy on development. Adolescent pregnancy is presented as a developmental interference impeding normative tasks of adolescents.

Harry Prosen, John Toews, and Robert Martin consider the life cycle of the family and examine the interaction of the adolescent's life cycle with the ongoing life-cycle experiences of his parents. The authors focus on several mutual dilemmas: time, sexuality, thought and action, the oedipal conflict, passivity and rebellion. They conclude that the adolescent's identity formation often occurs against the backdrop of his parents' midlife crises and involves conflictual solutions based on interlocking and inhibiting demands for crisis solutions.

In their second chapter, Toews, Prosen, and Martin consider the time dimension from a developmental point of view. Four patterns of maturational time distortions are examined: when parents attempt to retard the progression of their adolescent's life cycle at the same time the youngster is accelerating, when both parents and adolescent collude to delay maturational progression, when parents and adolescent attempt to accelerate finishing tasks and involvements of the nuclear family, and when parents accelerate passage and the adolescent, anxious about independence, attempts to delay maturation. The authors found that recognition of the developmental aspects of the conflict and consideration of the future as a perspective in transitional problems led to improved tolerance and respect within the family.

In their third study, Toews, Martin, and Prosen apply the epigenetic principles of Erikson to life-cycle theory and psychotherapeutic efforts with adolescents. They believe that life-cycle theory, which views the individual at a point along a developmental or maturational life course, with a past, present, and anticipated future within a constantly changing familial-social matrix, adds to the developmental perspective. The authors illustrate how a life-cycle approach integrates and highlights the particular life stages and tasks of the patient. They emphasize the importance of time focus in therapy, particularly with the adolescent whose difficulty may be in elaborating an image of himself as a person competent and able to face the future. The authors bring together a life-cycle theory which allows them to structure therapeutic interventions that recapitulate developmental sequences in a life-cycle sense. They believe this helps the patient conceptualize, experience, and actively engage in normal maturational process.

Lili Lobel studies characteristics of play during the childhood of borderline adolescents. Part of the symptom picture in severely disturbed children was a history of an inability to play happily. Lobel compares this with the inability of borderline adolescents to become genuinely interested in schoolwork or hobbies and their preoccupation with grandiose fantasies or self-destructive actions. She found that borderline adolescents have little or no history of transitional object use in childhood because of a paucity of pleasurable experiences with the mother or because of the mother's brushing aside those objects the child seeks to cathect with maternal memories. Additional findings were a barren sense of the future; history of abuse; a mother whose history included deprivation, brutality, and suffering; and a father described as ineffectual, unavailable, self-centered, often punitive, and sadistic. Lobel concludes that there are substantial differences in the development of normal versus borderline adolescents. Visible antecedents, illustrated by the existence of a transitional object, are significant determinants of adolescent development.

Perihan Aral Rosenthal describes a group of midadolescent girls who were having difficulties dealing with physiological changes and resurgence of their sexual and aggressive instinctual impulses. These adolescent girls could not separate and individuate but instead returned to the use of transitional objects (now drugs, alcohol, unacceptable boyfriends and friends) because of intense anxiety, depressive affect, and feelings of loneliness. Rosenthal contends that the return to transitional objects is not only a regression to a preoedipal stage but is in the service of mastery. It is the task of the therapist to build a bridge between the adolescent's object relationship and transitional object. When the adolescent is able to understand what the transitional object means, the therapist will then be able to help the patient with the individuation process.

Harold A. Rashkis and Shirley R. Rashkis explore parental communication and its effects on adolescent development. They wondered if the truth value of parental messages correlated with the success of the adolescent's moving out of the family into the community. They discovered that this group of disturbed adolescents did not receive adequate preparation for separation in the area of communication. Vagueness, contradictions by actions, lying, statements without truth value, and misrepresentations were characteristic of parental communication. Rashkis and Rashkis, in a continuing study of this group, further clarify the important parameter of parental competence at making true statements in a relevant context. They believe that parental appropriateness is a key concept in understanding emotional disorder, and they find distinguishing patterns of interaction in therapy that correlate with developmental achievement of readiness to undertake tasks associated with adulthood.

Adrian D. Copeland surveys the impact of pregnancy on adolescent psychosocial development. He reviews the demographical rise of the problem, the biological consequences, and the sociological ramifications. He discusses the failure to develop self-reliance, the arrest in personality development, the interferences in the development of stable heterosexual relationships, and the diminishment in life direction and role development. Copeland concludes that early pregnancy and subsequent maternity seem to interfere with the completion of the developmental tasks of adolescence.

HARRY PROSEN, JOHN TOEWS, AND ROBERT MARTIN

It has become increasingly common in recent years for conceptualizations of the human life span to be organized into systems
based on a recognition of a series of life stages, each with its own
age-related developmental tasks and its characteristic conflicts. Basically these conceptualizations stem from the life-cycle model
popularized by Erikson (1959). While the major focus of the literature
related to the life cycle is on specific developmental stages, in our
studies we are reexamining Erikson's original concept of the life cycle
as an entity which, despite discrete stages, has a certain sense of
wholeness.

The emphasis of life-cycle theory so far has been more on an individual's experience of his or her own life cycle than on the interaction of
an individual's life cycle with that of others, particularly in a family
setting. Family members are at different developmental stages which
interplay and interrelate. The maturational tasks of different family
members are continuously at variance, and the conflicts are often
clearly evident, although perhaps not recognized in developmental
terms. The purpose of these chapters, therefore, is to discuss life-stage
interrelationships with particular reference to some of the problems
encountered by middle-aged parents and their adolescent children.

Midlife Crisis and Adolescence

Because of the demands for reevaluation and change brought about
by the maturational transitions that are required of both adolescents

and their middle-aged parents, the upset and turmoil of a life crisis may occur. A life crisis can be defined as a critical problem that disrupts the life style of the individual or family and threatens their physical, emotional, or economic well-being.

Our particular interest in life-span psychology arose from several clinical issues relating to the midlife crisis specifically. The first significant clinical issue was our noting that a number of our middle-aged male patients suddenly and unpredictably became promiscuous, even though they had seemed to have lived rather stable and happily married lives. What we explored originally as a concern about a sexual matter became an exploration of normative ego aspects of midlife.

Self-examination includes a review of one's attainments in life, the awareness that early ambitions and plans embodied in the ego ideal may never be totally met, and the recognition that aging occurs without enough opportunity to achieve a sense of true ego mastery. This sense of frustration and disappointment provides a background for sexual acting out as well as the many impulsive characteristics of the midlife period.

An adult, now struggling with a midlife crisis, may make sudden changes in direction in order to make up for lost time and to realize as much achievement as possible. While impulsivity is characteristic of the adolescent stage of development, basic to both an understanding of midlife and adolescence is a sense of the use of time. Midlife is characterized by a realization that time has become short. There is a change in time perspective that comes with aging and is described by Neugarten (1970) as "a particularly conspicuous feature of middle age. Life is restructured in terms of time left to live rather than time since birth. Not only is there a reversal in directionality but an awareness that time is finite."

Another view of the transition in midlife has been described by Gutmann (1971). This begins with the transition from the stage of "alloplastic mastery," in which the emphasis is on control of outer world affairs and on pursuit of achievement through independence, to the stage of "autoplastic" or internal mastery, where the emphasis is on accommodation to the outer world and on changing the self rather than the external domain. In this stage thought is said to substitute for action, and philosophic resignation begins to substitute for drive toward achievement and autonomy. A later stage, more related to the shift toward older age, is "omniplastic" or magical mastery. This stage involves the maintenance of security and self-esteem by regressive, defensive strategies of denial and projection rather than through action against the external world or accommodation.

Characteristic of midlife is the life review (Butler 1963). The life review stems partly from the realization of the shortness of time left to live, and it is made possible by the shift to thought and reflection rather than action as a dominant mode of mastery. It is difficult to achieve change even through the expenditure of forceful energy, and it is therefore natural to become more contemplative and thoughtful. The need to take a more passive and reflective stance usually comes into conflict with the aggressive seeking for mastery of adolescents in the same family, although there are also times when the contemplative motive of a parent might complement the temporary contemplative moments of an adolescent child.

In those originally described midaged males who resorted to action in order to find an idealized younger mate, there was evidence of marked midlife crises and difficulties in midlife transition. Our theoretical explanation of this onset of promiscuity was based on the concept of the "remembered mother and the fantasized mother" (Prosen, Martin, and Prosen 1972). The essential hypothesis was that as the wife ages, the husband is reminded increasingly of his own mother. We suggested that he may start off in a quest to find a person embodying the younger more attractive image of his earlier and more erotically interesting mother, that is, the mother of his childhood. This quest usually ends disastrously because the middle-aged man is distorting time by attempting to turn it back to regain, through active mastery, that which is already long past. Promiscuity in this case is a reaction to the aging, a defense mechanism which also includes another important dynamic force, the reawakening of the oedipal conflict.

While it is well recognized that the adolescent must deal with the resurgence of the oedipal conflict at the time of puberty (Blos 1962, 1972), yet another resurgence of the conflict can be conceptualized to occur in middle age, particularly when it was inadequately resolved in adolescence. Possible stimuli for this resurgence are the retreat from the aging mate; having sexually stimulating adolescent children who once again awaken the incestuous strivings characteristic of the oedipal conflict; the memory of the younger mother; the subjective sense of the shortness of time; the pressure to act and to risk before it is too late; as well as the reawakening of the oedipal conflict through jealousy by fathers of daughters and by mothers of sons.

As with the earlier oedipal awakenings, in this rekindling there may be renewed pressure to prove one's role, one's competence and prowess. When this occurs in the family setting, the ordinary issues of control and family leadership become distorted by issues of jealousy and competition. There results much opportunity for misidentification of the adolescent by the adult and the adult by the adolescent. There arises also the opportunity for a fluctuating variety of age-related roles adopted by the parents and adolescents in the family. These roles may switch on a momentary basis, ranging from adult-parent and adolescent-child to adolescent-parent and adult-child.

To come to terms with midlife and to arrange a realistic accommodation with one's ego ideal, to take responsibility for living the way one has lived until midlife, and to take power over the rest of one's life means that one must accept passivity and helplessness in certain situations by using autoplastic mastery. It may be impossible by this time of life to make fundamental changes in a work situation or to make major changes in a family situation that would not ultimately be destructive. Of course, in some cases, dramatic and good changes can be made, but the prospect of making such changes is often frightening and risky.

While much of the early consideration of midlife issues involves clinical descriptions of men, it is now apparent that the same issues apply to women as well and are evident in the family context. In older midlife, the woman's reactions are made more complex by the fact that the impending cessation of menstrual function and reproductive capability add a definite pronounced reminder of aging. The effects are many and may vary from a feeling of decreased sexuality and more limited feminine identity to a sense of freedom, an explosion of oedipal feelings, and a resurgence of adolescent sexuality. The latter, in some cases, leads to a syndrome called "postmenopausal promiscuity" (Prosen and Martin 1979). In these situations one sees the concerns of mothers about their daughter's sexuality in adolescence, the possibility of fostering daughter's sexual acting out, or the creation of inhibitions and conflict about the expression of sexuality in adolescent female children.

Adolescence and Midlife Crisis

While the middle-aged parent may experience a certain passivity and helplessness, their adolescent children tend to experience opposite feelings. They are in rebellion, actively questing for their own identity and the right to control and determine their own future in line with their own goals and dreams. They resent parental authority and control and indicate to the parents that the parents are helpless. As a result, the midlife feelings of helplessness and passivity experienced by the parent are intensified. Added to the passivity of not being able to control one's own life is the distress of not being able to control one's own children; added to the anxiety about the uncertainty of one's own future now is the anxiety about the uncertainty of the adolescent's future.

It is evident then that some of the life-stage tasks and conflicts of the adolescent complement those of the parents. Both the youth and parent are involved in working through issues of identity. The youth's task is to form an identity that is secure enough to carry through to adulthood. The parent is concerned with the examination of his or her own identity and achievements in light of their own ego ideals. The adolescent experiences concerns about sexual intimacy and sexual adequacy. Both adolescent and parent may experience the fear of impotence or of sexual failure. Youths' fear is based on uncertainty at the beginning of a new and vulnerable aspect of their lives, but the parents' (particularly the father's) fear is based on the realization of declining sexuality and on the apprehension that sexuality as it represents and symbolizes youth will be sacrificed to advancing age.

In addition to these particular fears there is also a curiosity about the other's sexual life. The adolescent may often deny that the parent has a sex life. By the same token, parents may attempt to prepare themselves for the sexuality of their adolescents but may find it difficult to accept. There may well be a reciprocal relationship between the strength of the incestuous impulse that has existed between the adolescent and the parent of the opposite sex and the strength of their own sexual drives. The parents, in reaction formation to the blossoming sexuality of their teenage child, may become jealous of the sexual relationships of their adolescent children and attempt in various ways to interfere with their friendships, an interference that is often difficult to see and not readily admitted.

Since identity formation in the adolescent occurs usually against the backdrop of the parents' midlife crisis, parents and adolescents are both engaged in modifying their views of themselves and each other. Adolescents struggle with deidealization of their parents, and parents often attempt to force their adolescents to behave in such a way that the idealization of the younger child can continue. Part of the modification that is required has to do with the idealization, each of the other, that may have existed relatively unchecked by reality until this period of family life. The adolescent is expected by parents to conform to an idealized expectancy while, at the same time, this is the period during which the adolescent is often most ashamed and disappointed in his parents and sees them as least understanding. Both parents and adolescents find themselves in conflict, sometimes to the point of death wishes or suicidal thoughts. We see expression in families of desires to separate; and through fighting and threats of separation sometimes actual separation does occur. The more subtle loss, however, is that of the deidealization. The parent in midlife, already suffering from the damaging effects of deteriorating self-esteem, due to the loss of active ego mastery, is especially vulnerable to disappointment.

Ambivalence has long been recognized as a keynote in the feelings of adolescents toward their parents. We should also acknowledge that the parents' ambivalence toward their adolescent children is just as unpredictable and tumultuous. One would wish to see a healthy admiration available between adolescent and parent at the end of the adolescent turmoil and its complimentary midlife phase in the parent, but the opposite of admiration is too often present.

Adolescents often rebel against gratifying parental wishes but play out the rejected parental wishes with their own friends. In our clinical work with families of professionals it is common to see the adolescent who rejects learning, fails in school, and drops out in an effort to avoid compliance with parental wishes, an example of Erikson's (1962) concept of negative identity. In other situations, where the adolescent appears to be completely rejecting and different from the parent, one may actually see that the teenager, rather than express a negative identity, is hostilely identifying with the parent and is participating in a microsociety which replicates in parody the society of the parent. The society discovered and created by the teenager is reinforcing and protective, making it most difficult for the parents to make inroads on the adolescent's defenses. At the same time, it produces struggles within the family context that can be particularly reflected with other children who are directed to turn out differently from the disappointing adolescent. This produces further rejection of the adolescent, who then forms a greater tie to his or her own peer group. This type of identification is illustrated in the following case example.

Jane, age seventeen, was seen at the request of her parents, who had become concerned when she precipitously dropped out of senior high school. Jane's grades had been deteriorating for some time, although previously she had performed well in school. Despite coming from a home where alcohol was used in strict moderation, Jane had taken to returning home grossly intoxicated most weekends. The parents were concerned and confused by her actions. She refused all attempts to talk about her behavior and angrily accused her parents of not understanding her and of trying to live her life for her.

Jane's father, a high school principal, placed great value on education. He and Jane's social worker mother had been encouraging Jane to get a university education leading to a profession. During the initial interviews Jane described feeling parental pressure to perform up to their expectations. She felt pushed toward a university education, but was confused about her own plans for the future. She saw her failure at school as a statement of her disinterest in continuing her education and her use of alcohol as acceptable and usual by the standard of her friends. She realized her behavior worried her parents, but she protested that she had to determine her own future.

During the interviews she talked of many conversations with her friends, who also were failures of various sorts. In effect Jane related to these friends as though she were a high school counselor who encouraged education and future planning. She had rejected her parents' encouragement, but had at the same time taken a parental role with her peers.

Other conflicts are the ambivalence and resentment of the teenager toward the parents' material resources. The teenager, in rejecting the values of the parents, often denounces the desire and need for material wants and, as a result, is derisive of parental possessions or values. This is the use of the ascetic defense as described by Freud (1966). Parents, on the other hand, examine their own resources as they approach older age and use the counting of resources as some sign of success.

To this description of parallel and complementary conflicts between parent and youth we would also like to add some thoughts about the timing of maturational events as they occur in both the youth and the parent. The basic conflicts tend to involve an idea of the fullness of time for the youth as compared to the increasing shortness of time for the parent. In these situations, it is natural for the parent and the child to become out of phase with each other in their approach to the timing of maturational trends and events. The obvious example is the situation in which the midaged parent attempts to deny and retard the progression of the life cycle of their adolescent, who at the same time is attempting to accelerate his or her own progress. The parents wish to slow the child down, to keep him dependent, under control, and in what they see as a secure family environment; whereas the adolescent wants the freedom to have his or her own experiences. As one would expect, the families in which this happens experience sharp and continued conflict.

Another pattern occurs in families in which both parents and children collude in an attempt to delay the progression of the life cycle. In this case we see a dependent child afraid of the demands of independence in adulthood and dependent parents concerned about the implications of their own aging in terms of their roles as parents. On the surface in these families everything appears agreeable and there is often little conflict. However, close scrutiny of these families often shows neurotic and sometimes even psychotic symptomatology.

Discussion

The various developmental tasks of the middle-aged parent and adolescent child are of a magnitude that demand the utmost in accommodation and resiliency. Families in which parents are in midlife crisis and in which a parent is acting out in some way may find the destruction and chaos worsened by the adolescent's rebelling and acting out at the same time. The helplessness of the parents may only reinforce the adolescent turmoil, and it is not infrequent that the expression of this turmoil is ego alien to the parents. A previous example noted that parents often find their children responding negatively to the parental wishes and yet creating or living in a microsociety in which they take on their own parents' role. Parents with a strong academic achievement orientation often find their bright children failing academically. When reputation is important to the family, the adolescent may threaten its loss through some form of antisocial behavior. When parents are concerned about social propriety, the adolescent may act out sexually or through drugs. These reactions can arise developmentally, but there is often a direct connection between the unconscious impulses and fantasies of the parents and the acting out of the teenager (Johnson and Szurek 1952).

In the same way we may see parents acting out their own conflicts engendered by the reactions of their adolescent children. The helpless anger arising from the midlife changes and the action of the children may be projected upon the marital partner with further deterioration of a suffering marriage. Promiscuity of a parent may have as one of its etiological components erotic feelings for an attractive child. In these instances, and others, family members may foster the acting out of others in order to hide or avoid the real developmental issues and tasks. That these should be played out in the family is no surprise when one considers that collectively within the family a major threat results from the transitions required of its members. This threat is the threat to the continued existence of the family itself.

Conclusions

How then, can we help the midage parent and the adolescent child, caught as they are in their life-stage clashes? As clinicians we are all familiar with how difficult it is to give parents wise counsel in dealing with the issues they face with their struggling adolescent children. Similarly, those of us interested in the treatment of adolescents know how difficult it is to help the adolescent child to understand the reactions of the parent struggling with his or her own life tasks.

Perhaps the best approach to these problems is a combination of individual and family therapeutic interviews focused on the tasks and reviews necessary for both parent and youth to make the transitions required of them at their own particular ages. The concept of life stages and life tasks helps to give some understanding and strength in dealing with these issues, particularly in terms of the helplessness we so often encounter in these parents and families.

In order to help with these problems it is necessary to diagnose accurately the situation not just from an individual perspective, but from a family perspective as well. Both parents and youth should be assessed from the point of view of their own life tasks and the difficulties that they each encounter with them. One must then assess how the life tasks of the parent and youth complement each other and where their attempts at the solution of their life-stage problems bring them into inevitable conflict. In opening up the family to the review of what it is like to be the other family members at their life stage and with their life tasks one also hopes to open up an awareness and appreciation within the family each for the other. If this can be done, life tasks can be encountered in an open and supportive environment, in which, ideally, both parents and adolescents will be more tolerant of one another and will demonstrate more understanding with less recourse to panic reactions which are on the parents' part calculated to demonstrate authority, control, and a degree of active mastery and on the youth's part to demonstrate autonomy and independence from the parents.

One would then summarize by saying that the solution involves describing and discussing the maladaptive attempts of both the midlife parent and the adolescent to solve their individual problems as well as to show them the way in which they have negatively reinforced and yet paradoxically mimicked the other's solution.

REFERENCES

Blos, P. 1962. *On Adolescence*. New York: Free Press.

Blos, P. 1972. The epigenesis of the adult neurosis. *Psychoanalytic Study of the Child* 27:106–135.

Butler, R.N. 1963. The life review: an interpretation of reminiscence in the aged. *Psychiatry* 26:65–76.

Erikson, E.H. 1959. Identity and the life cycle. *Psychological Issues*. Vol. 1. New York: International Universities Press.

Erikson, E.H. 1962. *Young Man Luther*. New York: Norton.

Freud, A. 1966. *The Ego and the Mechanisms of Defense*. New York: International Universities Press.

Gutmann, D.L. 1971. Cross-cultural research on human behavior: a comparative study of the life cycle in the middle and later years. In N. Kretchmer and D.N. Walcher, eds. *Environmental Influence on Genetic Expression*. Fogarty International Center Proceedings, no. 2. Washington, D.C.: Government Printing Office.

Johnson, A., and Szurek, S. 1952. Genesis of antisocial acting out. *Psychoanalytic Quarterly* 21:323–343.

Neugarten, B. 1970. Dynamics of transition of middle age to old age. *Journal of Geriatric Psychiatry* 4:71–87.

Prosen, H., and Martin, R. 1979. Postmenopausal promiscuity. *Medical Aspects of Human Sexuality* 13(6):26–34.

Prosen, H.; Martin, R.; and Prosen, M. 1972. The remembered mother and the fantasized mother. *Archives of General Psychiatry* 12:791–794.

11 II. THE LIFE CYCLE OF THE FAMILY:
THE ADOLESCENT'S SENSE OF TIME

JOHN TOEWS, HARRY PROSEN, AND ROBERT MARTIN

A most stressful period in a family life cycle occurs when a developmental crisis in a child coincides with a developmental crisis in a parent. Such an event occurs in families in which parents face their midlife transition at the same time that their children experience the transitions of adolescence. Both of these transitions occur as a result of the individual's maturational progression through the life cycle. Each of these transitions involves a roughly comparable period of review, reworking of identities, and planning for the future. For the parent, the midlife transition results from a recognition of the shortness of time while, for the adolescent, the transition in part results from the need to prepare for an open, seemingly unlimited future. Normally, both parent and child understand and accommodate each other. However, if either the parent or child has particular problems with a life-cycle transition, the other, because of the interplay of a parallel and contrasting life-cycle transition period, may become involved in conflict.

It is no surprise to us that time, in a life-cycle sense, figures prominently in family conflicts arising out of the superimposition of the parents' and youths' life tasks, particularly as they apply to the speed with which one progresses through maturational events. Clinically, we notice parents attempting to retard or accelerate the passage of time as measured by maturational events in both their own and their children's life cycles in response to their conflicts about their own midlife transition. Adolescents, ambivalent about their own maturational thrust, attempt as well to accelerate or to retard their passage through time, being in the role of a young child at one moment and in the role of a mature adult the next.

This chapter will attempt to isolate and categorize some of these clinical patterns as seen in family interactions. In these situations, it is possible for both the parent and clinician to oversimplify the problem and to see the adolescent difficulties exclusive of their interplay with the parental crisis.

Generational Strain

One way of conceptualizing the stress experienced by family members during this superimposition of individual life-cycle crises is as a strain arising from the impending shift of generations. This shift brings with it a total shift in the ordering of life by age-related role in that a child becomes a parent, a parent a grandparent, and so on. Recent life-cycle studies indicate the significance of the generational span and list the major transition periods: early adult transition (ages seventeen to twenty-two); the midlife transition (ages forty to forty-five); and the late adult transition (ages sixty to sixty-five) (Levinson, Darrow, Klein, Levinson, and McKee 1978). While it is possible to disagree with the restricted time periods that Levinson et al. describe, it is interesting to note that these transitions correspond roughly to the periods of impending shift between generations, or in other words, the shift between the family of origin, parenting, and grandparenting.

In a sense, both parent and youth experience crises in their reactions to the threat or promise of the passage of maturational time and to the reordering of life and relationships that this implies. For the parents facing midage this means, as Neugarten (1970) has pointed out, that time is now measured in time left to live, rather than in time lived. This realization forces the life reviews, reevaluations of goals and directions, and the mourning of unattainable dreams that are characteristic of the midlife transition. This is in sharp contrast to the adolescent child who also sets goals, but with the dream of finally becoming big enough and old enough to be adult.

Thus some of the parents in the midlife transition find that time progresses too rapidly, while the impatient youth perceives time as moving too slowly. The youth faces an expanding future, the parent looks toward a time of consolidation, reexamination, retrenchment, and eventually failing health and death. These are certainly different generational parameters which are often difficult for the parent and adolescent to appreciate in each other.

The impending change in the nuclear family itself can contribute to reactions that may distort life-cycle time for family members. Children will leave home and the nuclear family as it has been known will disappear—a transition that is tantamount to the death of the family as it has been experienced during the years of parenting and maturation of the children. This impending change may be mourned in an anticipatory way. A natural tendency for both youth and parents would be to hold onto the family and thus, in a sense, to retard time. At best this holding onto the family is ambivalent because of the natural forward thrust of the maturation of both parents and child. Normally, this ambivalence allows time for working through the relationships and the formation of identities that are necessary for both youth and parent in order to separate. When the adolescent child or the parent cannot accept the fact that separation is necessary or cannot agree on the timing or the process of separation, maturational time distortions result.

Maturational Time Distortions

For the purposes of this discussion four patterns of maturational time distortions will be discussed. The first occurs when parents attempt to retard the progression of their children's life cycle at the same time that the adolescent may be attempting to accelerate his or her own life-cycle progression. A second pattern occurs in families where both parents and child collude to delay maturational progression. A third pattern occurs when parents and child both attempt to accelerate their life cycles and thus finish too rapidly the tasks and involvements of the nuclear family. A fourth pattern occurs in families in which the parents attempt to accelerate the passage of the life-cycle events while the adolescent child is anxious about independence and works to delay his or her own maturation.

CASE 1

Lynn, age sixteen, is the older of two adolescent children. Her parents state that in the last six months they have had severe conflict with Lynn whenever they disagreed with her actions. She started keeping late hours, often coming home well after midnight. They suspected that Lynn might be drinking. They worried because she was dating a man who was in his midtwenties and that she would be hurt in the relationship. Recently her grades in school have deteriorated. As a result of their concerns, Mr. and Mrs. Brown felt that as parents they must control Lynn's behavior. They demanded that Lynn not date, that she choose a quieter group of friends, and that she stay home evenings and study. They were even opposed to her involvement in school social activities in that they felt that Lynn would likely misuse these activities. With the imposition of these restrictions, Lynn's unacceptable behavior escalated. The precipitant for the consultation was a violent argument with her parents after a school report in which she did poorly. Lynn stated that she wished to be free of her parents. She wished to live by herself, away from all their silly rules and, if she could not be independent, she asked to be placed in a foster home.

Mr. and Mrs. Brown are both in their early forties. Mr. Brown felt his employment had become routine, and he was depressed at the thought of continuing his job as a banker until he retired. Mrs. Brown had elected to stay home with the children and appeared very involved in her role as a mother and homemaker.

The Browns each saw the period when they had a young family as the most enjoyable period in their lives. Much to Lynn's disgust, they repeatedly recounted stories of how cute Lynn was as a little child as they mourned the passing of this period. They stated that they particu-larly dreaded the prospect of the children leaving home. It was apparent during the interview that the Browns' marriage had lost its excitement. While both said that their marriage was satisfactory, it was noted that there was very little interaction between husband and wife except on the topic of the children. It was apparent that the Browns wished the children to develop normally, while at the same time they wished that the children would not mature and would remain at home.

In this example the parents attempted to retard maturational time while the adolescent needed to accelerate it. Here the adolescent attempts to be independent and mature beyond her years and abilities. To the youth this means independence and complete freedom from parental direction. The ambivalence in the reactions to the implications of the separation from home is seen in involvements, behavior, and relationships that are beyond the maturational equipment. The desire is to be mature and autonomous more rapidly than is possible. The parents try to delay the passage of time as welcome evidence that their adolescent cannot really function autonomously. As a matter of fact, this preoccupation allows them to abandon their own task of examining their lives and roles and facilitating the transition of their nuclear family through its changes in structure and function. When they strengthen their attempts to directly parent their adolescent child, the youth feels treated as a child. This causes a further escalation of the conflict since independence must now be displayed even more desperately. The vicious circle continues with youth and parents continuing out of phase with the life cycle of the other. The parents hold onto a parenting model more appropriate to years earlier, while the youth demands independence from the direction and support of home before she can successfully manage her independence. The result is marked conflict, desperate behavior, and drama for all involved.

CASE 2

Sara, a thirty-year-old single female, requested therapy because "I have to make a number of major decisions in my life if I wish to keep on developing." The particular shift she wished to make was to be able to live separately from her mother, with whom she shared a bedroom in a large house. The thought of leaving mother alone caused her great anxiety, ever since her father died when Sara was fourteen years old. During Sara's childhood, she felt a desperate need to please her mother. She worked hard at school and consciously selected friends and activities in such a way as to please her. During midadolescence, Sara began to experience depressive episodes and became suicidal. As a result, she spent a number of lengthy periods in psychiatric hospitals. Here, the underlying dynamic problem was felt to be her difficulty individuating from her mother. Eventually Sara was released from the hospital on the condition that she live separately and that she maintain contact with her own individual therapist. When Sara's therapist terminated her treatment she moved into her mother's house "for a few months"; now eight years later she still cannot separate.

Sara is the oldest of five children and at least two others have had difficulty separating. Relatives on the mother's side repeatedly compliment Sara on being a good daughter for keeping her aging mother company. Mother, for her part, urges Sara to leave if it will make her happy and if Sara's "illness will permit it." She is warned by mother not to be concerned that her mother faces failing health and eventual death all alone with no one to support her. In therapy, Sara's major gains have been made during extended periods in which mother travels to visit other family members. As mother returns, the struggle for separation intensifies.

This example illustrates the tendency toward a symbiotic relationship between one or both parents and the adolescent. In such a family, adequate individuation and separation of the youth cannot occur. There is instead a covert collusion between parent and child to retard the passage of time and delay the attainment of maturational goals. This allows the youth to relieve anxiety about the approaching independent existence of young adulthood. The parents contribute to the collusion in a way which relieves them, if only temporarily, of their own need to face a number of midlife issues, particularly those involving the change in the function and structure of the family and their own role as parents.

This pattern of family interaction also has been implicated in the development of schizophrenia. The concept has been broadened by Stierlin (1974) in his consideration of these families as the extreme of a continuum of families who are basically centripetal in style. The defensive stance of such families is to be overly cohesive and to hold family members firmly within the nuclear unit. In our view family members in this situation appear to defend against the anxiety present during the shift to the next period of the life cycle.

As both youth and parents distort the timing of maturational events in the same direction, there may be little overt familial conflict. The result may be the denial of a problem until quite late; help is not looked for until the youth has passed into young adulthood, by which time severe problems may be encountered in either setting a life course or achieving independence from the parents.

The third pattern of life-cycle time distortions in families with adolescents appears to be an attempt to accelerate the passage of maturational time by both generations agreeing to the early cessation of direct parenting and the youth leaving home. Stierlin (1974) labels such families as centrifugal and points out that many of the difficulties experienced in these cases may come to attention only as a result of the youth's sociopathic behavior.

There are a number of life-cycle dynamics that may explain the parents' desire to accelerate maturational time. In the face of midlife stresses, one or both of the parents may wish to resume the relative freedom and independence of their childless days. The process of separation of the youth from home then allows this freedom. Another dynamic may be the parents' wish to deny aging by living vicariously through the blossoming independence and vigor of their adolescent child.

185

The youth, for his or her part, may eagerly grasp the independence offered by the parents. Independence is, after all, a maturational goal. The danger in achieving independence too early is that the youth may encounter adult maturational tasks well before there is a maturational readiness for them. The teenager may then demonstrate this lack of readiness for adult responsibilities by innocently or almost deliberately running into difficulties with these tasks. Uncorrected, this process may result in an antisocial reaction, shallow and disturbed relationships, and a growing feeling of failure.

A fourth category of distortion in the timing of maturational events appears in families in which parents attempt to accelerate the attainment of maturational goals for their adolescent child while the youth holds back. In these situations the parent often tries to relive an aspect of his or her life through the life of the child. One of the responses to the midlife crisis may be to live vicariously through the adolescent child in order to obtain a sense of timelessness through identification with the youth. The area selected by the parent for the youth's accelerated achievements reflects the parent's own dreams or conflicts.

Examples of this are found in adolescents who are pushed prematurely into the world of heterosexual involvements and thus give evidence of the parents' own doubts or fears concerning their own continued sexual involvement in midlife. Parents then need not worry about continued sexual ability since the child can carry it for them. The child of a gifted parent may find himself pushed to achieve. Again, the parents' substantial fears concerning the shortness of time can be allayed by the immortality available in continuing through the child. The youth as the recipient of these pressures may respond by attempting to comply with the parents' wishes. However, the youth may hold back. Thus, the one who is to be bright may fail at school, the one who is to achieve may be characterized by a lack of achievement, and the one who seems mature and separates rapidly fails to leave home.

While these four patterns have been discussed as mutually exclusive and absolute, they are, in fact, only infrequently expressed in pure form. Instead there may be areas in which there are specific attempts to accelerate or retard maturation, while other areas may show the reverse pattern or may be proceeding normally at the same time. In addition there are various developmental arrests and role distortions that complicate the picture further and that appear throughout one's progression through the life cycle. These particular patterns have been described in order to stress the point that the overlap of the midlife and adolescent crises within the family can produce major patterns of distortion in the timing of maturational events.

Developmentally Based Therapy and the Timing of Maturational Events

Most current therapies utilize a much thinner concept of time than that which is applicable to the life-cycle issues just discussed. Many therapies, such as family and behavioral therapy, focus on the present tense often without enough consideration for the fact that the individual is at a point in the life cycle which is the result of many developmental and life experiences in the past and does have, as well, an anticipated and predicted future. Other therapies, such as dynamically oriented psychotherapy and psychoanalysis, tend to focus on the past-in-present by considering the reworking of the past in terms of the present therapeutic relationship as the significant aspect of therapy. Few therapies, if any, consider time as it is experienced in the human life cycle with an emphasis on the importance of considering the future or what can be expected in the life cycle as well as the past and present.

Developmentally based therapy in families in which difficulties arise out of the combination of life-cycle stresses of both parents and children should utilize the broad time focus that best approaches life itself. Both the therapist and family must recognize that in these situations much of the distortion in the timing of maturational events arises out of the juxtaposition of developmental stresses. If the individual or family can be helped to understand their part in this necessary transition it is possible that there may be more tolerance or respect for each other's reactions. We have observed that if these families are asked to view their goals for the family ten years hence, after both parents and youth have completed the transitions that are currently troubling them, both tend to agree on the model of the family that they wish to see. It is one in which the youth has successfully separated from home and can come and go freely, relating to the parents on a more equal friendship basis.

Conclusions

The therapist engaging in developmentally based therapy with these families must help both parents and their children come to terms with their own life tasks and to respect the life tasks and transitions required of the other. Parents must experience both support and assistance in their midlife review and must be helped to understand how their reactions to aging have affected their adolescent offspring. Youth may then feel more understanding of parents and may be helped to look forward to the demands and uncertainties of adulthood with more equanimity. In this way, the therapist can aid both parents and youth in their particular transitions. The strain encountered in the anticipated passing into new life stages and the reactions to shifting roles or functions can be explored and the young people and parents freed to work together to achieve both individual and family goals.

REFERENCES

Levinson, D.J.; Darrow, C.N.; Klein, E.B.; Levinson, M.H.; and McKee, B. 1978. *The Seasons of a Man's Life*. New York: Knopf.

Neugarten, B. 1970. Dynamics of the transition of mid age to old age. *Journal Geriatric Psychiatry* 4:71–87.

Stierlin, H. 1974. *Separating Parents and Adolescents*. New York: Quadrangle.

188

III. THE LIFE CYCLE OF THE FAMILY:
PERSPECTIVES ON PSYCHOTHERAPY
WITH ADOLESCENTS

JOHN TOEWS, ROBERT MARTIN, AND HARRY PROSEN

Life-cycle theory, as elaborated by Erikson, describes life as progressing through a series of stages, each with its characteristic tasks and crises. The order of these stages is seen to be determined by an internal maturational plan, the "epigenetic principle," which states "that anything that grows has a ground plan, and . . . out of this ground plan the parts arise, each having its time of special ascendancy, until all the parts have arisen to form a functioning whole" (Erikson 1959). This whole was seen as being the human life. The elaboration of this idea within a stage theory of tasks and crises stimulated attention to the human life cycle, particularly to the developmental tasks of adolescence and midage. Despite interest in the life cycle, the implications for psychotherapy of a life-cycle theory applicable to many stages of life have seldom been considered. The purpose of this chapter is to summarize the unique contributions of life-cycle theory to psychotherapy with adolescents. While the therapeutic principles discussed will be applicable to psychotherapy utilizing life-cycle principles at any period of life, the discussion will make particular reference to therapy with adolescents.

Life-Cycle Theory

Life-cycle theory, as we conceptualize it through our own psychotherapeutic research, entails a view of the individual at a point along a developmental or maturational life course with a past, present, and anticipated future contained within a constantly changing familial-social matrix. The theory adds to the purely developmental point of view in that while the developmental perspective could permit a view of oneself in a relatively isolated environment, playing out essentially innate capabilities in response to environmental stimuli, the life-cycle perspective adds that this development occurs within a social matrix with which one interacts, participates, and sees future and past images of who one was, is, and could potentially be. It is a theory that places more emphasis on the elaboration of one's constantly changing and evolving identity.

The internal model of an individual life, past and future, is not fully represented by the epigenetic principle, which appears to have more to do with an innate unfolding of various tasks and potentials throughout the course of one's development. In addition to this, in life-cycle terms, the sensing of one's ground plan or the view of one's life through time is elaborated by seeing images of one's past and future life course in the innumerable views of one's parents, grandparents, and eventually one's children. These images of both self and others are roughly ordered along a sense of one's personal time as images recalling one's past, present, and future. These images recall or point toward the tasks, conflicts, and opportunities at each particular period of development.

The internalized model is further ordered by a perception of the significance of generational differences, likely starting at about the time of the oedipal period. It must be emphasized that the oedipal conflict is but a small part of this period of life. It's greater significance lies in that it is here that the child begins to see within its parents a representation of its own personal future. The classic resolution of the oedipal crisis, that one must bide one's time in the hope of eventually becoming like one's parents and functioning as they do, speaks to the successful ordering of images along one's personal, internalized life-cycle time line. It is also apparent that this constellation does not rest entirely with the four- to six-year-old or even with the reawakening of the oedipal conflict during adolescence (Blos 1962) or in midage but continues as an active and dynamic force throughout one's life.

Adolescents, for example, can see a series of images of themselves in their memories of infancy and childhood. They become aware of these recollections spontaneously and also by comparison with others younger than themselves. The images of their future lives reside in their memories and current perceptions of their now midaged parents and grandparents. While adolescents can determine whether they wish to be like their parents in specific ways, they cannot escape the basic realization that in a sense, in the completion of their own life course and in the families that they will create, they will of necessity recapitulate in part the same basic life-cycle experiences and stresses that they note in their parents.

The adolescent's internal life-cycle model is further structured by the boundaries of birth and death, both realizations of which in a personal sense the adolescent is intensely aware. Both perceptions arise during the latency period of development. The startling realization of one's own sexual development and reproductive potential becomes dominant in adolescence. Kastenbaum (1959) has demonstrated that while most adolescents do not use death imagery as an organizing concept in their lives, preferring instead to think of their own generativity and boundless future, death is never far from awareness as evidenced by the profound anxiety evoked by death imagery in projective psychological studies.

The internal representation of one's life cycle is further organized into the realization of passing through various broad life-cycle phases, each with specific demands. This area has received the greatest attention in the developmental literature and will not be developed further here.

It is commonly considered that, as Erikson (1959) indicated, the task of adolescence is to form an identity which is considered basic to the adult personality. There is a growing realization that one's identity continues to be modified throughout life. When seen in terms of life-cycle theory, one's sense of *who one is* is the sum total of one's life experience to date and its potential within an anticipated future. In a sense, the unique perception of one's individual life cycle is the basic statement of one's identity. Viewing identity in this way, we see adolescence as a period of identity formation involving the basic tasks of separation and individuation (Blos 1962) but holding no more unique claim to identity formation than any other life stage.

Another characteristic of life-cycle theory is the series of life previews or anticipations and reviews or memories of periods of one's life that occurs throughout the passage through the life cycle. There is a changing ratio of preview to review as one moves through life, with the major division occurring during midage. The life preview of adolescence is a function of the life cycle's dynamic qualities, just as is the review of old age noted by Butler (1963). The older person reviews a life that has almost been completed; the midage person, realizing the shortness of time, reviews the past in terms of the anticipated future; and the child and adolescent previews a life that is to be largely anticipated. The child normally makes many statements about his or her personal future and indeed, in play, rehearses the future. The adolescent can be seen trying on many roles, often to the confusion of parents and teachers, in an attempt to anticipate possible futures, roles, and relationships. We would suggest that this anticipatory preview is as essential to the formation of the individual identity as the review of the past. Life reviews or anticipations at all of the different stages of life head to a further elaboration of individual identity.

The juxtaposition of various life-cycle stages within the family can lead to periods of intense stress and crisis. We have described the tensions of the juxtaposition of adolescence, midlife, and old age within the family of the adolescent. While this combination of life stages within the family may create some difficulties for the individuals concerned, within it are the forces for further examination and elaboration of each individual's life course, in effect, the impetus to further development.

Distortions can occur through one's passage through the life cycle. There may be distortions in the timing of developmental events. Certain tasks may be attempted before maturational readiness or there might be developmental arrests that create specific stresses. These may be biologically determined, for example the stresses related to the delayed onset of puberty. They might be psychosocially based, as for example in attempting the intimacy of marriage at a chronologically appropriate age without the emotional readiness for marriage because of a failure in the separation and individuation process (Toews 1980).

In our elaboration of life-cycle theory we have noted the distortions in the timing of maturational events that occur as a result of specific stresses. We have noted how maturational events can be anticipated and attempted too rapidly or delayed too long. We have also noted how dimly remembered images of the past may affect the behavior of an individual at very different periods of life, often leading to quests to recapture the past which are almost certainly doomed to failure (Prosen, Martin, and Prosen 1972). The juxtaposition of various life-cycle crises within the family may augment the stress experienced by any one person as a result of where they are in their own lives and increase the likelihood of these distortions in time-related images. These various elements of life-cycle theory also contribute to the therapeutic understanding of patients and may add an often unrecognized dimension to therapy.

Therapeutic Implications

A clinical example will be used in order to highlight various contributions of life-cycle theory to psychotherapy with adolescents.

CASE EXAMPLE

Jack, an appealing eighteen-year-old, requested therapy for a depression that had begun in the final year of high school and became markedly worse as he entered the final term and could contemplate graduating. He had never considered himself capable of completing high school, expecting with each grade to fail. The origin of this fear appeared to be related to a move from a neighboring city when he was in the primary grades. At that point he felt very alone, confused, and did fail his grade. He viewed the time prior to that move as the happiest period in his life. The dominant memory of the period before moving was feeling contented and playing in the sun with a friend.

Jack was the youngest child, the only male in a family with three sisters. The whole family was very intensely involved in church activities, and each child appeared to have received the parental expectation of living a near perfect life. Jack believed that he carried an added expectation since he was the only male child and, in effect, received many of father's admonitions. In this environment Jack gave clear evidence of an obsessive personality with a well developed, relatively rigid superego.

Other factors were important in Jack's current difficulties. He wished to develop relationships with girls but found himself inhibited and became guilty about his sexual fantasies. He responded to this anxiety by withdrawing from social contacts with women whenever he could. He wished to leave home and assume responsibility for himself but rationalized that while he was depressed he really could not establish himself independently. A further interaction, likely adding to Jack's own uncertainty about his future was that his father, at age forty-seven, had recently resigned from his practice of law to take additional courses in what he called a sabbatical year. Jack described that many of his father's days were now spent at home pondering different directions open to himself.

In addition to psychotherapy, Jack was treated with antidepressants to which he seemed to respond only partially. Early in treatment he became phobic about attending school and could not force himself to attend. His past performance was sufficient to receive credit for the year and to graduate from high school.

Initially the focus in therapy was to outline with him where he felt himself to be in relation to his own developmental tasks. His anxiety concerning that earlier image of himself as a school failure was reviewed and compared to his performance in school throughout high school. We wondered whether that part of his identity could change. The concern about leaving home and his anxiety about potentially developing heterosexual relationships was viewed in the light of his current life tasks and his anxiety concerning his own need to assume responsibility for himself and his own relationships was acknowledged. The fact that he remained dependent on his parents when his primary desire was to become independent was examined.

Father's difficulties in determining his own future was discussed with Jack as a parallel process, but with certain key differences based on the fact that father, at a different life stage, needed to examine the feasibility of earlier goals while Jack had time to set goals and experiment. Father's quest was not viewed as pathological but as a normative life crisis with considerable potential for growth. Jack was then helped to focus on his own need for growth in the transition he himself was facing.

After approximately six months of therapy Jack determined to leave home, travel, and then find work. A few weeks following these decisions, Jack brightly reported that he felt tremendously freed after his father had determined his own future course. As well, at this point he started recounting a developing relationship with a young woman. It was clear that in emerging from this period of his life-cycle conflict Jack had resolved a large portion of the remainder of the depressive symptomatology.

Discussion

The life-cycle approach to psychotherapy is not a new form of psychotherapy. Instead it integrates and highlights much of what we already know and practice in our daily work with patients. Its contribution is in allowing us to focus on the particular life stages and tasks of

194

the patient and to interpret many of our observations and even therapy itself in that light.

The time focus of therapy is important. Too often there appears to be an overfascination with the past to the exclusion of an adequate consideration of what one might anticipate in one's future. The stated time focus of many of the psychotherapies are either past-in-present or present with little consideration of the future. In a life-cycle sense, however, the time focus changes with patients of different ages in that the elderly will focus largely on the past or the life as lived while the adolescent anticipates the future. In therapy with Jack much time was spent in discussing his anticipation of the future. It was apparent that the experience of the past in the image of himself as a somewhat dislocated and lonely young boy failing grade two was still very real. We reviewed this perception of the past in terms of the present reality and discussed his difficulty in elaborating an image of himself as a person competent and able to face the future. We examined his depression and failure to attend school as an attempt to recapitulate the past, partially out of fear of the future, and looked at its destructive effects.

A great deal of time was spent in anticipating the future. This was not seen as an avoidance of dealing with reality or with the psychodynamic issues based on his past, but instead as a way of previewing future images of himself. We noted earlier that the scanning of the life cycle done by the adolescent is mainly future directed while those of older people will be mainly directed toward the past with the major division in its time focus occurring some time in midage. The therapist who is conscious of these tasks can assist the patient's life survey process in both of its forms: review and anticipation.

It is often helpful early in therapy to help patients elaborate a framework within which they can view and understand their reactions. For example, this is often done in crisis therapy and some of the shorter term, dynamically oriented psychotherapies. In psychotherapy from a life-cycle perspective, the understanding of the stages and tasks of the life cycle can provide just such an organizing model. The life-cycle model is a convenient one in that it allows the patient to elaborate a framework based on recollections and images of the past, on current tasks, and on an anticipation of the future in a task-specific way. While emotional understanding is a necessary development within therapy, the life-cycle framework developed early on in the course of therapy can help reduce anxiety and ally the patient's observing ego with the therapist in the process of change. Much behavior that would be otherwise unintelligible to the patient early in treatment can now be relatively easily interpreted in terms of one's reactions to the various demands of one's internalized life cycle. In this example, Jack's anxiety about becoming involved in a sexual relationship was discussed in terms of his wish to develop sexually, his fear and anticipation of a sexual relationship, and his need to anticipate and rehearse these areas within his own mind. We discussed his concern about his own identity and how he felt about sharing intimately with another. Likewise, his dependency on home was discussed in terms of his concern about his own growing independence and guilt about leaving home, especially when he saw, mirrored in his father at a different stage of life, difficulties which he perceived to be similar to his.

The juxtaposition of various life-cycle stages within the family can create some difficulty. In therapy with Jack this was discussed by clearly noting father's difficulties in terms of his own life cycle while we contrasted them to the specific life task that Jack was anticipating. We pointed out how his father's need to review his goals in life, in the light of where he was in his own life cycle, was a parallel process to Jack's need to start his adult life by affirming his own goals and directions. We discussed how the process was not strictly parallel in that Jack also saw in father an image of his own future, of what was in store for him just as we anticipated Jack's father would view Jack's current difficulties in the light of his own transition from adolescence to adulthood. We viewed father's confusion as normal and potentially helpful in that he was looking for a change of direction that he felt would be helpful. When father's confusion could be seen in this light Jack felt a greater sense of freedom. In these instances of the juxtaposition of various life crises in the family a combination of individual and family therapy may be indicated. We were planning this when father's crisis began to resolve and he obtained employment in another law firm, one which would allow him to develop along directions he wished.

A knowledge of life-cycle theory allows therapy to be structured in ways that resemble the demands of a particular stage in life and, in that way, obtain added congruence in considering developmental issues. This thesis of the structure of therapeutic interventions recapitulating developmental sequences in a life-cycle context has been developed in relation to marital therapy with young adults who have not yet completed the tasks of separation and individuation of adolescence (Toews 1980). In our example the active focus on the images of the future and

196

on Jack's need to assume responsibilities for his own life indicate this approach as well. Basically, the life-cycle perspective in therapy deals with helping the patient conceptualize, experience, and actively engage in the normal maturational process.

A word must be said about the role of the therapist lest we fall into the trap of viewing the contribution of the life-cycle perspective to therapy as a simplistic perception applied to the patient in treatment. The life-cycle basis for the therapist's and patient's understanding of each other is of fundamental importance here.

The therapist is an active participant in this approach to therapy in that the patient reminds the therapist of images, countertransference reviews, and previews of his own life cycle. This collage of images may in part form the basis for an empathic understanding of the patient, with each recognizing in the other a similar life process. Of course, many of the patient's transference reactions may in part be determined by the therapist's position in life. The therapist is viewed as someone who at times, or in certain aspects, is one to emulate or with whom to differ. These images, both positive and negative, combined with the many evoked images of one's childhood and one's future as seen in one's parents and grandparents, help to define what one's sense of identity is as represented by their view of one's life. The therapist too is forced as a participant to view internally his or her own personal understanding of life. If the patient evokes in the therapist images that the therapist has not yet become comfortable with in his or her own model of a life course, the therapist may lose the empathic understanding or become confused. This is particularly so when young therapists treat patients older than themselves (Martin and Prosen 1976) and must therefore attempt to help someone at a stage in life which they as yet have not experienced. For a young therapist it is difficult to deal with aspects such as sexuality, despair in aging, and a limited future in an older person. In a similar view the therapist may also experience difficulty in the treatment of adolescents when the therapist, forgetting or regretting his or her own position in life as an older person, seeks to be one with the adolescent in a process of overidentification.

Conclusions

This discussion has highlighted some of the essential observations that derive from a view of the life cycle in therapy. They do not alter other theories, observations, or therapeutic approaches. Instead, they provide an additional context within which therapy can be viewed. Life-cycle theory can, however, help the therapist and patient conceptualize their work together as mutually participating in bringing about the normative life tasks and unique experiences within the patient's life course.

REFERENCES

Blos, P. 1962. *On Adolescence*. New York: Free Press.

Butler, R.N. 1963. The life review: an interpretation of reminiscence in the aged. *Psychiatry* 26:65–76.

Erikson, E.H. 1959. Identity and the life cycle. *Psychological Issues*. Vol. 1. New York: International Universities Press.

Kastenbaum, R. 1959. Time and death in adolescence. In H. Feifel, ed. *The Meaning of Death*. New York: McGraw-Hill.

Martin, R., and Prosen, H. 1976. Psychotherapy supervision and life tasks: the young therapist and the middle-aged patient. *Bulletin of the Menninger Clinic* 40:125–133.

Prosen, H., and Martin, R. 1979. Postmenopausal promiscuity. *Medical Aspects of Human Sexuality* 13:26–34.

Prosen, H.; Martin, R.; and Prosen, M. 1972. The remembered mother and the fantasized mother. *Archives of General Psychiatry* 12:791–794.

Toews, J. 1980. Adolescent developmental issues in marital therapy. *Adolescent Psychiatry* 8:244–252.

13 A STUDY OF TRANSITIONAL OBJECTS IN THE EARLY HISTORIES OF BORDERLINE ADOLESCENTS

LILI LOBEL

An inability to play happily at an age-appropriate level is striking in the lives of severely disturbed children. In our therapeutic nursery the three- and four-year-olds begin to play with toys, but within a short time their play is interrupted by tantrums, agonizing screams, and bitter tears. Some of the children use their motor skills in ritualized, compulsive manipulation of puzzles and mechanical toys, oblivious to the pandemonium around them. There is a poignant contrast between this nursery and a place where playing is "normal and universal, facilitates growth and leads into group relationships" (Winnicott 1971).

There is a similarity between troubled children and the severely disturbed adolescents treated on the ward and in the outpatient clinic, specifically those not considered psychotic but given a diagnosis of borderline personality organization. These adolescents with a variety of symptoms, such as anorexia nervosa, suicidal behavior, and severe forms of acting out, all share an inability to become genuinely interested in schoolwork and hobbies. In the treatment of these patients, we became increasingly aware of the emptiness of their lives, which they sought to fill with grandiose fantasies or self-destructive action. Like the children in the therapeutic nursery, they seemed to have no inner resources to help them cope with frustrations and disappointments, nothing to offset their sense of loss.

Severely disturbed children and adolescents, frequently diagnosed as borderline, are generally portrayed in the literature as showing low tolerance for frustration, intense oral need, and impulsivity. Geleerd

(1958) described them as follows: "They were in contact with reality and not delusional. But when they were alone or when they felt frustrated, they very easily withdrew into fantasy life or had severe temper outbursts. . . . They did well and could relate when they felt loved by one adult, a mother substitute. As soon as this adult paid attention to someone or something else they felt unloved and would either withdraw or become hostile and aggressive."

Clinical encounters with our borderline adolescents provided many examples of such reactions. For instance, Tom, thirteen, an outpatient referred for violent behavior in school, seemed to have formed an attachment to his therapist, came regularly for his sessions, and was reported to be improving. One day he came a day early for his appointment. The doctor, however, could not see Tom for more than a few minutes, but he chatted with him briefly, expressing concern about Tom's smoking and his not having a warm enough jacket. Tom did not keep his appointment the next day. Instead, a social worker called his psychiatrist from a nearby hospital where he had been admitted to the medical ward after dipping his hand in sulphuric acid.

This type of behavior seems very much an adolescent version of the terrible tantrums we could observe in our therapeutic nursery. No inner resources seemed to be available to stem the onslaught of impulse. Indeed, the borderline patient is frequently described in the literature as not having achieved object constancy, a sense of self, or an identity.

Redl and Wineman (1951) describe the way relatively healthy children use previous satisfaction images as resources:

> It seems that normal children have a variety of possibilities to fall back upon spontaneously when confronted with moments of boredom, confusion, excitement, unhappiness, moodiness, or whenever the outside world fails to come through with adequate equipment or structural aid. If left to their own devices, most of them will simply "remember" something that had been fun before, or else a word, a piece of rope, an item of toy equipment, will remind them of something that could be done in a new combination, right now. They may remember, when a rainy day spoils their plans, that a book may offer the fun it had granted once before, they may dream up fantasy games out of pictures or stories they used to like, they may pull out an old abandoned toy and keep happy, varying old pleasurable themes with a new twist.

In contrast, highly disturbed children are described as "utterly destitute in situations like this." They may be pointing to the relatively neglected area in child psychiatry that Winnicott (1971) calls "transitional relatedness" or, in spatial terms, "the location of cultural experience." He states: "In the experience of the more fortunate baby (and small child, adolescent, and adult) the question of separation in separating does not arise, because in the potential space between the baby and its mother there appears the creative playing that arises naturally out of the relaxed state; it is here that there develops a use of symbols. . . . The child is now playing on the basis of the assumption that the person who loves and who is therefore reliable is available and continues to be available when remembered after being forgotten."

In an attempt to gain a better understanding of the painful sense of "nothing" in our patients, we considered the "something" that can be so visible in infancy and early childhood, the proverbial "blanky" or "teddy" that Winnicott introduced into the scientific literature as the transitional object. Somehow the infant acquires the capacity to imbue an inanimate object with the magical power to soothe him so that it becomes uniquely the infant's own and acquires lasting importance during early childhood. Winnicott (1953) postulates that its creation is made possible by "good-enough mothering at an early critical phase."

The disturbed children admitted to our therapeutic nursery had no history of transitional object use. Provence and Ritvo (1961) found that infants raised in institutions did not invest inanimate objects with meaning. In a study done with sailors and marines, Horton, Louy, and Coppolillo (1974) tested the hypothesis that persons with severe personality disorders will have little in their histories or their memory store to suggest a capacity for transitional relatedness. The authors interviewed the subjects who were up for a medical discharge and obtained reports from close relatives about childhood transitional object use and compared these findings with histories obtained from a relatively healthy comparison group. None of the individuals with personality disorders gave evidence of transitional relatedness in the present, and 84 percent had no history of transitional object use in childhood. This was sharply in contrast with the findings obtained from the comparison group; that is, 93 percent of well-adapted subjects demonstrated both past and present ability for transitional relatedness. The authors propose that the most useful piece of information in making a diagnosis of severe personality disorder is an absence of transitional relatedness, past or present.

201

Some disagreement exists as to how healthy transitional objects are. Sperling (1963) took the position that the existence of a transitional object denotes a certain insufficiency of unambivalent maternal attention and allotted to it pathological meaning by finding transitional object and fetish interchangeable. Eleven years later, another psychoanalyst, Bak (1974) stated: "There is a fair concensus that it is a nearly universal and healthy phenomenon in infancy. . . . The transitional object's warmth, fluffiness, and softness simulate not only the mother's breast and skin but her total ambience and provide satisfaction of the need for clinging."

Greenacre (1969) made an important distinction between the transitional object and the fetish. The former decreases excitation and provides soothing relief from anxiety and loneliness, while the latter increases excitation, leading to sexual discharge. Roiphe and Galenson (1975) note their observations of a normal child in their research nursery from ages eleven months to two years. It demonstrates the role of the transitional object (a Raggedy Ann doll) in coping with the normal strains implicit in the attainment of upright mobility, the separation-individuation thrust, and the anal-urinary and early sexual stages of development. It also shows in minutely observed detail the process of a transitional object being replaced by what the authors consider a fetishistic object in the face of unusual strains.

The transitional object is created by the infant as a substitute for the union with mother, but part of the phenomenon lies in the fact that he grows to prefer it to mother at times. Small children can be observed to become furious with their mothers and take solace in their favorite possession in her presence. The transitional object appears to allow children to maintain the representation of the good part of the mother while directing their rage against the frustrating "bad" mother. It is a magical device but the magic has its origin in reality; it depends on the real and continued availability of the mothering figure. However, the child's drive toward autonomy plays an equal part. We can postulate that by creating his own comforter he is not only reacting to disillusionment by the mother but also to his urge to outgrow the totally dependent relationship with her (Spock 1963). Thus, its use can be considered one of the visible demonstrations of the separation-individuation process (Mahler, Pine, and Bergman 1975).

Our hypothesis was that there would be little or no history of transitional object use in the infancy and early childhood of borderline adolescents. This could be attributed to a paucity of pleasurable and comforting experiences with the mother that could be internalized, or to the mother's need to brush aside those objects which the child seeks to render transitional, intruding on his fantasies and forcing herself to be a continuing presence out of her own needs.

The Study

In order to shed more light on this facet of infant behavior and maternal attitudes, we studied the early histories of twenty borderline and twenty relatively healthy adolescents. A requirement for inclusion in the study was that the mother or primary caretaker who had raised the child be available for an interview. In both groups there was a nearly equal ratio of boys and girls and a balanced ethnic mix. However, the socioeconomic level of the borderline group was lower than that of the relatively healthy group. The subjects in the first group came from predominantly lower-middle-class and working-class families, whereas a good proportion of the healthier group was middle class. However, this factor did not seem to affect the use of transitional objects since they were reported to have been widely used by siblings of the adolescents in both groups.

THE BORDERLINE GROUP

The subjects in this group were chosen from our clinic and ward population. All lived in our catchment area, a lower-middle-class section of the Bronx. Each patient had had a full diagnostic evaluation in our Division of Child Psychiatry.[1] The information given was obtained from interviews with the adolescents, from case histories, and from interviews with the mother of each patient. The ages ranged from eleven to sixteen at time of referral.

The reasons given for referral included one or more of the following: repeated running away, suicidal gestures, anorexia, severe anxiety attacks, prolonged school refusal, truancy, drugs, drinking, promiscuity, public exposure, stealing, vandalism, and aggressive acts at school and at home. Frequently there was a history of such behavior since puberty which had finally become intolerable.

Sometimes the early history would be in great contrast to the adolescent's presenting behavior. For instance, Jim, fourteen, was pleasant but shy and passive on the ward, tending to follow the younger patients around. In individual and family sessions he was markedly depressed.

His history belied his pleasant, cooperative behavior. At age eight he had had a psychiatric hospitalization because of "impossible" behavior in school where he tore the clothes of classmates and attempted to strangle a girl. After two months of treatment, his mother took him home via court action against medical advice. During the next six years at home he was described as "good," helping his mother to care for younger siblings but attending school erratically and remaining enuretic. His presenting problem on readmission was firesetting at home and sleeping with a knife under his pillow. His mother was afraid he might harm himself.

Two of the adolescents in this group had psychiatric hospitalizations before age ten for clearly disturbed behavior. A third was treated as an outpatient for one year at age five. The mother had brought her to the clinic at that time stating that she had always been a whiny, demanding child with many problems, but had become depressed following parental separation, not sleeping and eating well, and threatening to jump into the river. Another nine-year-old girl wrote a suicide note in school and was taken to see a child psychiatrist at the insistence of the school, but a recommendation for treatment was not followed by the parents.

Masterson (1972) comments that it is often difficult to get a good developmental history from families of borderline adolescents. The parents are often quite unaware of the fact that the child did not achieve autonomy at an appropriate age. I frequently heard the report that the patient was "a good baby," "a good child," "always very close to mother." In the case of two female patients with the presenting symptom of anorexia nervosa, both mothers described them as "the perfect child" before the problem started. In most cases, the past history given was a report of superficially compliant behavior interspersed with fighting, tantrums, running away; that is, submissiveness alternating with impulse-dominated behavior.

Tolstoi (1899) began *Anna Karenina* with "All happy families resemble one another; every unhappy family is unhappy in its own fashion." I found this to be at variance with the reality in the families of our borderline patients. They were all unhappy families. They each had at least one acutely disturbed child who served as a focus for their anxiety and anger, and they resembled one another in many other ways. These families seemed to be dominated by the mother even when the father lived in the household. Eight out of twenty children did not live with their biological fathers and had little or no contact with him. The fathers who were in the home were variously described in the protocol in such terms as: withdrawn from the family, withholding, ineffectual, alcoholic, strongly dependent on or subservient to his wife, sadistic, unpredictable. There were often indications of father's sadistic sibling rivalry with the child.

Sometimes there would be an early history of attachment to the father that had somehow been spoiled. On the other hand, the dependence on mother persisted into adolescence despite marked and chronic conflict. These adolescents were preoccupied with their feelings about their parents; anger, bitterness, longing, and anxious concern. When they did act out, it was invariably an activity (such as truancy, fighting, vandalism, promiscuity, drug use, running away) that would lead to renewed and persistent involvement of the parents. There were no reports of extended pleasurable family activities, such as joint vacations, that had gone well.

The adolescents in this group uniformly reported a lack of interest in school work, difficulty with concentration, and boredom. At least six out of twenty appeared to be of above average intelligence, the rest were average. Five had a history of erratic attendance in elementary school; school continued to be a major problem for them in puberty and adolescence. Fifteen had attended school without overt major difficulties until puberty. Only three out of fifteen continued to do reasonably well in school past puberty. In the remaining twelve cases puberty had brought with it the onset of provocative behavior with school personnel, failing grades, truancy, and a general withdrawal from academic competition.

As observed earlier, the adolescents in this group continued to be intensely involved with their families, albeit in a negative way. Their response to questions about peer relationships indicated that they seemed insignificant compared to the continued involvement with the parents. Some of the adolescents reported "hanging out with friends," but there seemed little in the way of meaningful friendships. In several cases, however, there was a history of a relationship with an "older protector" in elementary school or an intense symbiotic attachment to a boyfriend or girl friend. There was little or no involvement in special interests, sports, or hobbies. By far the most frequent reply to questions concerning leisure time activities was television.

In their mothers' accounts, childhood seemed to contain little in the way of pleasurable experiences, but much in the way of stress. There was not a single case where the adolescent or the mother reported an absorbing interest that led to further growth and development, although there was evidence of talent and dexterity in some cases. One child, later anorexic, was enrolled in dancing school at an early age and her potential career was of all-absorbing interest to her mother. Another, a boy, had developed the considerable mechanical skill involved in the process of stealing cars.

Out of twenty adolescents, only two acquired a transitional object during early childhood that could be recalled by the mothers. In these cases, the object was not relinquished during latency but remained important until puberty when the mother put an end to its use. The mothers were all familiar with what I meant by "a specially loved possession the child used to soothe himself " and sometimes described what apparently was transitional object use by other children in the family. With regard to our patients, the mothers frequently said something like: "No, he never cared about anything like that." They seemed to be very definite about the fact that this did not happen but—unlike the mothers described later on under the heading "The In-Betweens"—there was no indication that they actively prevented it. They remembered other ways their children were soothed at bedtime and in times of stress. Pacifiers were frequently given (one mother reporting that she never left home without several in her handbag). Many of the children remained attached to their bottle at bedtime until age five or six.

In keeping with the lack of transitional objects in their early history, these adolescents' sense of the future was equally barren. Borderline adolescents, like borderline adults, seem to spend a great deal of time preoccupied with secret fantasies of omnipotent control and self-glorification. We became familiar with their fantasies as they shared them with us in treatment. But when the young people in this study were asked specifically how they felt about their future, the answers revealed a profound sense of dread, pessimism, and lack of hope. One girl put it this way: "I'll probably get run over by a Mack truck." This sense of the future as a malignant force at worst and an empty chasm at best provided perhaps the most startling contrast between the two groups.

Many of the mothers in the borderline group reported that they had at times abused their children in early childhood. Predictably, the mothers' own history was frequently one of deprivation, brutality, and suffering. It was not to be expected that they could cancel their unmet needs and be ready to meet the rapidly changing needs of their growing children. However, it must be said that these factors by themselves are not sufficient to account for severe borderline pathology. Some of the siblings of the patients in this group seemed to suffer from neurotic symptoms, personality problems, depression, and learning disabilities, but were reported to compare favorably with the identified patient in regard to behavior, identity formation, and capacity for sublimatory channels.

The question would seem to be how mother and father combine in the rearing of a particular child. In some families, the parents seem to select one special child for their pathological needs and as these needs are discharged, other children may be spared to an extent. Thus, each child can be said to grow up in a different family.

THE NORMAL-NEUROTIC GROUP

There is controversy about what constitutes normalcy during the difficult period of adolescence. For the purpose of this study I chose twenty adolescents who seemed capable of establishing genuine and positive relationships with others, who were able to cope relatively well with school, and who were handling effectively the loosening of parental ties and the need to find new love objects. In addition, I was interested in their capacity for imaginative living, the quality that Winnicott (1953) calls "transitional relatedness" and that appears ultimately as a "capacity for cultural experience." For instance, the ability to feel a sense of belonging to one's school would indicate such a capacity in the adolescent. Conversely, a dislike of the school would not indicate a failure in transitional relatedness if there were indications of other areas imbued with genuine internal importance—sports, art, music, politics, a passion for the theatre. Anything that involved them in something other than direct gratification of primal needs would indicate a degree of health, a potential for growth.

When queried about special interests and hobbies, there was a particularly striking difference in the reports given by this group as compared with the answers of borderline adolescents who generally could not think of anything much they liked to do except watch television or "hang out." The subjects in this group were generally quick to respond, often enthusiastic and generally very specific. Twelve out of twenty listed sports as their most important special interest and pastime, two had a strong interest in music, one in art. Two had developed hobbies that required a good deal of time and effort, such as photography and the raising of tropical fish. One boy had spent five years learning about the subway system, researching how it was planned, designed, and built.

Eight adolescents remembered and described transitional objects. They had vivid memories of longtime relationships with a special bear, a little lion, a green nightgown that was kept after it was outgrown and had become ragged, a string of small Styrofoam animals that were one boy's friends in early childhood, replaced by the mother as they fell apart. Two boys remembered carrying a special blanket around with them. All these reports were later corroborated by the mothers, and three mothers reported transitional objects that the adolescents had forgotten or denied. No one reported continued use of such objects past the age of six. In all, eleven of the twenty adolescents had had transitional objects. Six of these were boys, five were girls.

THE "IN-BETWEENS"

In our search for normal-neurotic adolescents, we encountered three high school students, two boys and one girl, who seemed to belong in a space between the two groups compared in this study. They were able to cope with the demands of school and they made no complaints. Yet, they seemed to be fundamentally isolated young people who struggled hard, by role playing, false optimism, and numerous superficial relationships, to manufacture the feeling of being a worthwhile person. In interviews with their mothers we learned of considerable family pathology and marital unhappiness. However, in contrast with the borderline group, these mothers appeared to obtain major gratification from their present relationship with these particular children and had high expectations for them. When queried about transitional objects, two of the mothers reported that they had taken special pains to prevent them. One had changed blankets every day so that her infant son would not become attached to one in particular. The other cleaned out the crib every night and substituted a special doll of her own chosing for whatever her infant daughter might have selected. These accounts suggest the sparse beginnings of an attachment to a transitional object and the level of maternal anxiety aroused.

Discussion

Of the twenty relatively healthy adolescents, eleven had had transitional objects as defined by Winnicott (1953), that is, specially loved objects that acquire lasting importance in early childhood and in health lose their importance as the child's range of interest widens. No one reported an attachment to a transitional object past the age of five or six. Of the twenty borderline adolescents, there are only two reports of specially loved objects. These were acquired by two of the girls in early childhood and continued to be important until they were taken away by the mother during prepuberty.

MATERNAL FACTORS

The mothers of the adolescents in these groups were interviewed under very different auspices. The mothers of the relatively healthy students were aware that they had been approached because their children gave indications of being intact young people. The mothers of the borderlines agreed to be interviewed so that we could have a better understanding of their children's disturbance. Indeed, many of the mothers in the healthier group were pleased and proud to be asked to talk about their children, and some of the mothers of borderlines were clearly depressed. However, there was a good deal of variation of affect in both groups, and there were clear indications that these two groups of mothers differed in a great many ways that were not directly connected with the circumstances of our meeting.

In the healthier group, fourteen mothers held jobs; six mothers did not have paid jobs but were active in volunteer organizations. Among the mothers of borderlines, only one worked at a regular full-time job. Four did part-time work. The fifteen remaining mothers had worked sporadically in the past or were still involved in raising young children but for whatever reason seemed to live in a state of being cut off from the outside world. Nineteen mothers in the first group came from intact and stable families. Nine reported that their families had been close and loving as well as stable. A review of the childhood experiences of mothers in the borderline group revealed a number of glaring accounts of deprivation of parental affection. A reported lack of maternal and paternal love featured in the lives of most. Seven mothers had been raised by mother substitutes or in institutions because of their mothers' early death or illness. Virtually all the mothers reported difficulties during their own adolescence, sometimes attested to by the fact that they had dropped out of high school because of pregnancy. Some had had to assume early responsibility in their own families. Others had "run around." Seven had filled their lives with having children; one had taken in many foster children.

None of the mothers in the healthier group reported serious post-partum depressions. Twelve reported "good babies," eight mentioned various difficulties. The overwhelming majority acknowledged that they had needed support in their early childrearing days and had managed to find it—primarily from husbands but frequently also from family and friends. The mothers of the borderline adolescents recalled their early mothering with this specific child in a very different way; there seemed to have been little satisfaction in it for them. Some frankly reported extreme anxiety, depression, and occasional child abuse; others said babies were all right, but they could not stand it when the children started to "talk back" and "nag." Their lack of pleasure in childrearing was often at odds with the fact that many prided themselves at having produced many children, almost as though they had tried to make up in quantity what they had missed in the quality of the experience.

The importance of social factors in the family's life also cannot be overestimated. It would seem that a husband's support and his independent initiatives in child care which permit mother to relax her involvement, a warm and friendly neighbor who serves as a model, can make the difference between a "good enough" and an unrewarding experience with early mothering. For a number of complex reasons the mothers in the borderline group experienced their environment as cruelly disappointing and depriving.

PATERNAL FACTORS

Nineteen out of twenty relatively healthy adolescents interviewed lived with both parents. Only twelve of the twenty borderline adolescents lived with their biological father. The way in which the two groups of adolescents described their fathers provided one of the most striking contrasts of the study. The great majority of the relatively healthy adolescents, both boys and girls, stated that they would most likely turn to their mothers for understanding and sympathy in case of stress, but they spoke of their fathers with a mixture of affection, humor, and respect. Some said they had "learned to handle Dad." Almost all stated that they had "learned something from him." The borderline adolescents described their fathers with almost monotonous repetition in very different terms and with a very different affect. The fathers were described variously as ineffectual, unavailable, self-centered, and often punitive and sadistic. Human beings are in most instances raised by two parents in our society so that there is a certain

210

margin of safety—the failure of one parent may be prevented or rectified by the resources of the other. With our borderline adolescents, the margin of safety had been lost.

Conclusions

Comparing the two groups of adolescents, it became amply clear that the relatively healthy students had a capacity for investing their world with meaning. In developmental terms, they had through internalization of good enough object relationships acquired psychic structure they could employ for this purpose. They seemed to have a certain amount of confidence in their internal resources; thus, they could tolerate frustration in the interest of future benefits.

In contrast, the borderline adolescents were dependent upon outside stimuli, without which they tended to feel lost and empty. They defended against this by impulsive behavior and by grandiose fantasies that would permit them periodic feelings of elation. They had little or no investment in the future.

The three "In-Betweens" seem to me to provide a bridge between the two main categories. They maintained a facade of good functioning but turned out to be highly narcissistic, compliant young people whose actual sense of self appeared to be largely negative. However, they had learned to please the angry, disappointed women who mothered them. They had learned to cheer them up.

The major transactions between parent and child are basically not conscious and therefore not easily reportable. The early histories given by the mothers of the "In-Betweens" yielded some meaningful data when transitional-object use was explored. Two issues seem to be at stake there: the internal capacity of the child to create such an object, and the ability of the mother to release him for this purpose, to leave him in peace. The issue of separation-individuation, the issue of the father's role in childrearing all need to be considered in the light of these mothers' deep need to maintain a sense of control over their children, to resist unconsciously a loosening of the tie. Obviously, there can be difficulties with letting go in cases where a transitional object has been allowed to exist. The teddy bear is not a guardian angel on the road that leads from infantile dependence through a transitional stage to the stage of adult mature independence, but it is a start.

The links between childhood and adolescence are often difficult to discern because of one's need to forget the past. However, no link is more indissoluble. This study was based on the hypothesis that there can be visible antecedents in early childhood of the sense of healthy optimism that anticipates weathering successfully the developmental crises of adolescence. The data obtained would seem to bear out Winnicott's thesis that the existence of a transitional object is a visible index of a certain developmental achievement. When mothering has been "good enough," a transitional object may be created by the infant or small child to help keep intact an illusion of safety that permits the child to venture forward.

NOTE

1. This study originated in my participation in the Borderline Adolescent Study Group, Division of Child Psychiatry, Albert Einstein College of Medicine, Bronx, New York, under the direction of Robert Anderson.

REFERENCES

Bak, R. 1974. Distortions of the concept of fetishism. *Psychoanalytic Study of the Child* 29:195–213.

Geleerd, E. 1958. Borderline states in childhood and adolescence. *Psychoanalytic Study of the Child* 13:279–295.

Greenacre, P. 1969. The fetish and the transitional object. *Psychoanalytic Study of the Child* 24:144–164.

Horton, P.; Louy, J.; and Coppolillo, H. 1974. Personality disorder and transitional relatedness. *Archives of General Psychiatry* 30:618–622.

Mahler, M.; Pine, F.; and Bergman, A. 1975. *The Psychological Birth of the Human Infant*. New York: Basic.

Masterson, J. 1972. *The Treatment of the Borderline Adolescent: A Developmental Approach*. New York: Wiley-Interscience.

Provence, S., and Ritvo, S. 1961. Effects of deprivation on institutionalized infants: disturbances in development of relationship to inanimate objects. *Psychoanalytic Study of the Child* 16:189–205.

Redl, F., and Wineman, D. 1951. *Children Who Hate*. Glencoe, Ill.: Free Press.

Roiphe, H., and Galenson, E. 1975. Some observations on transitional object and infantile fetish. *Psychoanalytic Quarterly* 44:206–231.

Sperling, M. 1963. Fetishism in children. *Psychoanalytic Quarterly* 32:374–392.

Spock, B. 1963. The striving for autonomy and regressive object relationships. *Psychoanalytic Study of the Child* 18:361–364.

Tolstoi, L. 1899. *Anna Karenina*. New York: Crowell.

Winnicott, D. 1953. Transitional objects and transitional phenomena: a
study of the first not-me possession. *International Journal of
Psycho-Analysis* 34:89–97.

Winnicott, D. 1971. *Playing and Reality*. New York: Basic.

14   CHANGES IN TRANSITIONAL OBJECTS:
GIRLS IN MIDADOLESCENCE

PERIHAN ARAL ROSENTHAL

Adolescence is a transitional period when the resurgence of instinctual aggressive and sexual impulses accompanies reactivation of un-welcome preoedipal ties with the parents. The intensity of a girl's preoedipal feelings depends first on her mother's conflict about her own femininity (Benedek 1973) and then on the adolescent girl's negotiation and integration of these feelings through new identifications in order to achieve autonomy. When adolescents sever their re-lationships with their mothers or early caregivers, some return to use transitional object defenses, not to regress to the preoedipal stage be-cause of intense associated anxiety, depressive affect, and feelings of loneliness, but in the service of mastery (Galenson 1976).

Transitional objects (Winnicott 1953) bring back the infantile (and illusory) memories of being safe and comfortable in the absence of mother. According to Winnicott (Hong 1978), transitional objects are seen either as symbolically representing the mother or representing certain functional properties of the mother. The transitional object be-comes an "auxiliary soother" by innumerable minute internalizations and transforms into self-soothing psychic structures which assist the infant in the work of separation individuation and toward establishing a cohesive self. Winnicott emphasized the importance of "good enough" mothering during the earlier phase of infancy. With good enough mothering, fantasy coincides with satisfaction. The infant's use of tran-sitional objects results from the attempt to maintain the special dyadic relationship with the mothering person, especially when she is absent. Eventually, at the toddler stage, this phenomenon is displaced into toys, friends, and later still into academic achievement. In the absence of good enough parenting, the adolescent girl may again use transitional objectlike relationships which allow her to separate physically from her ambivalent mother.

Adolescence and Transitional Phenomena

Given the developmental progress of adolescence (Friday 1978), the female adolescent shows her ambivalence toward growth in her need to experiment with freedom while never wanting to lose the bond to her mother. The adolescent tries to resolve this ambivalence by substituting other things, also called transitional objects, for the mother. Transitional objects become important around early puberty for many girls between the ages ten and twelve. This is comparable to the first separation-individuation which takes place during the first three years of life. Mahler, Pine, and Bergman (1975) write that when a child becomes individualized and a separately functioning self, she keeps a constant and reliable internal image of her mother. The transitional object at the early adolescent stage is usually a girl friend of the same age. This close relationship is extremely helpful for mutual mothering; it is rarely a desire for explicit sex. During midadolescence, however, this phenomenon changes. Transitional objects then are usually boyfriends with whom the girls attempt to recreate the early heaven that existed between them as infants and their mothers. For these girls, falling in love means falling in love either with the memory of that mother-child relationship or with the fantasy of how they wish it had been. Even those suffocating affairs in which girls cannot bear to be away from their antisocial boyfriends for a moment recreate this infantile relationship. It is easy to see that the boyfriend is playing the role of surrogate mother. The relationships depend on the adolescent resolving the seeming contradiction of wanting freedom from mother, but also wanting to be close to the surrogate. The surrogate is not as fearful for the adolescent or as locked onto her as is the mother (Friday 1978). The surrogate thus gives the adolescent girl the old mothering security while also giving freedom to face the future.

The choice of transitional objects of the adolescent usually are more psychological than are infants' needs to be fed, held, and bathed. However, early and late transitional objects often similarly end in oblivion, forgotten by the children and adolescents who adopted them (Winnicott 1953). Whether the adolescent girl can resolve the transition and the use of somewhat pathological part-objects depends on the adolescent's earlier relationship with her mother (caregiver) and on whether she had "good enough mothering" (Winnicott 1953). If she experienced problems in nurturance or caring, the adolescent will have some problem giving up her transitional objects for she will fear, as a consequence of relinquishing them, regression to her earlier dependence on a depriving preoedipal mother. Because adolescent girls are increasingly aware of their mothers' growing lack of nurturing, the role of wife and homemaker becomes more interesting. The increasing antipathy which adolescent girls feel to the traditional female role (Galenson 1976) could easily lead to more acting out and an equivalent choice of transitional objects.

Winnicott (1953) assumes that the last of reality acceptance is never completed, that no human being is free from the strain of relating inner and outer reality, and that the transitional experience continues throughout life. The transitional mode appears in various forms at each stage of life, such as play, artistic creativity, mystical and religious experiences, and recreational activities. According to Anna Freud (1965), in the course of development, the child leaves behind the original transitional object, but not its qualities.

The increased appearance and heightened importance of transitional phenomena in the adolescent's emotional life marks an attempt by the adolescent to reinstate (Downey 1978) what had been in the toddler period a relatively satisfying mode of stabilization and to maintain the relationship to the object when the latter was absent or depriving. In adolescents, transitional phenomena spread over the psychological landscape between instinctual drives and external reality. This is where the adolescent spends so much time experiencing, reorganizing, and recreating the inner and outer world because bodily changes evoke sadness as they cut off familiar pleasures and safety of the past (Kestenberg 1975). The adolescent's transitional objects will have many of the same determinants as the infant's blanket (Downey 1978); all modulate inner and outer space, create a more delineated body boundary, and make separation from important objects tolerable, but also show the powerful identification with the parent.

Adolescent girls today are using more drugs and alcohol, and pregnancy and delinquency have increased alarmingly. One often sees middle-class adolescent girls intensely involved with motorcycle gangs or men with criminal records. For these girls, such involvements have transitional object quality. That is, they make the girls feel soothed and protected despite the negative qualities of the object (Wieder 1969). The adolescent girls will not easily give up these objects, but keep them at the expense of losing earlier important figures in order not to regress to the preoedipal stage (Kestenberg 1975). They feel soothed by the transitional objects. The transitional objects modulate the girls' aggression into something soft, something that helps her feel intact and differentiated as an individual from her mother (Downey 1978). These transitional objects, however, are important aids to therapy where the adolescent has to grasp what the transitional object means to her. It is important that the therapist be aware of whether the adolescent is dealing with oedipal or preoedipal issues (Meeks 1973).

Diagnosis and Treatment: The Study

Normal adolescent developmental fantasies can be tolerated and integrated, but in cases of pathological development, disturbing fantasies cannot be integrated and lead to fragmentation instead of structuralization. In normal development, defensive operations and external adaptations may be called into play to prevent the emergence of disruptive fantasies (Coppolillo 1976). Adolescents normally attempt to maintain contact with external reality through intimate contact with an external object. Transitional objects and phenomena, which focus on external perceptions, help avoid conscious disturbing fantasy. Transitional phenomena refer to an "intermediate area of experiencing to which inner reality and external life both contribute" (Weider 1969); that is, intermediate area between subjective and objective perceptions. The patient uses the transitional object to help avoid regression to illusion and hallucination while recognizing or testing the reality of the external object.

Winnicott (1953) thinks that the child's inanimate transitional objects are analogous to certain types of adult love relationships in which the relation of the subject to the object is primarily exploitive. The subject feels no concern for the needs of the object and the subject cannot acknowledge that the object has its own separateness and individuality. The child keeps the object between himself and his environment (Volkan 1976) in order to believe that he enjoys similar sovereignty over the environment itself and to entertain the illusion that the transitional object is under his absolute control, just as the infant believes he has the breast under magical control because immediately after birth the mother made herself available to him in a way that fosters the illusion of her breasts belonging to his own body. This illusion of control over the transitional object reassures the child that he has similar and absolute control over the external object (Burnham 1969).

Thus, for the adolescent, transitional objects, like an antisocial boyfriend, can become cherished and unrelinquishable possessions which enable the adolescent to confront and control her world. A new person may be endowed with the qualities of the mother and the child and thus can fulfill the function of the transitional object. This object, at times, becomes the prime target of aggression in the process of denigration of self and the object. She also creates transitional objects out of friends and reduces her mother to the state of an accessory object by accusing her of being merely the shadow of the oedipal father. The adolescent's renewal intimacy with the mother has oedipal features but is also an attempt to reach the father. That is, by excluding the father, the adolescent at once expels him and excites him, in a pattern reminiscent of the ambivalent relationship activity of toddlers (Kestenberg 1975).

The adolescent girls discussed in this chapter do well in academic achievements and peer relationships. They manifest socially acceptable behavior and activities until midadolescence, when they suddenly shift from their old mode of behavior to intense acting out. They become intensely involved with transitional objects; including alcohol, drugs, boyfriends, or an individual who has a long criminal record. Parents of these girls find themselves bewildered by this sudden change and in most instances lose control in handling their daughters' behavior. It does not matter how much pressure the parents put on their adolescent daughters; the girls' antisocial involvement with these transitional objects will continue despite the loss of parental approval, old peer relationships, and academic achievement.

We studied twenty such adolescent girls, 80 percent from intact middle-class families and 20 percent from divorced families. The group was ethnically and religiously mixed. The girls were between the seventh and tenth grades in school. The surface behavior of these adolescents manifested bizarre fluctuations in behavior, indicating psychological turmoil. The diagnostic process must differentiate whether the emotional problems reflect a basic pathology or a developmentally induced and time-limited side effect of the growth process (Masterson 1967). The outcome of the therapy greatly depends on the accuracy of the diagnosis.

Case Study

This case is representative of the twenty cases which we followed. N was a quiet and bright fifteen-year-old girl who was referred to us by the guidance counselor because of rebelliousness toward her parents, truancy from school, and running away from home. N's parents, in their early thirties, are middle class; the mother is a librarian and the father an ex-marine working as an executive at a computer company. N has one older sister who is described by the parents as a troubled child, but a good student who spent most of her time at school or in her room during the last two years. The sister is reported to have had hysterical blindness for which she received four to five years of psychiatric therapy.

DEVELOPMENTAL HISTORY

The mother's pregnancy and delivery of N were normal. However, when N was born, mother had a depression which lasted for eight months. During this time father and maternal grandmother performed the essential part of the child care, helping mother a great deal. N was a fussy but affectionate and good baby. She was a good precocious toddler who did well with autonomous tasks like self-care, toilet training, and dressing herself. However, the mother described N as always being an independent child who never took "no" for an answer. She made a strong attachment to her peers at nursery school and did not show any separation anxiety. The easy transition hurt her mother's feelings, making her feel left behind and abandoned. N did extremely well in elementary school and she was a very popular child and an A student.

However, she ran into problems when she started junior high school. At this time, N felt that she was rejected by her old friends, whom she described as "square." She was drawn toward an older group of wild adolescents who took drugs, were promiscuous, and engaged in antisocial behavior. N rationalized her involvement with this group saying that they at least accepted her when others did not. At this time N started to run away from home frequently, each episode lasting several days. N's parents were concerned about her disappearances from home and her intense involvement with boys who were considered delinquents. During this period, N and her boyfriends were using alcohol and heavy drugs. N was also involved in several fights in which she and these other adolescents used knives, and on other occasions, when hitchhiking, she defended herself with a knife.

PARENTAL HISTORY

N's mother, Mrs. L, always felt very close to her own father, who died four years before we saw N. Mrs. L now feels quite lonely and misses her father, with whom she was very close. She was her father's favorite, "daddy's little girl." Her mother was "the boss" who set the rules in the house. Mrs. L never felt close to her mother and felt rejected by her. She is overly critical of her, especially of her mothering of N and her sister.

Mrs. L suffered a long-standing chronic depression when N was five years old and started kindergarten. Around this time, Mrs. L returned to school and became a librarian. After returning from work each evening, she locked herself in her bedroom and withdrew from her husband and daughters. The older daughter also locked herself in her room every night. This behavior pushed Mr. L and N into an intense relationship. Mrs. L had difficulty seeing her contributions to this relationship and felt excluded from the family, lonely, and isolated. She complained that she found it difficult to show affection toward her daughters and her husband. At the same time she continued to recall her relationship with her father and to compare her other relationships unfavorably to it.

Mr. N, the oldest of three siblings was harshly treated by his father, who died seven years before. He had a good relationship with his mother and felt close to her. He now feels caught in a similar situation; his wife is being cold and demanding like his father, while his younger daughter is being warm and nurturant like his mother. At times, Mr. L loses his temper and hits N, but he is more kindly toward his children than his father used to be toward him. N's looks also reminded Mr. L. of his wife at a young age, a fact which complicated Mr. L's interaction with N.

DIAGNOSTIC EVALUATION

N is an attractive fifteen-year-old girl. During her interviews she appeared depressed but was able to relate well. She expressed a great deal of guilt about causing problems between her parents, but at the same time was very angry, feeling that no one cared for her. N felt that her mother always let her down by isolating herself every evening. As a result, N felt lonely and depressed, but also pushed toward her father. This situation created extremely uncomfortable feelings and restlessness for N because of her own incestuous anxiety. When her feelings escalated to an especially intense pitch, N found her answer in running away from home. N resented both parents—her mother for refusing to protect her from her father's intrusiveness, seductiveness, and restriction, and her father for finding out about her activities with her friends and then punishing her with beating or grounding.

At the same time, however, N was attracted to her father as the one person who really gave her attention and understanding. N's father was available to her. For instance, he sometimes took her hunting. However, he insisted on taking her alone. When N was fourteen, she began to object, saying that she would not go unless she could take one of her boyfriends with her. Mr. L refused, and also forbade N to see her boyfriends. N responded by bringing boys in front of the house and kissing them to tease her father. He would end up chasing N and her boyfriends around the neighborhood. N had an intense yearning for protection and mothering. Since N's mother had withdrawn and was unable to protect N from her incestuous and sexual feelings, N found the solution in running away to live with a poor family in town who had eight children. N enjoyed staying with this family and taking care of the small children for a few days before returning home. In providing mothering to these children, N felt that she was herself taken care of.

N felt that she was considered worthless at home because she was all alone or she had her father hovering over her. With her friends, especially her boyfriends, she felt important and loved. She believed her friends accepted her as she was, cared for her, and were not critical of her. N felt that her friends were very important in her life at this time, as important to her life as bread and water and insisted that no one could stop her from seeing them. Like the family N ran away to, her friends made her feel taken care of, loved, and safe.

THERAPY WITH N'S PARENTS

During therapy with N's parents, the therapist tried to engage both parents in the therapeutic process, helping them to negotiate and compromise with their adolescent daughter. Each parent resisted the therapy in some way. The mother broke several of her appointments and insisted that she could not take the time away from her job. The father came to every interview, but was unable to compromise with N because negotiation had become a matter of control. The mother's failure to be available for her daughter and the father's overinvolvement and intrusiveness hampered the therapy process. During therapy N's father was helped to see what her boyfriends meant to her. The therapist believed that if Mr. L could be a little more tolerant, N would eventually be able to give up the intensity with her boyfriends and stop running away. Unfortunately, the father was not consistent in handling N and continued to be overinvolved with his daughter. Mr. L remained rigid, punitive, controlling, and seductive throughout the time of the therapy. Eventually, he also stopped therapy.

THERAPY WITH N

N related positively to her therapist. She was depressed and, at times, anxious, but she was very open about her struggle around the issues of growing up and her interaction with her family. N remembered her early years as happy ones, but she recalled her feelings of loneliness, sadness, and an attraction toward her father when she started junior high school. She felt that her father cared about her but was very strict.

Because N's relationship with her father was sexualized, she became overly friendly with several boys whom she knew were not good for her, but whom she accepted as better than nothing. N needed to feel that she was taken care of. She recalled that taking pills and smoking pot make her feel better; as if she were on a cloud or in heaven where she was protected. Similarly, she felt that her boyfriends were like a drug. They made her feel assured. N felt that, unlike her relationship with her father, her intense relationships with her boyfriends were safe and that they would take care of her. She felt that her boyfriends accepted her as she was and made her feel good about herself. She continued these relationships at the expense of being beaten and grounded by her father and rejected by her mother. When I asked N what these relationships reminded her of, she spoke of uncomfortable feelings about her father; she felt her friends would protect her from an uncomfortable, close situation at home.

N's relationships with other girls was very ambivalent. She was suspicious of them, fearing that they depreciated her and would take away her boyfriends. N frequently got involved in fistfights with other girls and even had several fights with switchblade knives. She rationalized these relationships, saying that the other girls were no good anyway. N wanted mothering from her girl friends, but was so angry at her mother that she did not know how to get protection or nurturance from women. However, by the end of her therapy, N was able to relate positively with her therapist, which facilitated more positive interaction with other girls.

Since her parents were unable to make any changes in their marital relationship or the handling of their daughter, I continued to work with N alone. She became aware of her incestuous anxiety around her relationship with her father. When her father objected in a seductive manner to her relationship with boys, she ended up finding an older boy, who, however, was a school dropout, had long hair, and who smoked pot and drank. This boy was smaller and less intelligent than N. N's father was able to accept the boy because he did not find him a threat. N carried this boy as a security blanket, even bringing him to her therapy sessions. Following this, she stopped running away, settled down in her work at school, and became an honor student. N's explanation of her relationship with this boy was, "I don't know why I feel so good when he is with me. He reminds me of my teddy bear I had when I was two years old." N was still sad that her mother was not available for her, but she knew that her boyfriend was available and represented everything to her. At the same time, she questioned whether her boyfriend represented an unrealistic fantasy or a dream. N's therapy, about which her feelings were very positive, continued until the end of her high school years. She eventually stopped acting out but continued to have her boyfriend accompany her wherever she went. When she finished high school, she left her boyfriend and went to an out-of-state college. She wrote several letters to let me know that she was doing well.

DISCUSSION

N's mother, ambivalent about caring for N from the beginning, suffered from long-standing, chronic depressions. N, able to get some adequate mothering from her maternal grandmother and from her father, did well until she became an adolescent. When the resurgence of her earlier dependency needs were not met by her mother, who was very ambivalent about N's coming adolescence, she attempted to get the nurturance she needed from boys, drugs, and alcohol. When she reached midadolescence, N's increased anxiety about aggression and sexuality pushed her toward her rejecting mother and seductive father. She felt both these relationships were ambivalent and threatening and found a solution to the problems they presented by using transitional objects which could keep her safe from her parents, protect her from her incestuous sexual feelings, soothe her, and take care of her emerging needs.

Both parents were so involved with their own unresolved conflicts (although father showed some interest despite his wife's unavailability) that they could not empathize with N or help her work through her adolescent problems. They somewhat unconsciously fostered and pushed N toward unsuitable transitional objects. In this situation, N found solutions in her intense attachment to her boyfriends as transitional objects despite her intellectual awareness of their antisocial behavior.

During therapy, N became aware of her father's seductiveness, intrusiveness, and her mother's unavailability. She gained insight into her uncomfortable, sexualized interaction with her father. She found a solution with a boyfriend who was acceptable to her father. With this relationship she felt comfortable and protected from her regressive feelings toward her mother (which threatened N with severe depression) and her incestuous feelings toward her father. The boyfriend became the ultimate transitional object that protected her from her internal and external dangers and allowed further ego growth and development.

Conclusions

The psychological and hormonal changes leading to resurgence of sexual, aggressive, and instinctual impulses make adolescents extremely narcissistic (Kestenberg 1975). At the same time they have the task of integrating their ego ideals with their superego demands. They devalue their self-concept, confuse their sexual identities, and rigidly restrict their superego demands to conform to parental demands (Wieder 1969). With resurgence of instinctual sexual and aggressive feelings, the egos of adolescents are severely troubled (Galenson 1976).

During therapy with adolescents, therapists usually deal with the patient's self-representation and object constellation when the repressed material surfaces. When the primitive internalized object relations of adolescents are reactivated, they cannot tolerate loneliness, depression, or isolation, and at times consider suicide. They may turn to transitional objects to protect and soothe them.

Though the therapist must help the adolescent with the transitional object, he must not interfere with the relationship but rather help the patient understand the meaning of the transitional object. When the adolescent is able to understand what the transitional object means to her, she then develops her transference to her therapist, at which point the therapist will be able to help the patient with preoedipal and oedipal issues and facilitate separation individuation from her parents (Rosenthal 1979).

REFERENCES

Benedek, T. 1973. Parenthood as a developmental phase. *Psychoanalytical Investigations*. New York: Quadrangle.

Burnham, D.L. 1969. Schizophrenia and object relations. In D.L. Burnham, ed. *Schizophrenia and the Need-Fear Dilemma*. New York: International Universities Press.

Coppolillo, H.P. 1976. The transitional phenomenon revisited. *Journal of the American Academy of Child Psychiatry* 15:36–48.

Downey, T.N. 1978. Transitional phenomena in the analysis of the early adolescent males. *Psychoanalytic Study of the Child* 33:19–47.

Freud, A. 1965. *Normality and Pathology in Children*. New York: International Universities Press.

Friday, N. 1978. *My Mother, Myself*. New York: Dell.

Galenson, E. 1976. Psychology of women: late adolescent and early childhood. *Journal of the American Psychoanalytic Association* 24 (3):631–647.

Hong, K.M. 1978. The transitional phenomena. *Psychoanalytic Study of the Child* 33:47–81.

Kestenberg, J. 1975. Children and parents. In *Psychoanalytic Studies in Development*. New York: Aronson.

Mahler, M.S.; Pine, F.; and Bergman, A. 1975. *The Psychological Birth of the Human Infant*. New York: Basic.

Masterson, J.F. 1967. *The Psychiatric Dilemma of Adolescence*. Boston: Little, Brown.

Meeks, J.E. 1973. Nosology in adolescent psychiatry: an enigma wrapped in a whirlwind. In J.C. Schoolar, ed. *Current Issues in Adolescent Psychiatry*. New York: Brunner/Mazel.

Rosenthal, P.A. 1979. Delinquency in adolescent girls: developmental aspects. *Adolescent Psychiatry* 7:503–516.

Volkan, V.D. 1976. *Primitive Internalized Object Relations.* New York: International Universities Press.

Wieder, H., and Kaplan, E.G. 1969. Drug use in adolescence. *Psychoanalytic Study of the Child* 24:399–431.

Winnicott, D.W. 1953. Transitional objects and transitional phenomena. *International Journal of Psycho-Analysis* 34:89–97.

15

I. AN INVESTIGATION OF THE INFLUENCE
OF PARENTAL COMMUNICATIONS ON
ADOLESCENT EGO DEVELOPMENT

HAROLD A. RASHKIS AND SHIRLEY R. RASHKIS

If the principal developmental task of the adolescent is to move successfully out of the family and into the community—though this task may not necessarily be completed before the traditional period of adolescence has passed—it follows that parental behavior appropriate to this purpose must preserve what is useful in the parent-adolescent attachment while not sparing the adolescent the harshness of external reality. One of the parameters to be considered in evaluating parental behavior is parental communication. The present study is an attempt to organize case material in a way that will permit us to consider the truth value of parental messages as they relate to the success of adolescent children in adapting to extrafamilial reality.

One commonly hears adolescents complain that their parents have lied to them. Implicit in this complaint is the accusation of a breach of faith by the parent. It was suggested by Ekstein (1965) that "communication" has its origin in the "communion" that exists between parent and child. Wile (1942) observed that parents and children are mutually dependent on each other's statements. This dependency, of course, derives from the absence of an innate organismic mechanism for determining whether or not a statement is true. Lacking also an external means of verifying statements, parents and children are inevitably dependent on one another's good faith to maintain their "interpersonal organization."

Even if Chomsky (1972) is correct in his suggestion that syntax is innate in the human brain, the child would at best be able to recognize only the grammatical adequacy of parental statements but not their truth value. If the brain is programed to recognize the structures: A is on B, or A did B to C, it would not have the prior knowledge to distinguish these from: B is on A, or, C did B to A. Thus the child requires that the parent be correct in designating at least what is the subject and what the predicate. As the child moves into adolescence, there are increasing demands on the parents for meaning, accuracy, and adequacy.

Nutritive acts by parents feed the child both physiologically and emotionally. A dual function is accordingly served by communication. The content of the message provides information (cognitive "food"), while its form, modality, or ecology provides an emotional input. As the child's recognition of transitivity develops to replace an undifferentiating commutativity, the groundwork has been formed for the cathexis of truth. Once it begins to matter whether A or B is subject or predicate, it becomes possible for the child to compare statements with reality and to know whether or not the parent is in fact describing the structure and processes of the household and its environs.

We recognize that there is a considerable gap between the acknowledgment that parental communication serves a nutritive function and the demonstration that any direct relationship exists between the form and substance of such communications and the accomplishment by the adolescent of specific developmental tasks. In this chapter we hope to begin an organization of the space separating the communicative events from the intermediate evidence of maturity signaled by the adolescent's ability to separate from his parental home. We will not undertake to relate any particular kind of parental communication to any diagnostic category; correlational relevance may appear in subsequent more detailed analysis of our findings.

Method

SUBJECTS

Our subsequent observations are based on twenty-one patients equally divided as to adolescents, young adults, and adults; twelve male, nine female. Diagnostically more than half of the patients were neurotic or had character disorders; the remainder were borderline or had occasional psychotic episodes. Two had a history of multiple psychotic episodes. Since we plan to make no specific diagnosis-related statements, we consider this wide range desirable for exploratory purposes.

Two criteria determined our selection of patients: first, that they were well known to us and, second, that we felt quite familiar with the modes of parental communication. The typical patient in this group had had several hundred hours of therapy. About half the patients had had more than five years of intensive treatment.

GENERATION OF DATA

On the basis of our clinical observations we made two statements about each patient. The first statement was an appraisal of the patient's readiness as an adolescent to leave home. The second statement described the truth value of the parents' usual communications to the patient. The latter statement was necessarily based largely on the patient's appraisal of parental statements; in eight cases the patient's parents were also known to us either as a consequence of family therapy or of a number of parent interviews. Three of the parents had themselves been in therapy with one of us for several hundred hours. Accordingly we felt more than average confidence in the validity of the material about which our statements were made. It remains moot as to whether other therapists with the same experiences would have reached the same conclusions.

Results

OUTCOME CONDITIONS

We found that for each patient one of four conditions prevailed as the end of adolescence approached: (a) remaining emotionally bound to parents whether or not actually living at home; permitted to live at home or to live away and return; (b) having been forced out of the home prematurely without adequate emotional preparation; (c) having been forced out of the home prematurely but with their feelings largely worked through, effectively leaving their parents behind; (d) having had their leaving facilitated but with a continuing need for integration and extrapolation.

Some clarification of these conditions may be required.

1. Patients "emotionally bound" were consciously aware of preoccupation or overconcern with their parents and ultimately came to recognize the preeminent role of parental introjects in their daily behavior. Those living away from home frequently moved back to their parental home or kept in close contact with parents. When an adolescent is away at school, a judgment must be made with respect to the extent to which he or she is "truly away."

2. "Forced out prematurely" means that home conditions were so intolerable that either the patient or parents decided that the adolescent would have to move out at an early age. The patient's decision to move did not indicate that he was emotionally ready to make the move, and subsequent events demonstrated his continuing need for parenting.

3. Some patients were forced to move out of the home at an early age, before their formal education was completed. These people had to find ways to support themselves, both financially and emotionally, and were for the most part able to do so.

4. For some patients family circumstances were such that they developed an early sense of competence which they were eager to demonstrate. Rather than feeling forced out, these patients felt that their family was not permitting them sufficient opportunity for growth. Their need for psychiatric help was precipitated by problems associated with being overly ambitious. They in effect took on more than they could handle and had the good sense to look for help.

We judged nine of our twenty-one patients to have been in category 1 (emotionally bound). Of these, five had had at least one psychotic episode; two had had several. The other four had been neurotic or character disordered. Category 2 (forced out prematurely) included six patients. Four of these were neurotic or character disordered; the remaining two were borderlines who had never had psychotic episodes. In category 3 were four patients, one of whom had been psychotic, three neurotic or character disordered. In category 4 were one neurotic and one character-disordered patient.

No attempt will be made to make specific diagnostic statements. Those patients with psychotic episodes in their history tended to appear emotionally bound. The two most obvious borderline patients were forced out prematurely, totally unprepared. Neurotics and character disorders appeared in all categories.

PARENTAL STATEMENTS

What were these patients, with their various adolescent outcomes, told by their parents? For each of the four categories or conditions, the parental communications are as follows:

1. *Emotionally bound (nine cases):*
    a] Parents tell the truth but their plans are vague and the context of their statements unclear.
    b] Parents behave in contradictory ways from one situation to

another. They justify themselves by claiming distinctions among the situations, but these distinctions make no sense.

c] Father dead; mother talked nonsense.

d] Father absent; mother and grandmother talked nonsense.

e] Father a convicted criminal; mother told truth about him but not about herself.

f] The family lived a lie. The man believed by the patient to be her father was actually her grandfather; her mother and grandmother were in competition with one another.

g] Father dead; mother's behavior and statements did not correspond to each other.

h] Mother talked platitudes.

i] Mother talked religious nonsense.

2. *Forced out unprepared (six cases):*

a] Parental statements were literally true but misrepresented the situation.

b] Father does things his own way; independent; eccentric. Mother ran the home. Both accepted no truths other than their own.

c] Mother talked nonsense.

d] Father dominated. Made statements literally true but which were false when put in proper context.

e] Father "independent," with vague plans. Mother insecure, followed simple verbal, religious principles not thought through.

f] Both parents claimed to be always correct; merely tolerated patient who was "always wrong."

3. *Forced out prematurely, but somewhat prepared (four cases):*

a] Parents mostly make sense and tell the truth.

b] Father lies, beats mother, sarcastic to patient. Mother helpless.

c] and [*d*] (brother and sister to 2*e*). Father "independent," with vague plans. Mother insecure, followed simple verbal, religious principles not thought through.

4. *Departure facilitated (two cases):*

a] Mother talked affected nonsense.

b] Parents made sense, generally told truth, but were preoccupied and did not communicate much to patient.

TRUTH VALUE OF PARENTAL STATEMENTS

Only two of the patients had parents who actually lied. In one of these cases (1*f*) the family lied to cover up the fact that the patient had been, as she said, "born out of wedlock." Part of their motivation had been to protect her emotionally, letting her feel that she had a father. In the second case (3b), the father lied for his own convenience.

In seven cases (1c, 1d, 1g, 1h, 1i, 2c, 4a) the parent or parents talked nonsense, making statements without truth value.

In ten cases (1a, 2a, 2b, 2d, 2e, 2f, 3a, 3c, 3d, 4b) the parents more or less told the truth. In the remaining two cases (1b, 1e) it is difficult to tell how commonly statements turned out to be true; in both cases truth was used in a defensive, self-serving way, the parents never telling the truth about themselves. They could be said to have been lying by omission.

We could state at this point that, of the twenty-one cases, ten had parents who more or less told the truth while eleven had parents who did not, but that would misrepresent the situation. Of the ten truthful sets of parents, eight failed to put their statements in a useful context, one (4b) tended to be preoccupied with their own affairs and were insufficiently communicative. That leaves one set of parents (3a) who talked sense, told the truth, and put it in a useful relevant context. Their son, however, was on drugs, and it is questionable how much of their message he heard and absorbed as an adolescent.

Thus we are left with little useful parent-child communication as a preparation for life. It would be most interesting to study in depth parent-child communication in nonpsychiatric patients who meet the criteria for a control group.

RELATING PARENTAL STATEMENTS TO ADOLESCENT OUTCOME CATEGORIES

We can speak only of general trends. If we think of category 1 as the least favorable state as the patients moved on to adulthood, and category 4 as the most favorable state, we must conclude that our patients tended to be in less rather than more favorable states (1:9, 2:6, 3:4, 4:2). Generally those patients in less favorable states heard statements with less truth value than those in more favorable states, but only two of our patients had parents with the ability to make meaningful and useful statements about living.

OUTCOME OF TREATMENT

Two young adult patients were withdrawn from treatment by their parents. One of these was psychotic, the other borderline; one was in category 1, the other in category 2. Of the nineteen patients who continued treatment until a mutually agreed termination was reached, there were two adults (category 1) who did not achieve what we would consider a satisfactory result. They began treatment emotionally bound, though both were self-supporting, married and had children, and we considered them to be still emotionally bound to their parents on termination, though less so. The remaining seventeen have made satisfactory gains.

Discussion

To whatever extent our data reflect the actual state of affairs in our patients' families, it appears that adequate preparation for life in this series of disturbed adolescents was generally not provided. Nevertheless the patients in nearly all cases were able to use the experience of long-term intensive therapy to achieve gains in areas of self-understanding, mastery, and interpersonal relationships. These gains were not made easily, but it is noteworthy that they could be made at all.

As has been pointed out by others (Kirsh 1971; Wile 1942) lying is not the worst thing that the child and adolescent have to deal with. For the most part our patients had not been abused or neglected and most of them had been treated affectionately by their parents. Nevertheless they grew up without a very good understanding of family process or of interpersonal relationships outside the family.

The adolescent faces the developmental task of testing parental truths and introjects in his enlarging interpersonal community. His newly acquired conceptual abilities must be used to recognize extra-familial contexts and hence other truths. When parental use of truth is limited to object naming and giving orders, commonly without providing adequate example or verbal description of how the orders are to be carried out, the adolescent can learn little at home about the perception of meaning, emotion, context, or interpersonal systems. Concluding that only his parents can understand how life works, the adolescent remains dependent on them.

When parents deny reality, as by rationalizing contradictions, the adolescent may learn to reject parental truths, sometimes becoming prey to cults offering what may appear to be a superficially, at least, more consistent system of ideas. While family myths or white lies may serve to protect useful metaphors and provide feelings of hope and security, an excess of myth and metaphor can produce illusions within which the adolescent may hide.

Pathological lying by parents may result in the creation of secrets. When these secrets are shared, there may be created a libidinal bond between parent and child as a result of the paranoid excitement attending the exclusion of others. Often the utility of this bond is to gain support for weak parental egos. Lying from a position of strength has less dire consequences.

Many parental cognitive errors are not intended as lies, but result from innocence or ignorance, or from inability to discriminate among levels of analysis or systems of ideas, standards, or values. The adolescent, acquiring limited sophistication from outside the family, perceives these errors as lies; he is not reassured to learn that they are errors. While the resulting anger may be utilized for a creative outcome, the adolescent commonly continues to blame his parents, becomes hypocritical of himself, and remains locked in narcissism. Perceived lies may become an object for depression or obsessive rumination, truth having been equated with love and lies with manipulation.

Effective ego function requires an orderly interplay of cognitive maps and emotional energy. Gray and Gray (1977) have picturesquely likened it to the double helix of DNA. In the absence of an adequate set of maps and rules of the road, the adolescent facing the world is unlikely to make a wise distribution of cathexes. Fortunately, in the absence of useful parental guidance, he may sometimes be able to turn to peers or to important adults for guidance. Eventually, whether as adolescent, young adult, or adult, he may turn to a psychiatrist.

As noted, it is remarkable that people as ill-prepared for life as were our patients were able to benefit so much from psychotherapy. Having been raised by parents who made so little sense, what accounts for the existence of psychic structures that made the patients able to grasp the order of hierarchical organization and the dynamism of human interactions? Clearly these cannot be taught in therapy, and it may not be amiss to consider an ethological analogy in which psychotherapy serves as a releaser for an innate psychic mechanism.

Conclusions

We are exploring the relationship between the truth value of parental communications and the adolescent's readiness to separate from the home. Data on twenty-one patients and their parents are categorized and analyzed. Parental binding and premature separation prevail. There is little overt parental lying, but equally little life-task relevant truth telling. Yet nearly all of these patients are able to utilize intensive and extensive psychotherapy, indicating the presence of psychic structures capable of providing higher ego functioning despite inadequate parental communications.

NOTE

Based on a paper presented at the International Forum on Adolescence, Jerusalem, Israel, July 4–7, 1976.

REFERENCES

Chomsky, N. 1972. *Language and Mind*. New York: Harcourt.

Ekstein, R. 1965. Historical notes concerning psychoanalysis and early language development. *Journal of the American Psychoanalytic Association* 13:707–731.

Gray, W., and Gray, L. 1977. System precursors, emergents, reformulation, and blocking in therapy. In J. D. White, ed. *The General Systems Paradigm: Science of Change and Change of Science*. Louisville, Ky.: Society for General Systems Research.

Kirsh, C. O. 1971. The benefits of poor communication. *Psychoanalytic Review* 58:189–208.

Wile, I. S. 1942. Lying as a biological and social phenomenon. *Nervous Child* 1:293–313.

235

16

II. PARENTAL COMMUNICATION,
READINESS OF ADOLESCENTS TO LEAVE
HOME, AND THE COURSE OF TREATMENT

HAROLD A. RASHKIS AND SHIRLEY R. RASHKIS

We have been exploring for a number of years the relationship between what parents tell their children and the readiness of adolescents to perform that most important developmental task, leaving home. It is axiomatic in our culture that the offspring of any family is to grow up in his family of origin, leave it, and found a family of procreation. This is the most important act that most people accomplish in their lifetime, and it would follow that the most important parental task is to prepare children to carry it out. Accordingly we have studied what parents told children who later became our patients. Of course we do not know what parents of nonpatients tell their children, and we would be most interested in making the comparison when data are available.

Our population ranged from neurotics to severe psychotics with several hospitalizations. When we began treatment with them they were equally divided among adolescents, young adults, and adults. There were slightly more males than females (see Rashkis and Rashkis 1981).

We found that, during adolescence, nine of these patients had been emotionally bound to their home, though some of them lived away from home for varying periods of time; some as adults had established their own families while still bound to their parents. Six of the patients had been forced to leave home prematurely, unprepared. Four had to leave similarly, though better prepared. In two cases the family structure had actually facilitated departure of adolescent children from the home because of early acceptance of and demonstrated competence with responsibility.

We discovered that in only two cases had parents deliberately lied to their children, but only in two cases had they told them useful truths. In the remaining seventeen cases, parents had either talked nonsense or had uttered naive or literal truths that were found to be untruths when viewed in the larger context of their children's adaptation to extrafamilial reality, that which one of our patients unoriginally refers to as "the cold, cruel world."

We were reasonably pleased to note that while two patients had been withdrawn from treatment by their parents, seventeen of the remaining nineteen had persevered to a very favorable therapeutic outcome, although about half of them required more than five years to reach a mutually satisfactory termination.

Recognizing the contribution of extrafamilial supports, such as peers, school, and avocational and religious counselors, we have nevertheless wondered about the origin and nature of the psychic structures on which we were able to build in therapy. We wished further to explore the manner in which we identified these structures and the methods by which we were able to build on them.

The way we will conduct this exploration is by considering first the cases in the original study, from which we will extract certain principles. Following this we will test those principles with patients not included in the original study in order to determine the extent of their applicability.

Deriving Principles from Previous Study

EMOTIONALLY BOUND

In this group was the largest number of cases (nine) which included generally the most disturbed patients. Six had at one time been considered schizophrenic, but their recovery throws that diagnosis into doubt. The other three had severe personality disorders. Treatment was long and arduous.

A peculiarity of the group is that the six female patients had lost their fathers at an early age. The three males had living fathers who were described as very difficult, irrational men. The women immediately formed strong positive transferences to the male therapist, the men negative.

There were two simultaneous aspects to therapy. One of these was to respond to transference statements in an objective, straightforward way. The other aspect was continuously and unrelentingly to confront the patients with and to interpret their real world behavior, and to explain to them how they might have handled each situation better. In general, these patients had not had very good advice about living while at home, and prior to therapy had insufficient external support.

FORCED TO LEAVE HOME PREMATURELY, UNPREPARED

This group consisted of six patients: two borderlines and four moderately severe neurotics. The group was characterized by a number of breaks in therapy and by avoidance of transference. The therapeutic focus was on the patients' internal pain and their reality problems. Like the emotionally bound group, these individuals required much patience and tolerance from the therapist. On the other hand they needed less reality orientation and direction.

FORCED TO LEAVE HOME PREMATURELY, SOMEWHAT PREPARED

Three of the four patients in this group had symptoms associated with use of street drugs; all were adolescents, and all did well in therapy and in managing their own lives. Therapy required that they be reassured about their mental state and that drug effects be separated from emotional issues. All required guidance as they reentered the world following acute emotional crises. This group was in therapy the shortest time of all patients in the study.

DEPARTURE FROM HOME FACILITATED BY PARENTS

There were only two patients in this group; both were adults when they entered therapy. Both became self-reliant and ambitious in late adolescence. While reasonably successful, each had taken on more responsibilities than he could handle. Thus, while dealing effectively with the world, both in business and with wife and children, they had the feeling of having had insufficient parenting. In both cases the parents were very involved with each other and not with the children (Gunderson, Kerr, and Englund 1980). Therapy was largely reality oriented; the patients gained emotional support from having someone with whom to discuss how the world works, particularly in terms of interpersonal relationships. Truth or information received from the therapist seemed to be equated with love.

General Principles

Although we were originally interested in problems associated with parents who lie, we have generally abandoned truth value as an important parameter. Most of the parents in the study told the truth to their children; two parents lied, but that observation does not appear to be related either to the adolescent's readiness to leave home or to the outcome of therapy. The important parameter seems to be parental competence at making true statements in a relevant context. To be useful to the growing child, particularly when adolescence has been reached and conceptualizing ability attained, the parent must be able to designate the context of his remarks. If the child does not learn the correct frame of reference he can develop no sense of appropriateness either of thought or of action, since no statement can be correct in all contexts any more than any act can be considered proper in all situations. It is not simply truth, but appropriateness that must be learned. Failing this, it cannot be considered remarkable when any patient's behavior turns out to be inappropriate. And, indeed, appropriateness is the key concept in understanding emotional disorder.

Clinical data tend not to be as clear and sharp as one would like; nevertheless it is possible to construct hypotheses. We propose that the emotionally bound patients hear the fewest or smallest proportion of contextually related statements, and that at the other end of the continuum we find those whose departure was facilitated. In intermediate steps are those patients who left home prematurely, unprepared, and those who left home prematurely, somewhat prepared.

It is, then, not surprising that the emotionally bound patients developed immediate strong transferences, and that they needed the most instruction in how to deal with the world.

On the other hand, those who left home prematurely, unprepared, learned early to avoid emotional attachments, which may account for their frequently breaking therapy and then returning. We can also understand their awareness of inner pain and that it, along with reality problems, became the focus of therapy.

It is not difficult to understand why three of the four who left home prematurely, somewhat prepared, were involved with street drugs. We concluded that much of their preparedness came not from their parents but rather from their peer group, whence came also drugs. This group was still in need of good parenting to reestablish a positive relationship with authority.

The fourth group, those whose departure was facilitated, did hear some useful concepts at home, but suffered from emotional distancing. Determined to "make it on their own," they tended toward early excessive responsibility; to handle this they needed wise counsel, which they experienced as emotional warmth.

Summarizing these observations results in several general principles: (1) the emotionally bound patient develops the strongest transference, but, rather than providing emotional support directly, as through reassurance, the therapist is required to provide continuous interpretation of reality; (2) the patient leaving home unprepared avoids emotional bonding with the therapist, and requires much patience and tolerance, especially because of his tendency to break treatment; (3) the patients leaving home partially prepared require the most reassurance and "good parenting" by the therapist to win them back to acceptance of authority; and (4) those patients whose departure was facilitated and who are now in complex interpersonal and/or vocational situations require wise counsel, which they will experience as emotional warmth.

Thus we see that the first group requires principally cognitive development, the second patience, the third reassurance, and the fourth emotional support. To some extent, of course, all patients need all of these, but with different patients there is a difference in emphasis.

We have suggested that we sought psychic structures on which we might build. Our findings are at first puzzling since one might expect to build cognitive structures on top of other cognitive structures and emotional growth on an emotional base. It seems, rather, that our work was done from adjacent structures, as though from a scaffolding. With the emotionally bound group we worked through the distortions of transference, reaching to establish a solid block of fact. With the unprepared group we worked through time and distance, awaiting sufficient closeness to develop or redevelop beginning emotional ties.

With the partially prepared group we worked through the patients' fear and confusion, trying to establish trust and conversion to the adult world. With the departure-facilitated patients we were formal, professional counselors, working from the context of a contract, creating emotional warmth through our constancy, availability, and adherence to that contract. Thus we discovered no new psychic structures, but are describing, rather, four types of long-term therapeutic situations.

Application to Non-Study Patients

With the assumption that it is useful to predict the course of treatment, we sought to identify in patients not included in the earlier study where they had been in adolescence with respect to readiness to leave home. We then considered the course of treatment in these patients.

The authors selected from their practice a group of four patients for each of the four adolescent outcome categories (emotionally bound; forced out prematurely, unprepared; forced out prematurely, somewhat prepared; departure facilitated). It is on these sixteen additional patients that the following observations are based:

1. We were readily able to classify each of our patients into one of the four categories.

2. We confirmed that category 1 patients (emotionally bound) showed the strongest transference reactions to the therapist. These patients tended to see life through the eyes of their family and needed to be taught the more appropriate context of their lives, that is, the context in which they actually lived and worked. Their transference was not simply from parent to therapist; they also transferred their perceptions of home and family onto school, work, and interpersonal contexts.

3. Category 2 patients (forced out, unprepared) developed the strongest defenses against feelings and accordingly not only intermittently broke treatment but fought against the positive aspects of transference, using a variety of mechanisms, such as hysteria and manipulation, to avoid closeness. In time these patients, tired of their avoidances, sought ways of breaking through their own resistances to establish positive bonds with the therapist and with others.

4. Category 3 patients (forced out, somewhat prepared) demonstrated the most attractive personalities of the four groups. Requiring the support of others, they were pleasing and eager to learn from everyone, including, but not specifically, the therapist. Transferences were positive but dilute. In a negative sense, these patients tended to be opportunistic. For all of their seeming independence, they frequently required reassurance and clarification of the context in which they were operating.

5. Category 4 patients (departure facilitated) tended to be the most successful both vocationally and in establishing their family of procreation. Ambitious and goal directed, they were often narrow, rigid, and lacking in warmth. Because of their weak or limited transferences, these patients made good use of therapy when goals were specified. When therapy became more deep and dependency feelings approached, there sometimes occurred a phenomenon that might be termed "transference panic," manifested by anxiety and by phobic attitudes toward the therapist. If mismanaged by the therapist, the

241

anxiety and phobic behavior might well have escalated to paranoia. Accordingly, long-term supportive and reality directed therapy may in these patients be preferable to intensive uncovering.

6. We suspect certain similarities between category 4 and category 1 patients, though these are evidently the most and least successful individuals, respectively. The similarity derives from these patients, by definition, having spent more time with their family of origin than did category 2 and category 3 patients, and the nature of the continuing bond is often quite complex. While some aspects of the similarities are obvious or easily derivative from our observations, there is a definite suggestion of circularity deserving of further study.

Conclusions

Initially it was our intent to explore the relationship between the truth value and contextual relevance of parental statements and the adolescent's readiness to separate from his family of origin. In so doing we noted that our adolescent patients fell into four categories of readiness, considered without regard to diagnosis, degree of psychopathology, or underlying psychodynamics. In this chapter we have noted that these categories have distinguishing patterns of interaction with the therapist, with different kinds and degrees of transference; defenses and resistances; and needs for support, reassurance, information, and encouragement. These patient characteristics have elicited complementary therapeutic responses, and the course of treatment has accordingly been determined and followed usually to a successful termination. Thus it appears that the four categories have prognostic consequences, which may make them of interest as a system of classification.

Since it was not our intent to develop a nosography, having undertaken an empirical study, our findings are not coded to support or to deny any theoretical position. The following comments are accordingly of an ad hoc nature, and are subject to future empirical test.

Our four categories represent an evaluation of the patient's status at a certain point in his life; they consider his mastery of certain adolescent life tasks, and indicate his readiness to move ahead to undertake additional tasks associated with adulthood. This readiness reflects all of the known and unknown determinants of behavior and in itself cannot reasonably be attributed directly to constitutional endowment or family genetics; neither should it be considered clearly the result of family behavior or other environmental influences.

We do suspect that there are generational patterns with respect to these categories of readiness, but the unearthing of empirical relationships may not be expected to offer solutions to issues about heredity and environment. Certain questions inescapably arise. What is the relationship between the categorization of the adolescent and that of each of his parents? What are the consequences of the mating combinations made possible by the categories? Is there a relationship between categories and diagnosis or likelihood of hospitalization?

Whether or not we are able to pursue these questions farther, and regardless of their outcome, the suggested categories may be found useful in evaluating adolescents. The therapist treating young adults or older adults may also find it of interest to learn when, and under what circumstance, his patient left his family of origin.

REFERENCES

Gunderson, J. G.; Kerr, J.; Englund, D. W. 1980. The families of borderlines. *Archives of General Psychiatry* 37:27–33.

Rashkis, H., and Rashkis, S. 1981. I. An investigation of the influence of parental communications on adolescent ego development. *Adolescent Psychiatry,* this volume.

17

THE IMPACT OF PREGNANCY ON ADOLESCENT PSYCHOSOCIAL DEVELOPMENT

ADRIAN D. COPELAND

Adolescent psychiatry matured during the enormous problems of the 1960s. This was a period when the teenage population was considerably expanded by the post–World War II baby boom. This massive, agitated segment of society, with many of its needs unmet, explored new and sometimes destructive solutions, and suffered. Protest, rebellion, violence, homicide, suicide, running away, and drug abuse were among the major worries.

Fewer manifestations of countercultural protest characterized the late 1970s. An important problem of adolescence has appeared within the last decade, however, that has been somewhat insidious in its development. Having emerged with considerable destructive force, the problem of adolescent pregnancy is a complex issue that requires careful definition and perspective. It is part of the overall phenomenon of precocious adolescent sexuality, marriage, pregnancy, motherhood, and abortion that is currently so extant. The particular focus of this chapter is that of adolescent pregnancy per se and its impact upon psychosocial development and adaptation in adolescence.

Sexual activity in adolescence is not a new phenomenon. The United States has always had one of the highest teenage marriage rates (HEW 1976), especially notable in such rural groups as the southern black and the Amish. Nor has adolescent coitus always been linked inexorably to marriage. There had always been the proverbial high school senior not attending her graduation due to pregnancy.

But if adolescent sexuality is not new, there are clear indications that the incidence of premarital teenage coitus has increased greatly. This is true not only in the United States, but in a number of countries throughout the world, including England, the USSR, West Germany, and Japan (Chilman 1977; Settlage 1975). Adolescent pregnancy in the United States is now the fourth highest in the world (HEW 1976), increasing parodoxically at a time when the overall fertility rate has declined. It is estimated that half the population of fifteen- to nineteen-year-olds are sexually active and a fifth of the thirteen- and fourteen-year-olds as well (Dryfoos 1975). Currently there are just under 1 million American teenage pregnancies per year, resulting in approximately 600,000 births and 400,000 abortions (United Nations 1975).

At the same time, teenage marriage rates have been declining in the past decade, from eighty per 1,000 to sixty-seven per 1,000, while illegitimacy rates have continuously risen. In the fifteen- to nineteen-year group, there were forty illegitimate births per 1,000 in 1940, and this rate more than doubled to ninety per 1,000 in 1975 for blacks. For whites, the increase has been equally dramatic, though the rates were lower. In 1940, there were three illegitimate births per 1,000 and this rose to ten per 1,000 in 1975. Considering that the white population pool is many times greater, the absolute number of illegitimate pregnancies is considerable for both groups (Chilman 1977). This problem is especially acute in the United States, where the consequences are multiple and serious.

Biosocial Issues in Adolescent Pregnancy

From a biological point of view, pregnancy occurring at an age earlier than seventeen years is associated with an elevated mortality rate, toxemia of pregnancy, prolonged or precipitate labor (Stickle and Ma 1975), and anemia (HEW 1980). The babies of these young mothers are considered at risk. Stack (1974) indicates a higher incidence of prematurity characterized by a birth weight of under 2,500 grams. Associated with this low birth weight are a variety of congenital defects, mental retardation, cerebral palsy, and a 6 percent death rate in the first year (HEW 1980).

There are sociological ramifications as well. By virtue of an increased incidence of academic failure, repeat pregnancies, and a 50 percent divorce rate, many of these girls remain in the lowermost socioeconomic ranks of society, requiring enormous amounts of support both for themselves and their children for many years (Furstenberg 1976; Stack 1974). At this time, a comprehensive program of care for teenage mothers and their children is being developed that should expand these supports and services considerably (HEW 1980).

This paradoxical rise in early adolescent pregnancy in the face of a declining overall birth rate is difficult to explain. From a biological standpoint, Stack (1974) indicates that a rise in adolescent pregnancy is consistent with control of venereal disease inasmuch as it can be an important cause of abortion and sterility. It is not clear, however, how to evaluate this factor since it is uncertain how effectively this group has been diagnosed and treated. Rauh (1973) and others point out that earlier maturation, as evidenced by the earlier onset of menarche, may be significant. It has been documented that menarche occurs 1.5 years earlier than it occurred in 1900 in the industrialized nations of the world, with the average onset now at 12.5 years. A careful study would need to be made relating the incidence of pregnancy as a function of age of the adolescent, the adolescent population growth rate, and the decline in the average age of menarche.

To account psychologically for the increasing incidence of precocious adolescent sexuality, a number of authors relate this phenomenon with mental illness (Chilman 1977; Zelnik and Kantner 1974), which includes neurosis (Gottschalk 1974) and impulsive personality disorder (Poznanski and Blos 1975). A number of psychodynamic explanations are offered, including rebellion against parental authority, a covert manifestation of an incestuous wish, and the need for affirmation of a sense of feminine identity (Spiegel 1964).

In an attempt to embrace all of these possibilities, Copeland (1974) classifies adolescent pregnancy as (*a*) phasic, reflecting the result of the heightened sexual interest of adolescence and the contemporary societal values; (*b*) subcultural, reflecting sexual activity and resultant pregnancy that is compatible with the mores of a particular subculture (the more open sexuality of black ghetto youth is illustrative); and (*c*) psychopathological, reflecting sexual activity (and subsequent pregnancy) that is primarily the result of psychopathology.

Inasmuch as adolescent sexuality and subsequent pregnancy have been occurring with increasing precocity and frequency, it would be well to consider what impact, if any, there has been upon the psychosocial development of these girls. One approach to this question is to compare the status and accomplishments of these adolescents with prescribed developmental tasks as set forth by Katchadourian (1980) and others. Any set of developmental tasks is, to a certain degree, culturally and temporally relative (Joint Commission on Mental Health of Children 1973), and this relativity is of special significance when considering any particular group of girls in the pluralistic United States.

One psychosocial process that is ubiquitous and noted by most writers is "disengagement from infantile dependencies" (Blos 1977)—the development of a sense of personal identity with a clear sense of who I am and what I am (Freedman 1976), along with the development of a sense of personal values and goals (Erikson 1956; Rauh 1973). Gregory and Smeltzer (1977) point out the emerging primacy of the transitional group and the achievement of peer loyalties over family loyalties as another task at this phase.

The development of psychosexual roles during adolescence, as summarized by Freedman (1976), occurs when the individual begins to acquire a sense of direction for his/her libido. Blos (1977) adds that the development of this sexual identity ultimately functions in the service of stabilizing dyadic relationships. Hamburg and Adams (1967) point out the importance of finding direction for a life's work at this time as well as the acquisition of appropriate coping skills.

These, then, are the major tasks for the adolescent to accomplish at this phase of life. Of course, it is recognized that process and progress are the watchwords rather than mastery.

Transition from Infantile
Dependency to Self-Reliance

There is no evidence that precocious coitus and subsequent pregnancy reflect diminished infantile dependency, a loosened allegiance to the primary family unit, and an emotional shift to the peer group. Zelnik and Kantner (1974) point out that while adolescents are having sex at an earlier age, and Furstenberg (1976) indicates that many of them are pregnant before they are twenty, this behavior does not appear to be an indication of a declaration of emancipation. The vast majority of girls in these and other studies did not wish to become pregnant and many of them, as well as their mothers, were upset over the prospect. Those adolescents actively practicing contraception were doing so upon the explicit directions of their mothers (Zelnik and Kantner 1974). On the other hand, many of the girls becoming pregnant were encouraged by their mothers to keep their babies and remain at home. Many of these same parents were teenage mothers themselves (Copeland and Copeland 1980).

247

While peer-group involvement was notable, it was relatively superficial. There was little indication of primary allegiance to peers in general or to the fathers of their babies in particular (Chilman 1977; Copeland 1980). It would appear then that early coitus and pregnancy did not reflect a shift away from childhood dependency and towards emancipation and psychological growth. More probably, it was consistent with a maternal overidentification, producing a reinforced dependency.

Identity Development

If there is evidence of prolonged maternal dependency in this particular group, by virtue of pregnancy during adolescence, then what are the implications in terms of development of a sense of identity? This is a complex question because the concept of identity lacks sharp operational definition.

If one considers identity as a sense of self, answering the questions "who am I? what am I?" (Freedman 1976), then there is evidence to believe that repeat pregnancies are related to emotional deprivation, arrested personality development, and an incomplete identity sense (Copeland 1974). Little direct data, however, are available from which to make generalizations about identity development in the single-pregnancy adolescent. Of the thirty-eight girls studied by this writer, their feelings about themselves as people, about being female, and about their bodies, were consistently and strongly positive. Their projective tests were equally normative vis-à-vis identity sense. Thus, there is no real evidence that single pregnancy indicates failure of identity development. On the other hand, pregnancy may reflect restricted personality formation and "an early foreclosure of personal identity development" (Douvan and Adelson 1966) by virtue of overidentification with mothers and sisters who were, themselves, teenage mothers and who serve as limited role models (Bandura and Walters 1963).

Sexuality in the Service of
Developing Stable Relationships

Beginning with behavioral extremes, there is evidence that female promiscuity correlates positively with psychopathology and negatively with stable relationships with boys. On the other hand, there is also much evidence indicating that most adolescent coitus is monogamous (Copeland 1974).

From a quantitative standpoint, Chilman (1977) notes that one-fourth of white males and females are sexually active by age fifteen and 90 percent of black males and 50 percent of black females are equally active. Frequency of coitus varies from two to three times per week (Furstenberg 1976) to two to three times per month, with orgasm highly variable. Kinsey (1953) and Masters and Johnson (1966) indicated that the male was more orgastically motivated than the female during adolescence and it would appear that the female's participation in premarital coitus may not be solely the function of libido.

Regarding coitus, pregnancy, and relationship development, Furstenberg reports that one-quarter of the pregnant adolescents in his study were married at the time of the birth of the baby and one-third were married at the time of the five-year follow-up. He also indicates that 60 percent of these marriages ultimately were dissolved, indicating relational instability. Similar figures have been quoted for other groups of teenagers. In our two-generation study of teenage pregnancy, two-thirds of the girls' mothers were themselves pregnant teenagers and later married, but an insignificant number remained married. Of the girls under study, thirty-one of the thirty-eight were pregnant, and while they wished to maintain some contact with their consorts, only six intended to marry and few listed these boyfriends as their closest relationships. One may conclude that teenage coitus and pregnancy in this group did not seem to foster the development of stable heterosexual relationships.

Life Direction and Role Development

Adolescent pregnancy often influences life direction and life work. It must be remembered that most pregnancies at this phase are unplanned and, at least initially, unwelcomed. In addition, 40 percent of these pregnancies terminate in elective abortion (HEW 1976). It is the girls that are most successful academically and articulate realistic future plans who tend to seek abortion. On the other hand, the girls choosing to carry their pregnancies to term and keep their babies show much less evidence of going out into the adult world of self-reliance and competition (Furstenberg 1976; Stack 1974; Zelnik and Kantner 1974). No doubt, factors other than scholastic success are operant vis-à-vis the decision for or against motherhood.

However, once the decision is made for motherhood at this age, biology often becomes destiny and the life's work often becomes primarily that of mothering. Furstenberg (1976) notes further that the first pregnancy was frequently the harbinger of additional pregnancies, and in rapid succession. Once this occurs, all other options for a life's work rapidly diminish.

Thus, by default, adolescent pregnancy very frequently leads to only one major occupation, that of mothering. Often it is a single-parent motherhood; in some cases, it parallels the experience of the girls' own mother and is a role assumed by unconscious identificational processes. Finally, it is a role representing sociological default.

Conclusions

Adolescent coitus is more widespread, early adolescent pregnancy is rising paradoxically, and increasing retention of the newborn by the pregnant girl is irrefutable. From a developmental standpoint, and irrespective of psychopathological factors, it would appear that early coitus and subsequent pregnancy does not advance the female adolescent away from the primary family unit and towards the peer group, heterosexual pairing, and ultimate adult self-reliance. If anything, it would appear that precocious sexuality reinforces maternal dependency and, frequently, betrays a latent overidentification with a mother who was herself a teenage mother. Many times, pregnancy may, indeed, be wanted by the adolescent (Ryan and Sweeney 1980), albeit on an unconscious level.

It is difficult to generalize about the impact of precocious sexuality upon identity development because this is more an abstract concept than an operational term. Except for clearly disturbed girls, there is no evidence that coitus is related to failures of gender, sexual, or personal identity development (Money and Tucker 1975). But if the average teenager becomes precociously active sexually for reasons other than identity problems, there is reason to believe that motherhood occurring in early adolescence oftentimes inhibits the growth of individual identity and personality; there is evidence of a premature foreclosure of a process that is now believed to be lifelong. Thus, teenage maternity tends to limit personality development and one's sense of identity.

There is very little evidence that early coitus and motherhood fostered meaningful, long-term relationships with their partners, even though female sexual behavior was monogamous rather than promiscuous. Few expressed a desire for marriage, and statistics indicate a high degree of marital failure among those adolescents who did marry.

At a time in which so many educational and vocational opportunities are opening for women, there are strong indications that teenage mothers receive less education and occupy marginal jobs. And, inasmuch as teenage maternity often leads to second and third pregnancies, the development of a life's work other than mothering is remote. Two factors have been noted vis-à-vis the decision on the part of the adolescent to carry the pregnancy to term and to keep the baby. One is that of an unconscious identification with a single parent who, herself, was a teenage parent. Another factor was that of default, in which a number of the girls opting to continue their pregnancies were not succeeding in school and did not have any particular educational or career aspirations. The conclusion then is that pregnancy and subsequent maternity seems to interfere with the completion of the developmental tasks of adolescence.

REFERENCES

Bandura, A., and Walters, R. 1963. *Social Learning and Personality Development*. New York: Holt.

Blos, P. 1977. When and how does adolescence end? *Adolescent Psychiatry* 5:5–17.

Chilman, C. 1977. *Adolescent Sexuality in a Changing American Society*. Washington, D.C.: Department of Health, Education, and Welfare.

Copeland, A. 1974. *Textbook of Adolescent Psychopathology and Treatment*. Springfield, Ill.: Thomas.

Copeland, A., and Copeland, E. 1980. An in-depth psychosocial study of pregnant adolescents. Paper presented before the American Society for Adolescent Psychiatry Eastern Regional Meeting, Charleston, S.C., October 24.

Douvan, E., and Adelson, J. 1966. *The Adolescent Experience*. New York: Wiley.

Dryfoos, J. 1975. Women who need and receive family planning services: estimates at mid-decade. *Family Planning Perspectives* 7:172–187.

Erikson, E. 1956. The problems of ego identity. *Journal of the American Psychoanalytic Association* 4:56–71.

Freedman, A. 1976. *Modern Synopsis of Comprehensive Textbook of Psychiatry II*. Baltimore: Williams & Williams.

Furstenberg, F. 1976. The social consequences of teenage parenthood. *Family Planning Perspectives* 8:148–164.

Gottschalk, L. 1964. Psychosocial factors associated with pregnancy in adolescent girls: a preliminary report. *Journal of Mental and Nervous Disorders* 138:524–534.

Gregory, I., and Smeltzer, D. 1977. *Psychiatry*. Boston: Little, Brown.

Hamburg, D., and Adams, J. 1967. A perspective on coping. *Archives of General Psychiatry* 17:277–282.

Health, Education, and Welfare. 1976. *Vital Statistics of the U.S., 1974, Natality*. Washington: HEW National Center for Health Statistics.

Health, Education, and Welfare. 1980. *Draft Program Guidance Materials for Project Grants for Adolescent Pregnancy Programs*. Title VI, Sec. 603 of P. 95–626. Washington: HEW Office of Adolescent Pregnancy Programs.

Joint Commission on Mental Health of Children. 1973. *Mental Health for Infancy through Adolescence*. New York: Harper.

Katchadourian, H. 1980. Adolescent sexuality. *Pediatric Clinics of North America* 27:17–28.

Kinsey, A. 1953. *Sexual Behavior in the Human Female*. Philadelphia: Saunders.

Masters, W., and Johnson, V. 1966. *Human Sexual Response*. Boston: Little, Brown.

Money, J., and Tucker, P. 1975. *Sexual Signatures*. Boston: Little, Brown.

Poznanski, E., and Blos, P. 1975. Incest. *Medical Aspects of Human Sexuality* 9:46–76.

Rauh, J. 1973. The reproductive adolescent. *Pediatric Clinics of North America* 20:1005–1020.

Ryan, G., and Sweeney, P. 1980. Attitudes of adolescents toward pregnancy and contraception. *American Journal of Obstetrics and Gynecology* 137:318–356.

Settlage, D. 1975. Contraceptive practices of teenagers. *Medical Aspects of Human Sexuality* 7:171–172.

Spiegel, L. 1964. Identity and adolescence. In S. Lorand and H. Schner, eds. *Adolescents: A Psychoanalytic Approach to Problems and Therapy*. New York: Harper.

Stack, G. 1974. *All Our Kin: Strategies for Survival in a Black Community*. New York: Harper.

Stickle, G., and Ma, P. 1975. Pregnancy in adolescents: scope of the problem. *Contemporary Obstetrics and Gynecology* 3:12–15.

United Nations. 1975. Department of Economic and Social Affairs. *Demographic Yearbook, 1974.* New York: United Nations.

Zelnik, M., and Kantner, J. 1974. The resolution of teenage first pregnancies. *Family Planning Perspectives* 6:74–82.

PART III

PSYCHOPATHOLOGICAL ASPECTS OF ADOLESCENT DEVELOPMENT

EDITORS' INTRODUCTION

During the past several decades marked advances have occurred in the understanding of the diagnostic criteria, dynamics, and treatment of the borderline patient. There is a growing consensus that the borderline personality presents a structural disorder due to a developmental arrest with specific observable symptoms, ego defects, and impairment of capacities for object relations. Increased understanding of borderline psychopathology has enabled treatment to be more specific and effective.

Donald B. Rinsley reviews the development and endopsychic structure of borderline psychopathology, drawing particularly on his own conceptualizations and those of James Masterson. He documents the approaches of the pioneers of adolescent treatment and the gradual understanding that hospitalized young people manifested severe adolescent pathology and required a therapeutic milieu that fostered both reparenting and psychoanalytic psychotherapy. Rinsley establishes that the treatment process proceeds through several stages: resistance phase; definitive or introjective phase; and final resolution phase. Further, he discusses the borderline pathology: preoedipal transference; failure of separation-individuation; and the triad of aggression, depression, and identify diffusion. He believes that psychodynamic, developmental, and biological-genetic data are required for comprehensive diagnosis.

Minimal brain dysfunction has been the source of much confusion for both the clinician and the patient and his family. It is not surprising that a variety of approaches to diagnosis and treatment exist. Terms such as specific learning disability, hyperkinetic syndrome, minimal cerebral dysfunction, mild brain damage, and attention deficit disorders with and without hyperactivity all bear witness to this confusion.

In adolescence and young adulthood the diagnosis is often missed.

Many clinicians believe that most teenagers and young adults have "grown out" of minimal brain syndrome and thus the clinical index of suspicion is lessened. Only recently has there been an appreciation that minimal brain dysfunction may persist not only into late adolescence but also into adulthood, frequently contributing to an exacerbating serious personality disorder. In fact, some authors consider the sequelae of minimal brain dysfunction to be an alternative pathway to borderline psychopathology. There are too few long-term follow-up studies on adult patients with a history of hyperactivity in childhood. The chapters in this part should help broaden the adolescent psychiatrist's understanding of these important areas.

Harvey A. Horowitz considers that minimal brain dysfunction persists into adolescence and young adulthood and contributes to the development of specific disorders of behavior and personality. He presents a study of hospitalized adolescents and discusses those manifesting diffuse development disorder, affect-motor dyscontrol disorder, and discrete cognitive-social disorder as subgroupings of minimal brain dysfunction. Each group manifested unique characteristics, as did the family system in reaction. Horowitz concludes from his study that minimal brain dysfunction is a frequently missed diagnosis in adolescence and should be given extensive attention in the treatment of adolescents.

Lily Hechtman, Gabrielle Weis, Terrye Perlman, and Daphne Tuck consider a group of young adults with a history of hyperactivity in childhood. They cite four sources of study: follow-up studies, the families of hyperactive children, current clinical pictures in adults resembling childhood hyperactivity, and current prospective follow-up studies that are considering young adults, including their own. The authors conclude that about 10 percent of those with a history of hyperactivity present serious psychiatric and antisocial problems.

Loren H. Crabtree, Jr., delineates three types of minimal brain dysfunction (MBD) syndrome: hyperactive-dyscontrol disorder, hypoactive diffuse developmental disorder, and specific cognitive disorders that are found in adolescents and young adults. He determined that in such a hospitalized population over 50 percent had findings of clinical psychosis. He examines the impact of MBD on individual therapy, chemotherapy, the family, milieu therapy, and aftercare needs.

18   BORDERLINE PSYCHOPATHOLOGY: THE CONCEPTS OF MASTERSON AND RINSLEY AND BEYOND

DONALD B. RINSLEY

In 1975 James Masterson and I published a paper devoted to the development and endopsychic structure of individuals suffering from borderline psychopathology. Drawing heavily on our respective experiences in the treatment of severely disturbed adolescents, this study could be said to have represented the end result of a process of convergent evolution of the work of two clinician investigators who had reached remarkably similar conclusions while having proceeded independently and in different clinical settings. From both personal and scientific points of view, Masterson and I felt encouraged by independent validation and confirmation of each other's work. It may therefore be desirable to place that work in historical perspective and to consider its relationship to the ever-expanding literature devoted to borderline psychopathology and its relation to the psychoses and to other personality-characterologic pathology (related spectrum disorders) among preadults and adults (Rinsley 1981; Stone 1980).

I shall begin by looking back to the 1950s, that quiet decade when psychoanalysis reached the apex of its influence on American psychiatry. As is well known, psychoanalytic clinicians had come to view the adolescent years as a period of storm and stress, of proneness to what Erikson (1963) was to call "identity diffusion" such that the adolescent, buffeted by protean emotional fluctuations and ever susceptible to symptomatic and genetic-dynamic regression, was deemed a poor candidate for psychoanalytic treatment. Thus was the adolescent's purportedly weak ego cited as the basis for his unanalyzability, while his unanalyzability was cited as evidence of his ego weakness (Rinsley

1965). This rather pejorative view, sometimes termed the turmoil view, has long since been discredited in the wake of numerous later studies, the significance of which pointed to the conclusion that the normal, modal, or psychologically healthly adolescent is not turmoil-ridden and, conversely, that the turmoil-ridden adolescent is neither normal, modal, nor psychologically healthy (Rinsley 1972).

Among many studies was the important Symptomatic Adolescent Research Project conducted by Masterson and his colleagues (Masterson 1967a, 1967b, 1968; Masterson, Tucker, and Berk 1963, 1966; Masterson and Washburne 1966). It had become evident to Masterson that the symptomatic adolescents he saw and studied were not merely passing through some sort of time-limited, phasic "adjustment reaction"; rather, they were suffering from serious psychopathology, and "they didn't grow out of it."

I had already reached essentially the same conclusion regarding the psychopathology of adolescents disturbed enough to require admission to my own inpatient service (Rinsley 1963, 1965, 1967a, 1967b). Furthermore, Masterson's use and application of the inpatient or residential milieu bore a close similarity to the approach to inpatient treatment of the seriously disturbed adolescent that Hendrickson and his colleagues had been utilizing at Ann Arbor (Hendrickson 1957; Hendrickson and Holmes 1959; Hendrickson, Holmes, and Waggoner 1959) and to the one I had been applying in Topeka. All three, among others, emphasized the importance of the control of symptomatic behavior by means of firm limit-setting following the adolescent's admission into residence. By the same token, all three emphasized the totality of the milieu as the prime instrumentality of treatment, utilizing the gamut of individual, group, family, occupational, recreational, and educational modalities in accordance with the individualized treatment plan. The general assumption underlying such an approach was that the seriously disturbed adolescent emerged from a pathogenic, dysfunctional family nexus, so that the intensive, interpretive, and comprehensive treatment of the identified patient necessarily involved efforts directed toward the restructuring of the wider familial context in the direction of healthy communications, interactions, and relationships. Essential to this work was the initial removal of the patient from the dysfunctional family environment by means of inpatient or residential admission and providing him with both "ego support" and "ego interpretation" (Noshpitz 1962), thereby permitting the analysis of the patient's individual psychopathology and of the family's dysfunctionality to begin as soon as possible following admission. The attempt to provide a comprehensive diagnostic and therapeutic milieu was, of course, not novel. The specific features of Masterson's and my approaches bore a percipient relationship to the pioneering work of such clinicians as Noshpitz (1962), Bettelheim (Bettelheim and Sylvester 1952) and Redl (Redl 1959; Redl and Wineman 1951, 1952). Common to all of them is the concept of the "good enough" or "holding" environment (Modell 1968; Winnicott 1950–1955) as applicable within the inpatient or residential setting. For these seriously ill adolescents, therefore, appropriate reparenting was considered to be a fundamental accompaniment to analytic treatment, neither of which could be optimized without the other (Rinsley 1974a, 1980c).

The Residential Process

However dysfunctional the adolescent's family nexus has been, his removal from it and admission into full-time residence is invariably a traumatic affair. A major component of the patient's and the family's response to the separation is to mount a variety of resistances to the new milieu. These resistances comprise, in many cases, a protracted attempt to deny the fact and impact of the separation; thereby attempting to deny and undo the trauma associated with it. Both the patient's and the parents' patterns of resistance were noted to assume a variety of particular forms or manifestations (Rinsley 1968, 1974a, 1980c; Rinsley and Hall 1962; Rinsley and Inge 1961).

Our studies of resistance to treatment, including to the personnel and the physical features of the clinical service, and especially the collusive parent-child interactions that were noted to prolong it, led to an understanding of resistance behaviors as manifestations of preoedipal transference. We were, of course, applying the psychoanalytic concepts of transference and resistance to and within the wider residential context, taking departure from such prior workers as Stanton and Schwartz (1954) and, in modified fashion, William Menninger (1936a, 1936b, 1937, 1939). The clinical problem was to minimize or eliminate the transference-derived resistances in order to motivate the patient and the family to engage with the staff and the milieu, to get them into treatment as expeditiously and effectively as possible. Only when this had in significant measure occurred could the identified patient and the family begin to make lasting inner personality, group-communicative, and relationship changes. The preoedipal nature of the patients' and their families' transference-resistance paradigms was consistent with the increasingly evident fact that adolescents who needed admission into full-time residence were found to harbor major psychopathology.

But primitive, preoedipal transference and related resistance comprised only one of several phenomena that pointed toward our patients' longstanding and pervasive psychopathology. An associated phenomenon was their desperate clinging to and profound immersion in dysfunctional parent-child relationships that displayed the features of prolonged and unresolved symbioses, hence of failure of separation-individuation (Mahler 1968; Rinsley 1964, 1965, 1967a, 1967b, 1972, 1974a, 1974b, 1980b, 1980c). Another phenomenon consisted of the triad of deep-seated aggression, depression, and identity diffusion irrespective of diagnostic labeling. During the residential process, therefore, we found ourselves face to face with psychologically unseparated adolescents whose adaptive-coping mechanisms were in some cases episodically, and in other cases chronically and unremittingly, psychotic. These were not garden variety adolescent youth making their way toward adulthood via some sort of expected adolescent *Sturm und Drang;* rather, they were seriously developmentally deviant youngsters who had lost their way years before they came into treatment. In accordance with the nosology of the time, my staff and I diagnosed our inpatient adolescents as suffering from symbiotic psychosis or symbiotic (childhood) schizophrenia (Rinsley 1972). A minority who appeared never to have developed a need-gratifying mother-infant symbiosis, hence who were even more profoundly and pervasively disturbed and even more difficult to treat, we diagnosed as suffering from autistic-presymbiotic psychosis or (childhood) schizophrenia, following Fliess (1961) and Mahler (1952, 1958, 1965a).[1] As our awareness of the significance of the early transference-resistance manifestations developed, it became increasingly obvious that the major therapeutic task was the identification, exposure, and beginning resolution of the patient's and the respective parent's symbiotic "tie that binds" (Masterson 1967a, 1972b). The term "resistance phase" was accordingly given to that period following admission; Masterson (1972b) termed it the "testing phase."

Because our adolescent unit at Topeka State Hospital and Masterson's adolescent service at Cornell's Payne Whitney Clinic were long term and intensive, it was possible to study the ensuing course and natural history of the full-time inpatient or residential process both extensively and intensively and to observe and record the unfolding of lasting therapeutic intrapersonal and interpersonal-intrafamilial change in those cases that proved responsive. Once again, Masterson and I, now accompanied independently by Lewis (1970) at Timberlawn Hospital in Dallas, could agree concerning the phasic nature of the inpatient-residential treatment process. Following the successfully traversed resistance phase there emerged a second or middle phase, often prolonged, during which the immensely complex process of de-symbiotization could be seen to have begun and carried through. To it I accorded the label, "definitive" or "introjective phase" (Rinsley 1965, 1974a, 1980c), while Masterson (1972b) termed it the "engagement phase." In successfully treated cases, this middle phase was followed by a third, final "resolution phase" (Rinsley 1965, 1974a, 1980c) or "separation phase" (Masterson 1972b).

The initial presentation of this triphasic concept of the residential treatment process (Rinsley 1965) paid considerable attention to the vicissitudes of the middle (definitive, introjective, or engagement) phase of treatment with emphasis on the externalization of the adolescent's pervasive underlying depression *pari passu* the switching of good and bad objects. It seemed evident, at the time, that the clinical phenomena particular to this phase of treatment bore a discernible relationship to the triphasic natural history that Bowlby (1960a, 1960b, 1961, 1962) described in the case of prematurely separated infants. Our adolescents thus appeared to be recapitulating the elements of Bowlby's stage of protest during the resistance phase, and his stage of despair during the definitive or introjective phase; in unsuccessfully treated cases, they seemed to recapitulate Bowlby's stage of detachment as they bordered on, but appeared never to enter, the third or resolution phase of treatment. Thus, the process of admission into residence, of physical-geographical separation from the parent-child tie, appeared to have set in motion the latter-day manifestations of an otherwise healthy detachment process that had gone egregiously awry. The seminal writings of Mahler and her colleagues would further clarify what had early gone wrong in the case of our inpatient adolescents; they had remained essentially symbiotic, having never completed the process of healthy separation-individuation (Mahler 1952, 1958, 1965a, 1965b, 1967, 1968, 1971; Mahler, Furer, and Settlage 1959; Mahler and Gosliner 1955; Mahler, Pine, and Bergman 1975; Mahler, Ross, and DeFries 1949).

It was only later, however, when it also became evident that the depressive manifestations and introjective-projective switching that consistently characterized the definitive or middle phase of treatment had earlier been set down by Fairbairn (1941) as characteristic of his postulated transitional stage of quasi-independence. We seemed indeed to be witnessing, in the case of our inpatient adolescents, the beginnings of the "dichotomy and exteriorization" that Fairbairn had described, including their attendant differentiation of self and object, thereby endowing the external(ized) object with the quality of reality. In other words, we seemed to be witnessing the reinception of the complex process of separation-individuation within the residential or inpatient setting. In terms of Klein's (1940, 1946, 1955) view, we seemed to witness the patient's and the parent's beginning working through of the infantile depressive position with its attendant cessation of splitting, generation of whole-object relations, and onset of normal repression. Thus, the significance of the inpatient adolescent's rich variety of resistance metaphors and behavior could be understood in terms of the untrammeled operation of the primitive splitting defense typical of developmental arrest at the paranoid-schizoid position.

Object-relations theory had ineluctably entered our effort to understand the course and natural history of the intensive, reconstructive residential treatment process. The role of that process as a vehicle for the attaintment of lasting personality change could be understood in terms of its use to promote separation-individuation. Psychoanalysis, especially its object-relations offshoot, had provided a comprehensive understanding of the developmental pathogenesis of our patients' individual and familial psychopathology; that understanding would later be extended well beyond our earlier application.[2]

As noted, Masterson had been coming to a similar conclusion regarding the phasic nature of intensive inpatient treatment. He had been deeply impressed with the emergence of depression, once the resistance (testing) phase had been traversed, and he had been assimilating Mahler's developmental phase theory to his understanding of the clinical phenomena. Masterson (1972b) went farther in ascribing the emergent definitive or engagement phase depression, which he termed "abandonment depression," to early developmental arrest associated with failure of separation-individuation.

Diagnostic Considerations

Careful diagnostic study of the adolescents in need of hospitalization revealed a pattern of long-standing psychopathology with both thought and mood disorder. The mood disorders were usually expressed symptomatically in the form considered typical for adolescents (Rinsley 1965, 1967a, 1967b, 1972). They were, therefore, viewed as suffering from psychotic illness and, in conformity with the DSM II (1968), diagnosed as suffering from (childhood) schizophrenia, the two terms being then used roughly interchangeably.

To represent more than mere labeling, diagnosis has to serve as more than a catalog of symptoms. Rather, it should reflect the natural historical context within which the individual's psychosocial development had become arrested. The original developmental context was provided by classical psychoanalytic (psychosexual) stage theory (Rinsley 1981). Its full potential, however, was only to be realized in the epochal studies of Mahler and her colleagues devoted to the process of separation-individuation (Mahler et al. 1975). Mahler and her colleagues' ever-expanding contributions had by the late 1960s evolved into a comprehensive view of normal and deviant development, of the "psychological birth" of the human infant, based upon the observed phases of autism, separation-individuation, on-the-way-to-object-constancy, and the separation-individuation subphases of differentiation, practicing, and rapprochement (Mahler et al. 1975). Mahlerian phase theory added new and profound dimensions to classical stage theory (Rinsley 1980a, 1981), additionally incorporating into itself various components drawn from psychoanalytic object-relations theory and the psychology of mental representations (Jacobson 1964).

It was Mahlerian phase theory that was to provide workers such as Masterson and myself with the requisite understanding of the developmental etiology of our adolescent inpatients' psychopathology, not to mention the basis for their differential diagnosis.

In an important series of writings beginning in 1971, Masterson (1971a, 1971b, 1972a, 1972b, 1973, 1974, 1975) fruitfully applied phase-theoretical insights to a diagnostic and in-depth developmental understanding of the symptomatic adolescent, from which emerged his evolving concept of the borderline adolescent.

I moved in this direction rather more slowly. Thus, although the term "borderline" had appeared in my own writings on adolescents as early as the 1965 object-relations paper, I continued to apply to the majority of our inpatient adolescents the Mahler-derived diagnostic category symbiotic psychosis as essentially equivalent to borderline. When I became convinced, however, that Masterson's formulation of the abandonment depression and my patients' ineluctably emergent middle or definitive phase depression represented one and the same phenomenon, it became evident that we had been witnessing and writing about the major symptomatology accruing from subphase-related developmental arrest in our respective patients. It likewise became evident that, in our successfully treated cases, the triphasic process reflected the adolescent's progress from the paranoid-schizoid position to a successfully worked-through depressive position. Our experiences with the highly structured, intensive residential milieu had indeed provided us with a window into our patients' early developmental arrest or deviation.

Following Mahler's (1971) own suggestion, we could proceed to relate that developmental arrest to separation-individuation failure beginning in most of our cases during the practicing subphase (ten to sixteen months) and reaching its peak during the rapprochement subphase (sixteen to twenty-six months). For us, and for me in particular, the borderline concept had indeed come of age, especially as it could be employed to represent a particular form of internal object relations governed by the persistence of the primitive splitting defense (Masterson 1975), insight into which had been earlier provided by Fairbairn (1941). Masterson had been working on a manuscript in which all this might be put together, and he graciously permitted me to collaborate with him in bringing it to completion. The result was the 1975 paper (Masterson and Rinsley 1975), herewith described in condensed historical form.

The Developmental-Diagnostic Spectrum

It hardly needs to be restated here that American psychiatry, including its child and adolescent subspecialties, has undergone major and permanent change during the past twenty-five years. The earlier pivotal position of psychodynamic-psychoanalytic ascendancy has since given way to an enormous efflorescence of more biological, biochemical, and physiologic research representative of a recrudescent mind-is-brain view in the best tradition of Wilhelm Griesinger. Much of this conveys a behavioristic approach that either ignores or denigrates the vast body of what psychoanalysis has taught us. The complex determinants of this trend are embedded in the broader matrix of pervasive social change that has typified American and Western European culture throughout this same period (Lasch 1977, 1978; Rinsley 1978b, 1980b). The benefits accruing from this trend are, nevertheless,

266

significant, among which is an effort to understand the physico-chemical substrates of human behavior and psychopathology and an effort toward more accurate diagnosis and prognosis of the range of human mental disorders, as now reflected in the DSM III (1980).

This important diagnostic-prognostic effort, emanating in largest measure from biologically oriented psychiatrists, who are also interested in the hereditary transmission of mental disorders, has produced the important concept of the diagnostic continuum or spectrum (Rinsley 1981; Stone 1980). There are thus the schizophrenic spectrum (the various schizophrenias and closely related syndromes), the schizo-affective spectrum (combining primary cognitive and affective determinants and clinical features), the spectrum of the primary or major affective disorders (manic-depressive, unipolar, bipolar) and the spectrum of the personality or characterologic disorders (Rinsley 1981), within each of which are grouped a range of symptomatically and possibly genetically related syndromes.[3]

My own departure from child and adolescent psychiatry coincided with the publication of the Masterson and Rinsley (1975) paper. My new studies involved a deepening interest in the application of psycho-analytic object-relations and Mahlerian phase theories to an understanding of borderline disorder and, in turn, its relationship to the spectrum of other personality disorders and to the wider range or continuum of psychopathology. The result has been a series of papers that further explored and developed the concepts basic to the 1975 Masterson and Rinsley paper and extending beyond to include the major psychoses (Brende and Rinsley 1979; Carter and Rinsley 1977; Rinsley 1977, 1978a, 1979, 1980a, 1980b, 1981).

It had indeed seemed possible to attempt an integration of a number of apparently disparate but nonetheless related lines of research that pointed toward the spectrum concept. Emergent from such an attempt was the recognition, developed from psychodynamic, developmental, and biological-genetic sources, of the proximity of the borderline to the major affective disorders on one side of the developmental continuum, and to the more purely narcissistic personality disorders on the other (Kohut 1971, 1977; Ornstein 1974).

It also seemed possible to place the work that had led to the Masterson and Rinsley paper within a more rational diagnostic perspective. So far as the nosology was concerned (Rinsley 1972), symbiotic psychosis of adolescence could be seen to comprise no less than three diagnostically differentiable syndromes: a more regressive symbiotic process reflective of childhood schizophrenic disorder, akin to Mahler's original symbiotic psychosis (schizophrenia) of childhood manifesting predominant thought disorder; a group of dysthymic, schizoaffective psychotic cases, including some now recognized as adolescent-onset unipolar and bipolar affective disorder (Carlson and Strober 1979) manifesting predominant mood disorder; and finally a group of cases reflective of disordered internal object relations, considered borderline, as described in the Masterson and Rinsley (1975) paper. It now appeared that the earlier effort toward diagnosis had not been off the mark and that the attempt to ground it firmly upon a knowledge of development, specifically the separation-individuation process, had been both necessary and fruitful.

Conclusions

The sort of clinical cross validation provided by Masterson's and my own intensive work with seriously disturbed adolescents may thus be placed within the wider context of evolving research into the pathogenesis and treatment of the range of preadult and adult psychopathology. Within that context, psychodynamic, developmental, and biological-genetic data and inferences are required for a comprehensive view of how people become mentally ill and of the variety of mental illnesses from which they suffer. It is exciting to consider how much more is known concerning the diagnosis and treatment of mental disorder than was known twenty-five years ago, and to consider how contemporary multidisciplinary research will continue to add comprehensively to that knowledge.

NOTES

1. Because the great majority of the adolescent inpatients under consideration here were suffering from symbiosis-related psychopathology, this discussion will be devoted to them and not to the more developmentally primitive autistic-presymbiotic group, discussion of whom is presented elsewhere (Rinsley 1974a, 1974b, 1980c).

2. *Editor's Note:* In 1968, Dr. Rinsley was recipient of the Edward A. Strecker Memorial Award of the Institute of the Pennsylvania Hospital for this work.

3. This work is discussed and summarized in Stone's (1980) recent, comprehensive book.

REFERENCES

Bettelheim, B., and Sylvester, E. 1952. A therapeutic milieu. *American Journal of Orthopsychiatry* 22:314–334.

Bowlby, J. 1960a. Grief and mourning in infancy and early childhood. *Psychoanalytic Study of the Child* 15:9–52.

Bowlby, J. 1960b. Separation anxiety. *International Journal of Psycho-Analysis* 41:89–113.

Bowlby, J. 1961. Processes of mourning. *International Journal of Psycho-Analysis* 42:317–340.

Bowlby, J. 1962. Childhood bereavement and psychiatric illness. In D. Richter et al., eds. *Aspects of Psychiatric Research*. London: Oxford.

Brende, J. O., and Rinsley, D. B. 1979. Borderline disorder, altered states of consciousness, and glossolalia. *Journal of the American Academy of Psychoanalysis* 7:165–188.

Carlson, G., and Strober, M. 1979. Affective disorders in adolescence. *Psychiatric Clinics of North America* 2:511–526.

Carter, L., and Rinsley, D. B. 1977. Vicissitudes of "empathy" in a borderline adolescent. *International Review of Psycho-Analysis* 4:317–326.

DSM II. 1968. *Diagnostic and Statistical Manual of Mental Disorders*. 2d ed. Washington, D.C.: American Psychiatric Association.

DSM III. 1980. *Diagnostic and Statistical Manual of Mental Disorders*. 3d ed. Washington, D.C.: American Psychiatric Association.

Erikson, E. H. 1963. *Childhood and Society*. New York: Norton.

Fairbairn, W. R. D. 1941. A revised psychopathology of the psychoses and psychoneuroses. In *An Object-Relations Theory of the Personality*. New York: Basic, 1954.

Fliess, R. 1961. On the mother-child unit: its disturbances and their consequences for the ego of the neurotic adult. In *Ego and Body Ego: Contributions to Their Psychoanalytic Psychology*. New York: Schulte.

Hendrickson, W. J. 1957. Adolescent Service, Neuropsychiatric Institute, University of Michigan. *Bulletin of the Michigan Society for Mental Health* 13:1–9.

Hendrickson, W. J., and Holmes, D. J. 1959. Control of behavior as a crucial factor in intensive psychiatric treatment in an all-adolescent ward. *American Journal of Psychiatry* 115:969–973.

Hendrickson, W. J.; Holmes, D. J.; and Waggoner, R. W. 1959.

Psychotherapy of the hospitalized adolescent. *American Journal of Psychiatry* 116:527–532.

Jacobson, E. 1964. *The Self and the Object World*. New York: International Universities Press.

Klein, M. 1940. Mourning and its relation to manic-depressive states. In *Love, Guilt and Reparation and Other Works, 1921–1945*. New York: Delacorte, 1975.

Klein, M. 1946. Notes on some schizoid mechanisms. In *Envy and Gratitude and Other Works, 1946–1963*. New York: Delacorte, 1975.

Klein, M. 1955. On identification. In *Envy and Gratitude and Other Works, 1946–1963*. New York: Delacorte, 1975.

Kohut, H. 1971. *The Analysis of the Self*. New York: International Universities Press.

Kohut, H. 1977. *The Restoration of the Self*. New York: International Universities Press.

Lasch, C. 1977. *Haven in a Heartless World: The Family Besieged*. New York: Basic.

Lasch, C. 1978. *The Culture of Narcissism: American Life in an Age of Diminishing Expectations*. New York: Norton.

Lewis, J. M. 1970. The development of an adolescent inpatient service. *Adolescence* 5:303–312.

Mahler, M. S. 1952. On child psychosis and schizophrenia: autistic and symbiotic infantile psychoses. *Psychoanalytic Study of the Child* 7:286–305.

Mahler, M. S. 1958. Autism and symbiosis: two extreme disturbances of identity. *International Journal of Psycho-Analysis* 39:77–83.

Mahler, M. S. 1965a. On early infantile psychosis: the symbiotic and autistic syndromes. *Journal of the American Academy of Child Psychiatry* 4:554–568.

Mahler, M. S. 1965b. On the significance of the normal separation-individuation phase with reference to research in symbiotic child psychosis. In M. Schur, ed. *Drives, Affects, Behavior*. Vol. 2. New York: International Universities Press.

Mahler, M. S. 1967. On human symbiosis and the vicissitudes of individuation: an overview of human symbiosis and individuation. *Journal of the American Psychoanalytic Association* 25:740–763.

Mahler, M. S. 1968. *On Human Symbiosis and the Vicissitudes of Individuation: Infantile Psychosis*. Vol. 1. New York: International Universities Press.

Mahler, M. S. 1971. A study of the separation-individuation process and its possible application to borderline phenomena in the psychoanalytic situation. *Psychoanalytic Study of the Child* 26:403–424.

Mahler, M. S.; Furer, M.; and Settlage, C. F. 1959. Severe emotional disturbances in childhood: psychosis. In S. Arieti, ed. *American Handbook of Psychiatry*. Vol. 1. New York: Basic.

Mahler, M. S., and Gosliner, B. J. 1955. On symbiotic child psychosis: genetic, dynamic and restitutive aspects. *Psychoanalytic Study of the Child* 10:195–212.

Mahler, M. S.; Pine, F.; and Bergman, A. 1975. *The Psychological Birth of the Human Infant: Symbiosis and Individuation*. New York: Basic.

Mahler, M. S.; Ross, J. R.; and DeFries, Z. 1949. Clinical studies in benign and malignant cases of childhood psychosis (schizophrenia-like). *American Journal of Orthopsychiatry* 19:295–305.

Masterson, J. F. 1967a. *The Psychiatric Dilemma of Adolescence*. Boston: Little, Brown.

Masterson, J. F. 1967b. The symptomatic adolescent five years later: he didn't grow out of it. *American Journal of Psychiatry* 123:1338–1345.

Masterson, J. F. 1968. The psychiatric significance of adolescent turmoil. *American Journal of Psychiatry* 124:1549–1554.

Masterson, J. F. 1971a. Diagnosis and treatment of the borderline syndrome in adolescents. Paris: *Confrontations Psychiatriques* 7:125–155.

Masterson, J. F. 1971b. Treatment of the adolescent with borderline syndrome: a problem in separation-individuation. *Bulletin of the Menninger Clinic* 35:5–18.

Masterson, J. F. 1972a. Intensive psychotherapy of the adolescent with a borderline syndrome. (Buenos Aires) *Cuadernos de la Asociacion Argentina de Psiquiatria y Psicologia de la Infancia y de la Adolescencia* 3:15–50.

Masterson, J. F. 1972b. *Treatment of the Borderline Adolescent: A Developmental Approach*. New York: Wiley-Interscience.

Masterson, J. F. 1973. The borderline adolescent. *Adolescent Psychiatry* 2:240–268.

Masterson, J. F. 1974. Intensive psychotherapy of the adolescent with a borderline syndrome. In S. Arieti, ed. *American Handbook of Psychiatry*, Vol. 2. New York: Basic.

Masterson, J. F. 1975. The splitting defense mechanism of the borderline adolescent: developmental and clinical aspects. In J. E. Mack, ed. *Borderline States in Psychiatry*. New York: Grune & Stratton.

Masterson, J. F., and Rinsley, D. B. 1975. The borderline syndrome: the role of the mother in the genesis and psychic structure of the borderline personality. *International Journal of Psycho-Analysis* 56:163–177. Revised and reprinted in R. F. Lax, S. Bach, and J. A. Burland, eds. *Rapprochement: The Critical Subphase of Separation-Individuation*. New York: Aronson, 1980.

Masterson, J. F.; Tucker, K.; and Berk, G. 1963. Psychopathology in adolescence. IV. Clinical and dynamic characteristics. *American Journal of Psychiatry* 120:357–366.

Masterson, J. F.; Tucker, K.; and Berk, G. 1966. The symptomatic adolescent: delineation of psychiatric syndromes. *Comprehensive Psychiatry* 7:166–174.

Masterson, J. F., and Washburne, A. 1966. The symptomatic adolescent: psychiatric illness or adolescent turmoil? *American Journal of Psychiatry* 122:1240–1248.

Menninger, W. C. 1936a. Individuation in the prescription of nursing care of the psychiatric patient. *Journal of the American Medical Association* 106:756–761.

Menninger, W. C. 1936b. Psychiatric hospital treatment designed to meet unconscious needs. *American Journal of Psychiatry* 93:347–360.

Menninger, W. C. 1937. Psychoanalytic principles applied to the treatment of hospitalized patients. *Bulletin of the Menninger Clinic* 1:35–43.

Menninger, W. C. 1939. Psychoanalytic principles in psychiatric hospital therapy. *Southern Medical Journal* 32:348–354.

Modell, A. H. 1968. *Object Love and Reality*. New York: International Universities Press.

Noshpitz, J. D. 1962. Notes on the theory of residential treatment. *Journal of the American Academy of Child Psychiatry* 1:284–296.

Ornstein, P. H. 1974. On narcissism: beyond the Introduction, highlights of Heinz Kohut's contributions to the psychoanalytic treatment of narcissistic personality disorders. *Annual of Psychoanalysis* 2:127–149.

Redl, F. 1959. Life space interview techniques. *American Journal of Orthopsychiatry* 29:1–18.

Redl, F., and Wineman, D. 1951. *Children Who Hate*. Glencoe, Ill.: Free Press.

Redl, F., and Wineman, D. 1952. *Controls from Within*. Glencoe, Ill.: Free Press.

Rinsley, D. B. 1963. Psychiatric hospital treatment with special reference to children. *Archives of General Psychiatry* 9:489–496. Reprinted in *Treatment of the Severely Disturbed Adolescent*. New York: Aronson, 1980.

Rinsley, D. B. 1964. Psychiatric hospital treatment with special reference to children. *Current Psychiatric Therapies* 4:69–73.

Rinsley, D. B. 1965. Intensive psychiatric hospital treatment of adolescents: an object-relations view. *Psychiatric Quarterly* 39:405–429.

Rinsley, D. B. 1967a. Intensive residential treatment of the adolescent. *Psychiatric Quarterly* 41:134–143.

Rinsley, D. B. 1967b. The adolescent in residential treatment: some critical reflections. *Adolescence* 2:83–95.

Rinsley, D. B. 1968. Theory and practice of intensive residential treatment of adolescents. *Psychiatric Quarterly* 42:611–638. Revised and reprinted in *Adolescent Psychiatry* 1:479–509. Reprinted in *Treatment of the Severely Disturbed Adolescent*. New York: Aronson, 1980.

Rinsley, D. B. 1972. A contribution to the nosology and dynamics of adolescent schizophrenia. *Psychiatric Quarterly* 46:159–186. Reprinted in *Treatment of the Severely Disturbed Adolescent*. New York: Aronson, 1980.

Rinsley, D. B. 1974a. Residential treatment of adolescents. In S. Arieti, ed. *American Handbook of Psychiatry*. 2d ed. Vol. 2. New York: Basic. Reprinted in *Treatment of the Severely Disturbed Adolescent*. New York: Aronson, 1980.

Rinsley, D. B. 1974b. Special education for adolescents in residential psychiatric treatment. *Adolescent Psychiatry* 3:394–418.

Rinsley, D. B. 1977. An object-relations view of borderline personality. In P. Hartocollis, ed. *Borderline Personality Disorders*. New York: International Universities Press.

Rinsley, D. B. 1978a. Borderline psychopathology: a review of aetiology, dynamics and treatment. *International Review of Psycho-Analysis* 5:45–54.

Rinsley, D. B. 1978b. Juvenile delinquency: a review of the past and a look at the future. *Bulletin of the Menninger Clinic* 42:252–260.

Rinsley, D. B. 1979. Fairbairn's object-relations theory: a reconsideration in terms of newer knowledge. *Bulletin of the Menninger Clinic* 43:489–514.

Rinsley, D. B. 1980a. The developmental etiology of borderline and narcissistic disorders. *Bulletin of the Menninger Clinic* 44:127–134. Reprinted in *Treatment of the Severely Disturbed Adolescent*. New York: Aronson, 1980.

Rinsley, D. B. 1980b. Diagnosis and treatment of borderline and narcissistic children and adolescents. *Bulletin of the Menninger Clinic* 44:147–170. Reprinted in *Treatment of the Severely Disturbed Adolescent*. New York: Aronson, 1980.

Rinsley, D. B. 1980c. Principles of therapeutic milieu with children. In G. P. Sholevar, R. M. Benson and B. J. Blinder, eds. *Emotional Disorders in Children and Adolescents*. New York: SP Medical & Scientific Books.

Rinsley, D. B. 1981. Dynamic and developmental issues in borderline and related "spectrum" disorders. *Psychiatric Clinics of North America* 4:117–132.

Rinsley, D. B., and Hall, D. D. 1962. Psychiatric hospital treatment of adolescents: parental resistances as expressed in casework metaphor. *Archives of General Psychiatry* 7:286–294. Reprinted in *Treatment of the Severely Disturbed Adolescent*. New York: Aronson, 1980.

Rinsley, D. B., and Inge, G. P., III. 1961. Psychiatric hospital treatment of adolescents: verbal and nonverbal resistance to treatment. *Bulletin of the Menninger Clinic* 25:249–263. Reprinted in *Treatment of the Severely Disturbed Adolescent*. New York: Aronson, 1980.

Stanton, A., and Schwartz, M. S. 1954. *The Mental Hospital*. New York: Basic.

Stone, M. H. 1980. *The Borderline Syndromes: Constitution, Personality and Adaptation*. New York: McGraw-Hill.

Winnicott, D. W. 1950–1955. Aggression in relation to emotional development. In *Collected Papers: Through Paediatrics to Psycho-Analysis*. London: Tavistock, 1958.

19 PSYCHIATRIC CASUALTIES OF MINIMAL BRAIN DYSFUNCTION IN ADOLESCENTS

HARVEY A. HOROWITZ

Minimal Brain Dysfunction (MBD) is one of many terms used to describe a common and still controversial behavioral syndrome of childhood, also called Hyperkinetic Syndrome, Learning Disability, and, currently in the DSM III (1980), Attention Deficit Disorder. The syndrome is characterized by inattention, impulsivity, excitability, and emotionality. Its prevalence in the prepubertal population has been estimated by Wender (1971) to be 10 percent.

Originally, MBD had been considered to be a childhood behavior disorder outgrown by adolescence (Laufer and Denhoff 1957), but more recently, many reports have suggested that MBD may persist into adolescence and young adulthood and may, indeed, contribute to the development of specific disorders of behavior and personality. This relationship between childhood MBD and adolescent and young adult psychopathology is inferred from longitudinal, retrospective, drug response, and family studies.

Mendelson, Johnson, and Stewart (1971) studied eighty-three teenagers who had been diagnosed as having the hyperactive syndrome two to five years earlier. At follow-up, over 50 percent of the teenagers had persistent symptoms of restlessness, impulsiveness, excitability, and aggressiveness associated with poor school performance and low self-esteem, while 25 percent had significant histories of delinquent behavior. Weiss, Minde, and Werry (1971) studied sixty-four hyperactive children followed for five years into adolescence and found that while the hyperactivity has diminished, the social and intrapsychic difficulties and the affectional and learning disorders persisted. Heussy, Metoyer, and Townsend (1974), in a follow-up study of eighty-four children treated for behavior disorders, observed that eighteen manifested severe psychopathology, including sociopathy and psychosis.

Menkes, Rowe, and Menkes (1967) and O'Neal and Robins (1958), in retrospective follow-up studies, identified a group of adults who had been treated for behavior disorders as children and who today would likely be given the diagnosis of MBD. This group had an increased incidence of psychosis and sociopathy in adulthood. Healy and Bronner (1936) reported that symptoms suggestive of MBD were more common in the childhoods of delinquents than in their nondelinquent siblings, while Hartacollis (1968), in a study of fifteen hospitalized patients ages fifteen to twenty-five, described an association between neurologic soft signs, developmental history consistent with MBD, and a clinical diagnosis of impulsive or immature personality disorder. Quitkin and Klein (1969) selected a group of thirty-one patients from 105 nonchronic psychiatric inpatients under age twenty-five and reported an association between indicators of childhood brain dysfunction (including developmental delay, hyperkinesis, learning problems, and social disorganization) and current symptomatic behaviors, judgments of organicity in psychometric test battery, abnormal EEG, and diagnosis.

A variety of reports describing drug response suggests the persistence of MBD into adolescence and young adulthood. Hill (1944) reported the treatment of adult psychopaths with amphetamines, describing the pretreatment subject group as hostile, aggressive, alcoholic, and antisocial, with persistent enuresis. There was an amelioration of symptoms with those who could be maintained on amphetamine therapy. Morrison and Minkoff (1975) report the effective use of imipramine in a small series of patients with histories of childhood hyperkinesis and symptomatic behaviors in adulthood characterized by affective lability, explosivity, and episodic rage, while Mann and Greenspan (1976) described the use of imipramine chemotherapy in patients with "adult brain dysfunction," adults who had MBD as children and who presented in adulthood with attentional deficit and related behavior disorders.

Wood, Reimherr, Wender, and Johnson (1976) reported a series of fifteen putative MBD adults identified on the basis of current MBD-like complaints, self-description of MBD characteristics in childhood, and a parental rating on a standardized scale of "hyperactivity" in childhood. In a double blind study of methylphenidate and in an open trial of tricyclics and stimulants, a significant number showed a good to moderate response to chemotherapy as measured by changes in observed behavior including impulsivity, hyperactivity, frustration tolerance, affective disability, excitability, moodiness and distractibility, and short attention span.

Finally, family studies have suggested a relationship between MBD in childhood and sociopathy, alcoholism, and hysteria in adulthood. Morrison and Stewart (1971, 1973) and Cantwell (1972, 1973) studied the parents of hyperactive children and found an increased incidence of alcoholism and sociopathy in the biological fathers and hysteria in the biological mothers. Taken together, these studies also suggest that certain adult alcoholics, sociopaths, and hysterics may represent an adult expression of MBD.

From the above reports, it would seem reasonable to conclude that childhood MBD persists into adolescence, though perhaps symptomatically transformed by maturation, adaptation, and defense. This conclusion suggests several questions which this chapter will address: the incidence of MBD in a population of severely disturbed hospitalized adolescents, the clinical characteristics associated with adolescent MBD, and are clinically distinct groups present?

Methodology

Fifty consecutive psychiatric patients between the ages of thirteen and eighteen, admitted to the Adolescent Treatment Unit, a twenty-four-bed, long-term residential program in a private psychiatric hospital, were studied for the presence of minimal brain dysfunction. Sufficient data were obtained from forty patients who made up the sample population, while ten subjects were lost due to early termination from the treatment program. All forty patients in the sample group were middle class and thirty-nine were white. Evaluation of the sample group included extensive developmental histories, psychological testing, observations of current ward behavior, and psychiatric interviews of the identified patient and the family.

DEVELOPMENTAL HISTORY

Developmental histories were obtained from both parents, where available, using a parent response questionnaire followed by an interview to obtain a family psychosocial history. Factors from the questionnaire and interview considered to be suggestive of MBD included: (1) a history of encephalopathic events such as prematurity, neonatal anoxia, or infantile seizures, and subsequent abnormal development; (2) developmental delay or abnormality in the areas of speech, language, cognitive, perceptual, or motor behaviors; (3) the presence in childhood of hyperactivity, impulsivity, short attention span, low frustration tolerance, and emotionality; (4) the presence in the primary school years of global learning difficulties and/or specific skill deficits (as in dyslexia); (5) the presence of behavior disorders, continued achievement difficulties, and/or a growing resistance and antagonism toward the learning situation in later school years. A developmental history was considered consistent with MBD when at least three of the five factors were present.

PSYCHOLOGICAL TESTING AND EDUCATIONAL ASSESSMENT

A complete psychoeducational test battery was used to evaluate each of the subjects in this study. The Wechsler scales were administered to evaluate intellectual functioning, the Bender Gestalt to assess perceptual motor functioning, and projective techniques of personality were given, including the Figure Drawings, Sentence Completion, Thematic Apperception Test, and Rorschach. Normative data on the development of visual-motor functions were collected through the administration of the Berry-Bukstenica Developmental Test of Visual-Motor Integration.

A series of standarized and informal educational measures were used to delineate achievement status. The Wide Range Achievement Test provided quick estimates of basic skills in the reading (word recognition), spelling, and arithmetic areas. A more detailed, diagnostic assessment of the reading process was derived through the administration of the Woodcock Reading Mastery Test and informal reading inventories. Consequently, specific information regarding the subject's strengths and weaknesses in decoding and word recognition as well as comprehension of contextual materials was available. Informal writing samples were also collected to determine quality of handwriting, and the level of productivity and the quality and content of each subject's written skills.

A variety of factors were considered to be suggestive of MBD, including:

1. A significant basic skill deficiency in the rudiments of reading,

writing, or arithmetic. A significant deficiency was operationally defined as an achievement level two years or more below the grade level which might be expected based on the subject's chronological age.

2. An unusual degree of inconsistency or scatter in the subject's intellectual functioning based on a large discrepancy between verbal and performance IQ scores and/or an excessively erratic intellectual profile.

3. A significant deficiency in visual-motor functions. Again, a performance level finding two or more years below age expectations was considered significant.

4. A variety of qualitative, clinical signs obtained through the testing process:

   a) A variety of disturbances in behavioral and attentional control or focus. Such patients show evidence of diminished capacity for attention, concentration, persistence, and intentional control. Their work styles are impulsive, with little tolerance for the typical stress and frustration associated with mental effort.

   b) Impaired ability to assimilate and retain directions, particularly those of any degree of complexity. Short- and long-term memory functions are scattered, isolated, and poorly organized.

   c) Qualitative distortions in visual-motor integration noted in drawing and writing ability. In addition to a careless and haphazard approach, real deficits were noted in fine motor execution, eye-hand coordination, distortion in figure-ground relationships, and an impaired capacity to evaluate relevance of target stimuli across visual and/or auditory modes.

   d) In addition to the generalized educational skill deficiency, there is evidence of specific educational disorder associated with organic dysfunction, dyslexia, dysgraphia, or, more specifically, serious word recognition difficulty, letter and word reversals and letter transpositions, or marked impairment of handwriting skills.

Psychological testing and educational assessment were considered positive for MBD when factor 1, a significant basic skill deficiency, and at least two other factors were present.

CRITERIA FOR THE DESIGNATION MBD

Adolescents were assigned to the MBD index group when two criteria were met: (1) a developmental history suggestive of MBD and (2) psychological testing and educational assessment positive for MBD.

OBSERVATIONS OF CURRENT WARD BEHAVIOR

Observations of current ward behaviors were made daily by the author who was directly involved in the milieu therapy of all patients on the Adolescent Treatment Unit. Observations were organized into the following major areas: (1) motor behavior—including the rate and organization of motor behavior; (2) affects and arousal—including affective stability, reactivity, and regulation; (3) attentional processes—including concentration or the ability to sustain focus on relevant information; (4) social behaviors—including the degree of organization and the forms of interactions in large, complex groups as well as small, task-oriented groups; and (5) alterations in any of the above behaviors in response to changes in environmental structure.

PSYCHIATRIC ASSESSMENT

Open-ended psychiatric interviews of the identified patient were conducted by the author, who had access to the developmental and psychosocial histories but was without knowledge of the psychometric findings. The interview included a routine psychiatric history and mental status examination, with an additional focus on special aspects of mental functioning associated with MBD such as distractibility and concreteness of thinking. The interview of the identified patient was followed by a one-hour interview of the family to assess structure, communication, and dynamics in the family system.

Patients in the sample population were given two diagnoses on discharge from hospital: A DSM II diagnosis by the private attending psychiatrist, and a research project diagnosis made according to DSM III (1980) criteria.

Results

INCIDENCE

Fifteen patients or 37.5 percent of the sample population satisfied the criteria for inclusion in the index group, designated minimal brain dysfunction (MBD). The sex ratio in the index group, 13 males:2 females, is comparable to reported ratios in MBD populations, while the sex ratio in the sample population approximated 1:1.

CLINICAL CHARACTERISTICS AND CLASSIFICATION

Within the index group, clinical findings derived from psychiatric interviews, psychosocial histories, and observations of ward behavior defined three distinct clinical groups, which have been named descriptively for purposes of classification: (1) diffuse developmental disorder; (2) affect-motor dyscontrol disorder; (3) and discrete cognitive-social disorder. The clinical characteristics of patients in these groups are presented in Appendix 1. The data for age, sex, developmental history, intelligence, academic achievement, and organic indicators from psychological testing are presented in Appendix 2.

DIFFUSE DEVELOPMENTAL DISORDER

Adolescents in this group were characterized clinically by lifelong and diffuse developmental disturbances in attention, intellect, motor functioning, and social adaptation. The group represented four of fifteen patients in the index group with two patients having histories of encephalopathic event (i.e., neonatal anoxia), associated with subsequent developmental delay, while the remaining two had histories of delay in the development of motor and language skills, childhood hyperkinesis, and learning disability. Personality functioning during childhood was markedly abnormal and the children were described as asocial, infantile, behaviorally inappropriate, and socially incompetent. The clinical presentation in adolescence is of two varieties, one subgroup presenting with normal intelligence and overt psychosis, the second subgroup presenting greater intellectual impairment, borderline intelligence, and defective reality testing in the absence of psychosis. These patients are immature and childlike, dependent, egocentric, demanding, and unable to relate to adults in other than a need-gratifying manner. Relationships with peers shift through a cycle from extreme isolation to a passive-dependent mascot status, to overt hostility and scapegoating frequently precipitated by their egocentricity, intrusiveness, and differentness.

Intelligence in this group varied from dull normal to normal, and all had significant, severe skill deficiencies in reading, arithmetic, and spelling. Affect was labile, at times inappropriate, infrequently explosive with frustration and rage. Attention, concentration, and conceptual tracking were disturbed, as was cognition, where marked concreteness and severe deficits in comprehension, abstraction and generalization, reasoning, and judgment were demonstrated. In addition, all four of the patients in this group demonstrated transient but severe disturbances of reality testing with over-inclusive, referential, and personalized thinking. However, only two of the four were overtly psychotic, and these two did not have the bizarre, idiosyncratic, or systematized quality of schizophrenic thinking and language, nor was gross disorganization, regressive behavior, or autism present.

THE AFFECT-MOTOR DYSCONTROL GROUP

This group represents five of fifteen index patients, demonstrating clear disturbances in attention, affect, and motor control functions, the "hyperactive child" as adolescent. Each of the five patients within this group had a history of childhood hyperkinesis and learning disability with consequent interpersonal difficulties with peers, teachers, and family. In adolescence, these patients present with hyperactivity, distractibility, impulsivity, and extreme lability of affect. All five patients had histories of antisocial behavior leading to contacts with the police and courts, disciplinary suspensions from school, and often explosive violence at home, and it was this behavior disorder which precipitated hospitalization.

Adolescents in this group have significant deficits in cognition, most notably in abstraction and generalization, reasoning and judgment, deficits which give the clinical impression that they are unable to learn from experience, are unable to gain and benefit from insight, are unaware of the future consequences of their actions, and willfully repeat antisocial and self-destructive behavior patterns.

In the ward milieu, adolescents with this syndrome demonstrate social information processing deficits in addition to the dyscontrol syndrome. They are easily frustrated, intrusive, impulsive, and egocentric, qualities which quickly lead to isolation and hostility from peers. They are hypersensitive and hyperreactive to affective and social stimuli, thus peer group hostility and rejection generates a process which creates anxiety, volatility, and potentially affective violence. And yet, these patients are genuinely confused by interpersonal events, by the social expectations of the group, by the rules, and by the complexities of relationships, a confusion which reinforces their defective self-image and anger.

THE DISCRETE ATTENTIONAL-COGNITIVE GROUP

This group represents 40 percent of the index group (six of fifteen patients) and presents with more discrete, mild deficits in attention; cognition, including abstraction and generalization, concept formation, synthesis and integration, reasoning and judgment; and in memory functions such as short-term auditory and visual memory. Three of six patients in this group had histories of possible central nervous system insult, but none had evidence of developmental delay or abnormality. Five of six were described as hyperactive and restless in childhood, inattentive with learning difficulties and problems with peers. However, these adolescents are less impaired than groups I and II and were often thought of as underachievers. In fact, they are overachievers, developing compensatory intellectual mechanisms, and struggling to adapt socially and intellectually.

As adolescents, patients in this group present clinically without a primary motor or affect dyscontrol disturbance, without hyperactivity or affective lability, but rather, present a significant secondary dysphoria characterized by anxiety and depression. This dysphoria is directly related to a defective self-image, intense fears of failure, and a profound sense of helplessness and hopelessness concerning the issues of mastery, competence, and independence, issues which assume developmental primacy in adolescence.

In contrast to syndrome groups I and II, social function in this group does not appear blatantly disturbed, these adolescents appear able to process socially relevant and complex information, to cooperate with others in group settings, to assume leadership positions in peer groups, and superficially to form age-appropriate attachments. However, their dysphoric state, defective self-image, fragile self-esteem, and mild but real cognitive deficits combine to produce a disturbance of personality organization characterized by inhibition, ego restriction and avoidance, isolation and withdrawal, contrasted with occasional episodes of explosive rage and antisocial behavior, chronic drug and alcohol abuse, and a tendency toward self-injury.

CLINICAL CHARACTERISTICS OF THE INDEX FAMILIES

The fifteen index families manifested severe family system dysfunction. In two groups there appeared to be an association between the clinical syndrome presented by the individual index patient and a characteristic family pattern.

The diffuse developmental disorder family system was characterized by profound feelings of humiliation and narcissistic injury in family members precipitated by the index patient, who is seen as the defective child and the family problem. Parents in this group used massive denial concerning the reality of the child's deficits and, hypothetically, to defend against the depression and anger generated by the perception of shared defectiveness. They demonstrated great ambivalence toward the index patient, showing enormous concern, an exaggerated sense of responsibility and guilt, intrusiveness, and hostility toward staff for "not doing enough," yet keeping a distance and seeming unaware of the rejection and abandonment their child experienced.

The index patient in each of these families was seen as a "special" child, having developed a dependent relationship with the nurturing parent, the mother in all cases. Mother and child appeared in conflict around resolving their attachment, physical and psychological separation precipitating guilt, depression, and anger.

The affect-motor dyscontrol disorder family system was characterized by the response to the index patient's impulsivity, hyperactivity, and emotionality. These families were primarily concerned with control, aggression, and dominance-submission issues. Their inability to be effective in controlling their child and stabilizing family life left the parents with feelings of helplessness, impotence and rage, particularly in the fathers, all of whom related difficulty controlling their own aggressive impulses toward the index patient, and a majority of whom had been involved in physical violence with their sons.

Siblings in these families reported intense anger in response to the inordinate amount of parental time and energy demanded by their impulsive, troublesome sib. Parents in this group demonstrated conflict around authority and discipline, inconsistency and rigidity in determining family rules, and an inability to resolve parental conflict, leaving the children confused and without limits.

The discrete cognitive-social disorder family system presented a less consistent and characteristic pattern, demonstrating the range of family system dysfunction and psychopathology. However, there were several features in common in these families, including an orientation toward performance and achievement with high expectations of family members, and a tendency toward personalizing the child's underachievement, with consequent disappointment and covert criticism of the child, who was often seen as lazy, unmotivated, and uncooperative. This created a pattern which perpetuated the child's defective self-image, and intensified performance anxiety and avoidance behavior, while leaving the parents disappointed, frustrated, and ultimately distant. These families tended to be demanding, driven, detached, and depressed.

DIAGNOSIS

As can be seen in Appendix 3, discharge diagnoses of attending psychiatrists differed markedly from research project diagnoses concerning the presence of brain dysfunction syndromes. Of the fifteen patients satisfying the project criteria for brain dysfunction, only five were given diagnoses by attending psychiatrists suggestive of organic brain dysfunction (MBD, Learning Disability, ADD). Greater agreement was seen in diagnoses given to describe psychopathologic entities.

In group I, the two patients with borderline intelligence and marked intellectual deficits (patients 1 and 2) were seen by the attending psychiatrists and the research project as presenting organic dysfunction with developmental disorders in conjunction with a personality disorder featuring passivity, dependency, and maladaptive aggression. However, the patients with normal intelligence (patients 3 and 4) were described diagnostically by attending psychiatrists as psychotic without reference to brain dysfunction while research project diagnosis referred to both a psychotic process and brain dysfunction. There was disagreement as to the exact nature of the psychosis.

Group II was seen by the attending psychiatrists as manifesting MBD in two of five cases. Diagnoses relating to disorders of behavior and personality showed greater agreement, with both attending psychiatrists and project classifications focusing on the impulsive and delinquent behavior patterns. Group III, the group with discrete attentional and cognitive deficits, had only one patient receive a MBD diagnosis by attending psychiatrists. Diagnoses of personality disorders in the group focused, in both attending psychiatrists and project diagnoses, on the prominent depression and deficits in object ties, with primary affective disorders, borderline, paranoid, and schizoid personality disorders described.

Discussion

The major finding of this study is the presence of organic brain dysfunction in 38 percent of a sample population of psychiatrically hospitalized adolescents. This finding is consistent with those of Rutter, Graham, and Yule (1970) and Shaffer, McNamara, and Pincus (1974) in demonstrating that children with brain dysfunction are at risk to develop severe psychopathology in adolescence.

A second finding is the presence of distinct clinical groups within the heterogeneous index patient population. Group I in this study, designated the diffuse developmental disturbance, presents in adolescence with marked defects in reality testing and social incompetence, associated with a history of developmental delay in language, speech, and/or motor skills. Patients with a similar clinical presentation were reported by Quitkin and Klein (1969), who described a group of adolescents and young adult MBD patients with the "socially awkward, withdrawn" syndrome. These patients showed obvious intellectual defects, thought disorder, social incompetence, withdrawal and isolation, academic difficulties, and marked inability to organize their life. Each patient had a history of childhood asociality. Seven of twelve patients in this group were given the diagnosis of schizophrenia, had had no evidence of psychosis prior to adolescence, and had a poor response to phenothiazines and a poor prognosis.

Within group I, we have further described two distinct varieties of this diffuse developmental disturbance, a subgroup with borderline intelligence and marked social immaturity, and a subgroup with overt psychosis. While the Quitkin and Klein (1969) study does not distinguish between these subgroups, Menkes et al. (1967) found such a distinction in their outcome study of fourteen MBD patients first seen twenty-four years earlier as children. They reported four patients hospitalized as chronic psychotics, while two patients were classified mentally retarded and living sheltered lives with their families, although when first evaluated in childhood these two patients had IQs of 84 and 76.

Furthermore, the finding in this clinical group of a possible association of language and speech retardation, a strong indicator of MBD in childhood, a subsequent severe psychiatric sequelae in adolescence is consistent with the findings of Cantwell, Baker, and Mattison (1980) and suggests that this form of brain dysfunction in childhood, particularly if associated with childhood asociality, may be a specific indicator of social and cognitive incompetence in later life.

Group II in this study, the affect-motor dyscontrol group, includes patients who had behavior disorders with hyperactivity in childhood, and who emerged as delinquent adolescents. The relationship between hyperactivity and delinquency has been reviewed by Cantwell (1978), and the clinical descriptions of these patients in the literature resemble the syndrome described here. The Quitkin and Klein (1969) study previously cited, described a second group of adolescent and young adult patients with MBD having an "impulsive-destructive" syndrome. Patients in this group were relatively intact intellectually and socially, with infrequent thought disorders and some ability to organize their lives under very structured conditions. However, they were also characterized by destructive, impulsive behavior, low frustration tolerance, mood swings, overreactive emotionality, and temper tantrums. Mendelson et al. (1971) had similar findings in their study, in which over 50 percent of MBD patients at follow-up were described as hyperactive, impulsive, rebellious, and destructive, with low self-esteem, temper tantrums, failing one or more grades, and often being involved in lying, stealing, and fighting.

The predictive significance of childhood hyperactivity with behavior disorder in relation to adolescent psychopathology posited by Quitkin and Klein and supported by this study, is also substantiated by the findings of Offord, Sullivan, Allen, and Abrams (1979), who compared a group of hyperactive delinquents with a matched group of nonhyperactive delinquents. They found that the subgroup of delinquents with hyperactivity had more severe delinquency and a probable poor adult prognosis. Thus, we would conclude that MBD with hyperactivity in childhood is a strong, specific predicator of adolescent psychopathology, and that the predominance and continuation of affective and motor excitability into adolescence may contribute to the specific development of impulsive and antisocial personality disorders.

The third clinical group in this study, the discrete attentional-cognitive disorder, represents a clinical constellation of attentional deficits, impulsivity, and dysphoria without hyperactivity, which, in these patients, was either not present in childhood or outgrown by adolescence. The absence of hyperactivity in the presence of higher general intelligence, more circumscribed cognitive and memory deficits, greater social competence, and well developed compensatory

287

mechanisms, tend to conceal the organic components of a clinical picture dominated by dysphoria, disturbances in object-relations, and the impulsive, antisocial and self-destructive behaviors.

Patients in this group in our study are frequently seen as borderline personality disorders and resemble diagnostically and descriptively hospitalized patients described by Hartacollis (1968), who reported an association between neurologic soft signs, a developmental history consistent with MBD, and a clinical diagnosis of immature personality disorder. We would conclude then that residual disorders of attention and cognition in which hyperactivity diminishes over time in childhood remain predictive of adolescent psychopathology, and that attentional and cognitive deficits, the related impulsivity, and the resultant dysphoria contribute to the specific development of severe personality disorders including the borderline and dysthymic.

A third finding of this study is the presence of severe psychopathology in the families of all index patients, a finding consistent with Rutter et al. (1970), who reported in the Isle of Wight study that brain-injured children with psychiatric disorders had significantly more pathology in their family environment than did those brain-injured children free of psychologic disturbances. This finding lends support to the notion that MBD may be a significant contributor to severe psychiatric disorders in adolescence only in the presence of family system dysfunction. It remains for subsequent studies to evaluate the interaction between the organic substrate and the family system in the development of specific psychiatric syndromes.

Conclusions

The study demonstrates that MBD is a frequently missed diagnosis in adolescence. This may be due to the persistence of the myth of its disappearance in adolescence or to the prominence and severity of its psychiatric sequelae. However, it would seem that treatment of adolescent patients with MBD without attention to the underlying deficits and their developmental consequences is fraught with difficulties.

NOTE

The author wishes to acknowledge the contribution of the following members of the Learning Disability Project Group: Loren Crabtree,

M.D.; Barbara Cram, Ph.D.; Ben Geever, Ph.D.; Lisa Schell, B.A.; Alan Zaur, M.D. The author also wishes to acknowledge the invaluable assistance of Mark Forman, M.D., in the preparation of this manuscript.

APPENDIX 1

CHARACTERISTICS OF THE CLINICAL GROUPS

I. *Diffuse Developmental Disorder*

A. Affect: mild lability and dyscontrol with infrequent episodic explosive affect and violent behavior; inability to modulate or dampen affect ("affective perseveration").

B. Attention: difficulty in concentration, task memory deficient, internally and externally distractible.

C. Cognition: global cognitive impairment with marked defects in reality testing, including concrete, referential, egocentric, rigid and over-inclusive thinking with or without overt psychosis; intellectual impairment with borderline intelligence in some cases; disturbances in abstraction, conceptualization, reasoning and judgment.

D. Motor: awkward, uncoordinated, hypo- or hyperactive, restless.

E. Social: global social dysfunction, markedly age inappropriate and immature, imitative, dependent, demanding; significant defect in processing and comprehending socially relevant information leading to intrusiveness, social perseveration, inappropriateness.

II. *Affect-Motor Dyscontrol Disorder*

A. Affect: marked lability, hyperreactivity.

B. Attention: disturbance in attention, concentration and conceptual tracking; distractible, particularly to external stimuli.

C. Cognition: moderate concreteness of thinking, disturbance in abstraction, reflection, generalization, reasoning, judgment, and comprehension.

D. Motor: hyperactive, fragmented, disorganized behavior.

E. Social: intrusive, egocentric, impulsive, destructive, unable to tolerate reasonable authority or limits; often violent and explosive, antisocial.

III. *Discrete Attentional-Cognitive Disorder*

A. Affect: mild lability; marked dysphoria with anxiety, depression; infrequent rage.

289

B. Attention: subtle disturbance, seen only with anxiety in demand situations.

C. Cognition: mild disturbance in association, generalization, conceptualization, and comprehension.

D. Motor: no overt disturbance.

E. Social: able to process and comprehend socially relevant information, function in peer groups, and form superficial affective attachments; tend to be restricted, inhibited, and avoidant, with episodic explosive or delinquent behavior, and often chronic drug and alcohol abuse; may be self-destructive, suicidal.

APPENDIX 2

IDENTIFYING DATA

Patient	Age	Sex	Developmental History	Intelligence WAIS	Academic Achievement WRAT	Qualitative Signs of Organicity from Psychological Testing
			Diffuse Development Disorder			
1	18	M	Neonatal anoxia, hydrocephalus, developmental delay, hyperactivity, learning disability, dependency, temper tantrums	V 83 P 94 FS 87	R 5.3 S 5.0 M 4.5	Global cognitive deficits, expressive language disorders; attention-concentration, perceptual-motor disturbance
2	15	M	Motor, language developmental delay; learning disability; hyperactivity; peer difficulty; dependency	84 80 82	3.9 4.1 4.6	Impulsivity-disinhibition, attention-concentration disturbance, severe visual-motor deficits
3	17	M	Language developmental delay; hyperactivity, learning disability, peer difficulty	95 105 99	5.8 6.5	Impulsive, disinhibited, syntactical problems, attention deficits, concrete reasoning, letter transpositions
4	17	M	Neonatal anoxia with motor, language developmental delay; hyperactivity, learning disability	112 108 111	9.6 7.8 6.5	Inconsistency in intellectual functioning, attention-concentration, impulsive-disinhibition, concreteness in thinking
			Affect-Motor Dyscontrol Disorder			
5	15	M	Respiratory infection (infancy) hospitalization (O_2 therapy); developmental delay, hyperactivity, learning disability, temper tantrums, hyperaggression	70 80 73	3.1 3.0 3.4	Inconsistency in intellectual functioning, impulsive-disinhibited, attention deficits, sequencing disturbance, letter reversals

Patient	Age	Sex	Developmental History	Intelligence WAIS	Academic Achieve-ment WRAT	Qualitative Signs of Organicity from Psychological Testing
			Diffuse Development Disorder			
6	18	M	Hyperactivity, learning disability, hyper-aggression, peer difficulty, dependency	100 99 99	5.2 6.5 8.5	Attention, visual sequencing, concrete reasoning, kinetic reversals, perceptual persev-eration, reading disability
7	13	M	Hyperactivity, learning disability, destructiveness, runaway, truancy, stealing, enuresis, encopresis	105 104 105	7.0 6.1 5.3	Visual-motor disturbance, perseveration, angulations, poor organization, reversals, deficient short term visual memory
8	14	M	Hyperactivity, learning disability, runaway, stealing, destructive, hyperaggression, peer difficulty	72 105 86	7.8 6.7 2.9	Impulsive-disinhibition, attention-concentration disturbance, low frustra-tion tolerance, auditory sequencing disturbance, memory deficit, IQ discrepancy
9	15	M	Hyperactivity, learning disability, truancy, lying, stealing, drug abuse	104 95 100	10.5 7.4 5.3	Impulsive-disinhibition, low frustration tolerance, IQ discrepancy, poor visual-motor matching, attention-concentration disturbance
			Discrete Attentional-Cognitive Disorder			
10	16	F	Prolonged labor, maternal infection and neonatal jaundice, peer problems, over dependency	108 104 107	12.9 10.5 8.0	Attentional deficit, long-term memory-retrieval difficulty, perceptual perseveration
11	14	M	Chronic allergic otitis media (to age 2½) 10 hospitalizations, general anesthesia, surgical drainage; hyperactivity, learning disability, enuresis, encopresis (age 11), lying, stealing, temper tantrums	106 95 101	8.6 8.3 3.3	Inconsistency in intellectual functioning, impulsivity-disinhibition, attention-concentration disturbance, mixed laterality, short-term auditory and visual memory disturbance
12	14	M	Restless, hyperactivity, stealing, peer difficulties	117 114 118	12.0 7.6 5.3	Inconsistency in intellectual functioning, short-term visual and auditory memory disturbance, low frustration tolerance, visual-motor deficit
13	18	M	Prematurity (3 lbs. 3 oz.), respiratory distress, hyperactivity, learning disability (methylphenidate responsive)	114 106 111	12.0 9.6 9.5	Concreteness, disturbance in recall of spatial arrangements, difficulty in organization and conceptualization

291

Patient	Age	Sex	Developmental History	Intelligence WAIS	Academic Achieve- ment WRAT	Qualitative Signs of Organicity from Psychological Testing
			Diffuse Development Disorder			
14	15	M	Chronic otitis media, surgery (age 2), hyperactivity, learning disability (reading), stealing, lying, destructive, temper tantrums	101 121 111	7.8 6.7 6.3	Impulsivity-disinhibition, conceptual difficulty, letter reversals, short-term auditory memory disturbance, WAIS discrepancy
15	16	F	Attention disorder, learning disability, hyperactivity (methylphenidate responsive)	95 102 98	10.9 9.9 6.7	Attention-concentration, short-term auditory memory, inconsistency in intellectual functioning

APPENDIX 3

ATTENDING PSYCHIATRIST AND RESEARCH PROJECT DIAGNOSES

Patient	Discharge Diagnosis (DSM II)	Research Project Diagnosis (DSM III)
1	Chronic Brain Syndrome due to hydro-cephalus Passive aggressive personality disorder	Pervasive Developmental Disorder Passive aggressive personality disorder
2	Minimal brain dysfunction Passive dependent personality disorder	ADD w/o hyperactivity Passive dependent personality disorder Pyromania
3	Schizophrenia, paranoid	ADD with hyperactivity Atypical Psychosis
4	Psychotic depression Drug abuse, Cannabis Schizoid personality	Atypical bipolar disorder ADD with hyperactivity Schizotypal personality disorder
5	Adjustment reaction of adolescence Learning disability Impulsive personality disorder	ADD with hyperactivity Conduct disorder, socialized, aggressive Impulsive personality disorder
6	Situational adjustment reaction of adolescence Depressive reaction	ADD with hyperactivity Paranoid Personality Disorder
7	Minimal brain damage Learning disability Adolescence adjustment reaction	ADD with hyperactivity Conduct disorder, undersocialized, non-aggressive Antisocial behavior disorder
8	Impulsive personality Situational adolescence adjustment reaction	ADD with hyperactivity Conduct disorder, undersocialized, non-aggressive Antisocial behavior disorder
9	Depressive neurosis Adolescence adjustment reaction	ADD residual type Cannabis, alcohol abuse Conduct disorder, undersocialized, non-aggressive Antisocial behavior disorder
10	Adolescence adjustment reaction	ADD without hyperactivity Borderline Personality Disorder

Patient	Discharge Diagnosis (DSM II)	Research Project Diagnosis (DSM III)
11	Situational adjustment reaction of adolescence Sociopathic personality	ADD without hyperactivity Atypical paraphlia vs. exhibitionism Paranoid personality disorder
12	Depressive neurosis Schizoid personality	ADD residual type Dysthymic Disorder vs. Borderline Personality Disorder Cannabis abuse
13	Anxiety neurosis with depression	ADD without hyperactivity Dysthymic Disorder Obsessive Compulsive Disorder
14	Adolescence adjustment reaction	ADD without hyperactivity Cannabis abuse Conduct disorder, undersocialized, non-aggressive Dysthymic Disorder
15	Psychotic depression with agitation Hyperkinesis Syndrome	ADD residual type Borderline Personality Disorder

REFERENCES

Cantwell, D. P. 1972. Psychiatric illness in the families of hyperactive children. *Archives of General Psychiatry* 27:414–417.

Cantwell, D. P. 1973. Genetic studies of hyperactive children: psychiatric illness in biologic and adopting parents. In R. R. Feve, D. Rosenthal, and H. Brill, eds. *Genetic Research in Psychiatry*. Baltimore: Johns Hopkins University Press.

Cantwell, D. P. 1978. Hyperactivity and antisocial behavior. *Journal of the American Academy of Child Psychiatry* 17:252–262.

Cantwell, D. P.; Baker, L.; and Mattison, R. E. 1980. Psychiatric disorders in children with speech and language retardation. *Archives of General Psychiatry* 37:423–426.

DSM III. 1980. *Diagnostic and Statistical Manual of Mental Disorders*. 3d ed. Washington, D.C.: American Psychiatric Association.

Hartacollis, P. 1968. The syndrome of minimal brain dysfunction in young adult patients. *Bulletin of the Menninger Clinic* 32:102–114.

Healy, W., and Bronner, A. F. 1936. *New Light on Delinquency and Its Treatment*. New Haven, Conn.: Yale University Press.

Heussy, H. R.; Metoyer, M.; and Townsend, M. 1974. Eight to ten year follow-up of 84 children treated for behavioral disturbances in rural Vermont. *Acta Psychiatrica* 40:230–235.

Hill, P. 1944. Amphetamines in psychopathic states. *British Journal of Addiction* 44:50–54.

Laufer, M. W., and Denhoff, E. 1957. Hyperkinetic behavior syndrome in children. *Journal of Pediatrics* 50:463–474.

Mann, H. B., and Greenspan, S. I. 1976. The identification and treatment of adult brain dysfunction. *American Journal of Psychiatry* 133:1013–1017.

Mendelson, W.; Johnson, N.; and Stewart, M. 1971. Hyperactive children as teenagers: a follow-up study. *Journal of Nervous and Mental Diseases* 153:273–279.

Menkes, M. M.; Rowe, J.; and Menkes, J. 1967. A twenty-five year follow-up study of the child with minimal brain dysfunction. *Pediatrics* 39:393–399.

Morrison, J. R., and Minkoff, K. 1975. Explosive personality as a sequel to the hyperactive child syndrome. *Comprehensive Psychiatry* 16:343–348.

Morrison, J. R., and Stewart, M. H. 1971. A family study of hyperactive child syndrome. *Biological Psychiatry* 3:189–195.

Morrison, J. R., and Stewart, M. H. 1973. The psychiatric studies of the legal families of adopted hyperactive children. *Archives of General Psychiatry* 28:888–891.

Offord, D. R.; Sullivan, K.; Allen, N.; and Abrams, N. 1979. Delinquency and hyperactivity. *Journal of Nervous and Mental Diseases* 167:734–741.

O'Neal, P., and Robbins, L. M. 1958. The relation of childhood behavior problems to adult psychiatric status. *American Journal of Psychiatry* 114:961–969.

Quitkin, F., and Klein, D. F. 1969. Two behavioral syndromes related to possible minimal brain dysfunction. *Journal of Psychiatric Research* 7:131–142.

Rutter, M.; Graham, P.; and Yule, W. 1970. *A Neuropsychiatric Study in Childhood.* London: Heinemann.

Shaffer, D.; McNamara, N.; and Pincus, J. H. 1974. Controlled observations on patterns of activity, attention, and impulsivity in brain-damaged and psychiatrically disturbed boys. *Psychological Medicine* 4:4–18.

Weiss, G.; Minde, K.; and Werry, J. S. 1971. Studies on the hyperactive child. VIII. Five-year follow up. *Archives of General Psychiatry* 24:409–414.

Wender, P. 1971. *Minimal Brain Dysfunction in Children.* New York: Wiley.

Wood, D. R.; Reimherr, F. W.; Wender, P. H.; and Johnson, F. E. 1976. Diagnoses and treatment of minimal brain dysfunction in adults. *Archives of General Psychiatry* 33:1453–1460.

20 HYPERACTIVES AS YOUNG ADULTS: VARIOUS CLINICAL OUTCOMES

LILY HECHTMAN, GABRIELLE WEISS, TERRYE PERLMAN, AND DAPHNE TUCK

In recent years there has been a growing interest in adults with a childhood history of hyperactivity or, according to DSM III (1980), Attention Deficit Disorder. In fact, this classification lists a residual type of attention deficit disorder which one suspects was included to accommodate this adult group of hyperactives. The interest in adults who were hyperactive in childhood comes from four main sources.

The first is follow-up studies which attempt to identify, trace, and assess adult subjects and how they are functioning. These subjects are usually selected from available childhood medical records. Notable in this retrospective category are the studies of O'Neal and Robins (1958) which indicated that many disturbed children (some of whom had symptoms of hyperactivity) do not outgrow their problems and that this applied particularly to those children who showed antisocial behavior.

Menkes's (Menkes, Rowe, and Menkes 1967) twenty-five-year retrospective follow-up study of eighteen hyperactive patients indicated that fourteen had relatively poor outcomes as adults. However, the inclusion of subjects with IQs of 70 may have affected the results. Unfortunately, no control group was used, which could have been matched for IQ. Somewhat less negative results were obtained by Laufer (1971) and by Borland and Heckman (1976).

Laufer (1971) followed, via mailed questionnaires to the parents, 100 hyperactives aged fifteen to twenty-six years (mean 19.8 years). Only sixty-six returned the questionnaire. Among other findings, 30 percent (sixteen subjects) had had some trouble with police, but none were in jail. Again, no control comparison is available and the results may have been positively skewed by the portion of the subject population which returned the questionnaire.

Borland and Heckman (1976) compared twenty men (mean age: thirty years) whose childhood medical records conformed to diagnostic criteria for a hyperactive child syndrome twenty to twenty-five years ago, with their brothers (mean age: twenty-eight years). They found that a large majority of the men who were hyperactive had completed high school and each was steadily employed and self-supporting. However, half the men who were hyperactive continued to show a number of symptoms of hyperactivity; restlessness, nervousness, impulsivity, and being easily upset. Nearly half had problems of a psychiatric nature and despite normal IQ scores and levels of education these men had not achieved a socioeconomic status equal to that of their brothers and their fathers.

A second group of studies has focused attention on the families of hyperactive children. Morrison and Stewart (1971) interviewed parents of fifty-nine hyperactives and forty-one control children and found a high prevalence of sociopathy, hysteria, and alcoholism in the parents of the hyperactive children. They also showed that significantly more parents of hyperactives than control children had been themselves hyperactive as children. This was not the case for adopting parents of hyperactive children (Morrison and Stewart 1973).

In a similar study, Cantwell (1972) did psychiatric examinations of parents of fifty hyperactive children and fifty matched control children. Again, increased prevalence rates for alcoholism, sociopathy, and hysteria were found in the parents of hyperactive children. Ten percent of parents of hyperactive children were thought to have been hyperactive children themselves and of this 10 percent all were psychiatrically affected by alcoholism, sociopathy, or hysteria. All these studies hint that childhood hyperactivity may be a precursor for certain adult psychiatric illnesses.

A third group of studies involves looking at adult patients and identifying in them a current clinical picture which is similar to childhood hyperactivity as well as a past history consistent with the syndrome. Thus, Morrison and Minkoff (1975) suggested that the explosive personality characterized by sudden intense outbursts of verbal or physical aggression and general inability to control one's over responsiveness to environmental pressures, may be a sequal to the hyperactive child syndrome.

Mann and Greenspan (1976) hypothesized that adults who had minimal brain dysfunction as children constitute a distinct diagnostic entity: Adult Brain Dysfunction (ABD), which may exist alone or with a variety of other psychiatric syndromes. The main characteristics outlined by this group which are necessary to make the diagnosis of Adult Brain Dysfunction include a history of early learning disorder with short attention span; diffuse severe symptoms in adulthood, with elements of anxiety and depression or their equivalent; a rather remarkable, dramatic alteration in the symptom picture with imipramine; and a mental status exam characterized by rapid flow of speech and many shifts of subject, but without overt indicators of psychotic thinking (e.g., circumstantializing ideas of reference).

Wood, Reimherr, Wender, and Johnson (1976) also attempted to make a case for the diagnosis of Minimal Brain Dysfunction in adults. Clinics were asked to refer patients aged twenty-one to sixty who had prominent complaints of impulsivity, irritability, inattentiveness, restlessness, and emotional lability in the absence of schizophrenia, primary affective disorder, organic brain syndrome, or mental retardation. The patients were given self-report forms which tapped most common characteristics of childhood MBD as well as current extentions or manifestations of this condition. A second party report (parents) was also used. Eleven of fifteen subjects were given a double blind trial of methylphenidate; eight showed significant positive response. All fifteen subjects were given open trials of pemoline, imipramine, or amitriptyline. Of these, eight showed good response to stimulants or tricyclic antidepressants.

Other authors, Arnold, Strobl, and Weisenberg (1972) and DeVeaugh-Geiss and Joseph (1980), have also suggested the existence of adult hyperactivity on the basis of "paradoxical" (calming) effect of amphetamine on some selected patients showing similar "hyperkinetic" clinical pictures in adulthood. This, however, has been questioned by Rapoport, Buchsbaum, Zahn, Weingartner, Ludlow, and Mikkelsen (1978), who found similar responses to amphetamines in normal subjects. Nonetheless, there is some support for a clinical entity in adulthood which is similar to childhood hyperactivity.

The last group of studies which has focused attention on adult hyperactivity have been long-term prospective follow up studies. Most such studies to date have followed hyperactive children into adolescence, but not beyond. Generally, they (Ackerman, Dykman, and Peters 1977; Blouin, Bornstein, and Trites 1978; Huessy, Metoyer, and Townseld 1974; Mendelson, Johnson, and Stewart, 1971; Stewart, Mendelson, and Johnson 1973; Weiss, Minde, Werry, Douglas, and Nemeth 1971) have found that hyperactive adolescents continue to have significant scholastic, antisocial, and emotional problems. Stimulant treatment in childhood does not seem to affect this somewhat negative picture in adolescence. It has been suggested that the negative picture in adolescence is in part due to adolescent turmoil, which may be more severe for the hyperactives because of the additional stresses and handicaps they must face. Therefore, the need to follow these subjects beyond the turbulent years of adolescence into young adulthood is evident. Our ten- to twelve-year prospective controlled follow-up study was, therefore, undertaken.

Method

HYPERACTIVE SUBJECTS

The hyperactive subjects were first referred to the Child Psychiatry Clinic of the Montreal Children's Hospital some ten to thirteen years ago, when they were six to twelve years of age, predominantly for long standing symptoms of hyperactivity both at home and at school. They all had IQs of eighty-five or above, were free of epilepsy, cerebral palsy, or psychosis and were living at home with at least one parent. One hundred and four hyperactive subjects had initially participated in a short-term drug study involving chlorpromazine (Thorazine) (Werry, Weiss, Douglas, and Martin 1966) and dextroamphetamine (Dexedrine) (Weiss, Werry, Minde, Douglas, and Sykes 1968).

Ninety-one of the 104 children were reevaluated in a series of follow-up studies during their adolescence five to six years after initial assessment (Minde, Weiss, and Mendelson 1972; Minde, Lewin, Weiss, Lavigeur, Douglas, and Sykes 1971; Weiss et al. 1971). In the present study seventy-six of these ninety-one subjects agreed to participate once more; nine subjects refused. The most common reason for refusal given on the telephone was that they were "doing well" and did not wish to be reminded of their problems. All nine who refused to come for follow-up stated that they were living at home and were working or going to school. Six subjects could not be traced; one subject was dropped from the analysis in order to facilitate matching.

THE CONTROL GROUP

Forty-five normal subjects were selected for the control group. Thirty-five of these were selected in 1968 at the time of the five-year follow-up study of hyperactive children. At that time, notices were posted in three high schools asking for volunteers who would partici- pate in some studies on adolescents in which they would be required to talk with a psychiatrist and do some pencil-and-paper tasks. Payment was offered for volunteers who were selected. The three high schools were selected to represent a range of socioeconomic classes. Many students volunteered, and we included those who met all the following criteria: (1) they matched individually with a hyperactive subject on age, IQ, socioeconomic class, and sex; (2) they had never failed a grade; (3) nor had they ever been a behavior problem at home or at school.

At the beginning of the present ten-year follow-up we decided to enlarge our control group from thirty-five to forty-five subjects. Ten additional subjects were included, generally referred to us by another control subject as being someone they knew at work or school (high school, college, or university). The same inclusion criteria already de- scribed were used to select the additional volunteers. Thus the overall group for the ten-year follow-up study consisted of seventy-five hyperactive and forty-five control subjects matched for age, sex, and socioeconomic class. The control group had a slightly higher mean IQ (table 1).

ASSESSMENTS

Subjects had comprehensive psychiatric (Weiss, Hechtman, Perlman, Hopkins, and Wener 1979), physiological (Hechtman, Weiss, and Perlman 1978), psychological (Hopkins, Perlman, Hechtman, and

TABLE 1
BIOGRAPHICAL DATA: BACKGROUND VARIABLES

Variable	Controls (N=44)		Hyperactives (N=75)		
	Mean	Range	Mean	Range	Significance
Age	19.0	17–24	19.5	17–24	. . .
Socioeconomic status (Hollingshead Scale)	3.4	1–5	3.4	1–5	. . .
WAIS (IQ)	108.1	87–129	105.0	89–136	<.08 (trend)
Sex (%):					
Male	88.64	. . .	90.66	. . .	. . .
Female	11.36	. . .	9.33	. . .	. . .

Weiss 1979), electroencephalographic (Hechtman, Weiss, and Metrakos 1978), and biographical assessments reported on elsewhere.

Details of antisocial behavior, particularly drug abuse and court/police involvement, were obtained during a semistructured open-ended psychiatric interview only after a fairly good rapport had been established with the subjects and confidentiality was assured. The two psychiatrists (LH and GW) had interviewed a number of subjects together and correlated highly ($R = .9$) on interview technique and scoring. One of the interviewers (LH), who was initially blind, quickly became aware of who had been hyperactive in childhood by the nature of the history spontaneously given by the subject.

From the detailed comprehensive assessment outlined, one is left with certain overall clinical impressions.

RESULTS

The clinical outcomes of the hyperactive young adults fall roughly into three distinct categories. First, there are those hyperactive young adults whose functioning is fairly normal. Second, there are those hyperactive young adults who continue to have significantly more social, emotional, and impulsive problems than the matched controls but whose problems are not sufficiently severe to reflect marked psychiatric or antisocial pathology. Finally, there is a third group of hyperactive young adults who clearly constitute a significantly disturbed group requiring psychiatric hospitalization and/or those who are in adult jails.

Even though one can clearly identify these three types of outcome groups at the margins or in the transition between one group and another, there is a great deal of overlap. Therefore, it is dangerous and inaccurate to quote what percentage of the hyperactive young adults fall into one group or another. Very rough estimates suggest that 30 to 40 percent fall into the fairly normal outcome group; another 40 to 50 percent fall into the group with significant social, emotional, and impulsive problems; and finally, about 10 percent are seriously psychiatrically and antisocially disturbed.

FAIRLY NORMAL OUTCOME GROUP

These subjects generally are working full-time or are still attending full-time school (usually at a post–high school level). Their work history is fairly stable and such that subjects see an opportunity for future advancement either in their company or in their general area. Some of the work situations involve mechanical or other technical type training rather than formal academic training. Occasionally work is combined with part-time evening school. Subjects in full-time school are often pursuing some particular training program as opposed to general liberal arts.

Subjects in this group are either living at home or with friends. Few live alone. Their living arrangements are fairly stable with moves not being particularly numerous or sudden. Hyperactive young adults with fairly normal adjustment seem to have some long-standing significant friendships with both sexes. They usually have one or more same sex friends whom they have known for at least several years. They feel close to these friends and can confide intimate problems. They may have also had one or more close heterosexual relationships lasting at least several months. They do not feel lonely or isolated from peers. They get along fairly well with both peers and supervisors at school or work and generally do not have any marked difficulty in their family relationships.

With regard to mood, they are not particularly depressed or anxious. The subjects have normal variations of mood depending on the circumstances and are able to enjoy positive things in their lives. Most will drink socially and have tried marijuana. However, there is no significant drug or alcohol abuse. Similarly, there is no current history of antisocial behavior. This includes the absence of stealing, aggressive acts, or significant numbers of car accidents. Generally, these subjects have fairly good self-esteem and are quite optimistic about their future.

GROUP WITH CONTINUING SOCIAL, EMOTIONAL, AND IMPULSIVE PROBLEMS

Hyperactive young adults are usually occupied with either work or school. However, their work or school history is much more unstable when compared to the control group, or the first group of hyperactives. They tend to change jobs or school programs frequently. Often these changes are made suddenly on impulse following some disagreement with a peer or supervisor. The jobs they occupy are often manual, with little chance for advancement or future career opportunity. There are general statements that the subject would like to get into something else with more of a future, but few specific plans as to how he would proceed. Few of these subjects are enrolled in evening training programs, though they express a vague wish to receive some specific training in the future.

Hyperactive adults in this group give a history of frequent moves. These moves are often characterized by moving in and out of their family home several times. The moves are often sudden and impulsive and occasionally as a result of disagreements with either family members or roommates. More subjects in this group eventually live alone.

This group of hyperactive young adults continues to have interpersonal problems. They often lack long-standing, close, or intimate relationships with either sex. They have more casual friendships, but these come and go. These tend to be recreational friends to go out with from time to time as opposed to people the hyperactive adults can rely on or confide in. Heterosexual relationships tend to be brief and not particularly significant. However, a subgroup does develop a significant dependent heterosexual relationship. Often this person has the role of structuring, organizing, and motivating the subject. When this happens, his functioning improves. Some of these hyperactive subjects feel lonely, but not totally isolated. They often give a picture of continued disputes with peers, supervisors, and family members.

Hyperactive young adults in this group also have more emotional problems. They are more apt to be depressed. Their use of alcohol and marijuana is greater than the control group or the hyperactive group having fairly normal outcome. However, they would not generally be classified as being alcoholic or significantly abusing drugs. Their antisocial behavior is not significant. However, they are more prone to physical aggressive acts and tend to get into more fights. These young adults describe themselves as being short tempered and as "flying off the handle" easily. They also have more car accidents than the control group and the accidents tend to result in costly damages. Generally, these subjects have poor self-esteem, are not happy with their current life situation, and are not particularly optimistic about being able to change it.

GROUP WITH MORE SERIOUS PSYCHIATRIC OR ANTISOCIAL DISTURBANCE

As the heading suggests, this group divides into two subgroups: the psychiatrically disturbed and the antisocially disturbed with occasionally some overlap. Hyperactive young adults in this group are usually not involved in either school or work on any regular basis. They may occasionally have a part-time or temporary job or begin a training program with which they rarely continue. Some have long histories of unemployment and drifting from one job to another. There may also be a history of one or more jail terms for the more antisocial or several psychiatric hospital admissions for the more psychiatrically disturbed. The jail terms are for crimes which include assault, robbery, breaking and entering, and drug dealing. The psychiatric hospital admissions are for suicide attempts, drug detoxifications, and borderline psychosis.

These subjects usually live alone. They also tend to move more frequently and impulsively. This is particularly true when they are living with others and interpersonal difficulties arise. Hyperactive young adults in this group have serious interpersonal problems. They tend to be socially isolated and friendless. They generally have no close intimate friendships and sometimes lack even casual acquaintances. These subjects often use their acquaintances for personal gains, for example, drugs, or become overly dependent on them and so lose even these contacts. There is usually little contact with their family. However, a small subgroup is overly controlled and enmeshed by the family with no contacts outside of family members. Generally, the relationships of this group of hyperactives are either nonexistent, superficial, or very disruptive.

This group of hyperactive young adults has serious emotional difficulties. Some have had serious depressions with suicide attempts requiring psychiatric hospitalization. Others are clearly borderline psychotic though none have presented with florid psychosis. Some subjects present a pleasant false facade which hides a great deal of hostility and despair. Subjects in this group tend to abuse alcohol and drugs, particularly marijuana and minor tranquilizers. Some have wide-ranging drug use which includes cocaine, methaqualone, etc. As described previously, the more antisocial subjects have histories of being jailed for assault, armed robbery, breaking and entering, and drug dealing. This group also has more car accidents which are more costly when compared to the control or other hyperactive group. Generally, these subjects have very poor self-esteem. They tend to live from day to day with little or no view of their future, perhaps because their present is often so bleak.

Conclusions

The foregoing clinical descriptions shed some light on the discrepant and divergent reports about the outcome of adults who were hyperactive as children. Some of these reports were quite negative (Menkes,

Rowe, and Menkes 1967; O'Neal and Robins, 1958) while others were more positive (Laufer 1971). As we see, the outcome is not homogeneous; some hyperactives do well while others do poorly.

Many of the studies on hyperactive adults (Mann and Greenspan 1976; Morrison and Minkoff 1975; Wood et al. 1976) dealt with patients who had come for psychiatric help. Since most of the well-adjusted group of adult hyperactives would be unlikely to seek psychiatric treatment, these studies may be dealing with a negatively biased group. This would account for the pessimism most people had about the adult outcome of this condition. Some of this pessimism can now be slightly modified.

However, what determines good versus poor outcome? In a recent study (Hechtman, Weiss, Perlman, and Amsel 1980), it was shown that no one factor or circumstance determines good versus poor outcome, but a number of key factors (for example, characteristics of the child, his family, as well as the number and severity of his problems) all act together to determine the outcome.

We are thus left with two challenges: one of identifying the various areas that require intervention, for example, family and work, and the other of offering social skills training and remedial teaching as well as prescribing medication, to secure a more positive long-term outcome for hyperactive children. We also need to address ourselves as to how best to help our hyperactive young adults with the more disturbed adjustments.

NOTE

The studies carried out at the Montreal Children's Hospital and referred to in this article were supported by grants to Dr. Gabrielle Weiss from Health and Welfare Canada and the National Institute of Mental Health (USA).

REFERENCES

Ackerman, P.; Dykman, R.; and Peters, S. 1977. Teenage status of hyperactive boys. *American Journal of Orthopsychiatry* 47:577–596.

Arnold, E.; Strobl, D.; and Weisenberg, A. 1972. Hyperkinetic adult study of the "paradoxical" amphetamine response. *Journal of the American Medical Association* 222:693–694.

Blouin, A.; Bornstein, R.; and Trites, R. 1978. Teenage alcohol use among hyperactive children: a five-year follow-up study. *Journal of Pediatric Psychology* 3(4):188–194.

Borland, H., and Heckman, H. 1976. Hyperactive boys and their brothers: a 25 year follow-up study. *Archives of General Psychiatry* 33:669–675.

Cantwell, D. 1972. Psychiatric illness in the families of hyperactive children. *Archives of General Psychiatry* 27:414–423.

DeVeaugh-Geiss, M., and Joseph, A. 1980. Paradoxical response to amphetamine in a hyperkinetic adult. *Psychosomatics* 21:247–252.

DSM III. 1980. *Diagnostic and Statistical Manual of Mental Disorders*. 3d ed. Washington, D.C.: American Psychiatric Association.

Hechtman, L,; Weiss, G.; and Metrakos, K. 1978. Hyperactive individuals as young adults: current and longitudinal electroencephalographic evaluation and its relation to outcome. *Canadian Medical Association Journal* 118:919–923.

Hechtman, L.; Weiss, G.; and Perlman, T. 1978. Growth and cardiovascular measures in hyperactive individuals as young adults and in matched normal controls. *Canadian Medical Association Journal* 118:1247–1250.

Hechtman, L.; Weiss, G.; Perlman, T.; and Amsel, R. 1980. Hyperactives as young adults: adolescent predictors of adult outcomes. Presented at the meeting of the American Academy of Child Psychiatry, Chicago, October.

Hopkins, J.; Perlman, T.; Hechtman, L.; and Weiss, G. 1979. Cognitive style in adults originally diagnosed as hyperactives. *Journal of Child Psychology and Psychiatry* 20(3):209–216.

Huessy, H.; Metoyer, M.; and Townseld, M. 1974. Eight to ten year follow-up of 84 children treated for behavioral disorder in rural Vermont. *Acta Paedopsychiatrica* 40:230–235.

Laufer, M. 1971. Long-term management and some follow-up findings on the use of drugs with minimal cerebral syndromes. *Journal of Learning Disabilities* 4:55–58.

Mann, H., and Greenspan, S. 1976. The identification and treatment of adult brain dysfunction. *American Journal of Psychiatry* 133:1013–1017.

Mendelson, W.; Johnson, N.; and Stewart, M. 1971. Hyperactive children as teenagers: a follow-up study. *Journal of Nervous and Mental Disease* 153:272–279.

Menkes, M.; Rowe, J.; and Menkes, J. 1967. A twenty-five year follow-up study on the hyperactive child with minimal brain dysfunction. *Pediatrics* 39:393–399.

Minde, K.; Lewin, D.; Weiss, G.; Lavigueur, H.; Douglas, V.; and Sykes, E. 1971. The hyperactive child in elementary school: a five-year controlled follow-up. *Exceptional Children* 38:215–221.

Minde, K.; Weiss, G.; and Mendelson, N. 1972. A five-year follow-up study of 91 hyperactive school children. *Journal of the Academy of Child Psychiatry* 11:595–610.

Morrison, J., and Minkoff, K. 1975. Explosive personality as a sequel to the hyperactive child syndrome. *Comprehensive Psychiatry* 16:343–348.

Morrison, J., and Stewart, M. 1971. A family study of the hyperactive child syndrome. *Biological Psychiatry* 3:189–195.

Morrison, J., and Stewart, M. 1973. The psychiatric status of the legal families of adopted hyperactive children. *Archives of General Psychiatry* 28:888–891.

O'Neal, P., and Robins, L. 1958. The relation of childhood behavior problems to adult psychiatric status. *American Journal of Psychiatry* 114:961–969.

Rapoport, J.; Buchsbaum, M.; Zahn, T.; Weingartner, H.; Ludlow, C.; and Mikkelsen, E. 1978. Dextroamphetamine: cognitive and behavioral effects in normal prepubertal boys. *Science* 199:560.

Stewart, M.; Mendelson, W.; and Johnson, N. 1973. Hyperactive children as adolescents: how they describe themselves. *Child Psychiatry and Human Development* 4:3–11.

Weiss, G.; Hechtman, L.; Perlman, T.; Hopkins, J.; and Wener, A. 1979. Hyperactives as young adults. a controlled prospective ten-year follow-up of 75 children. *Archives of General Psychiatry* 36:675–681.

Weiss, G.; Minde, K.; Werry, J.; Douglas, V.; and Nemeth, E. 1971. Studies on the hyperactive child. VIII. Five-year follow-up. *Archives of General Psychiatry* 24:409–414.

Weiss, G.; Werry, J.; Minde, K.; Douglas, V.; and Sykes, D. 1968. Studies on the hyperactive child. V. The effects of dextroamphetamine and chlorpromazine on behavior and intellectual functioning. *Journal of Child Psychology and Psychiatry* 9:145–156.

Werry, J.; Weiss, G.; Douglas, V.; and Martin, J. 1966. Studies on the hyperactive child. III. The effect of chlorpromazine on behavior and learning ability. *Journal of the American Academy of Child Psychiatry* 5:292–312.

Wood, D.; Reimherr, F.; Wender, P.; and Johnson, G. 1976. Diagnosis and treatment of minimal brain dysfunction in adults. *Archives of General Psychiatry* 33:1453–1460.

21 MINIMAL BRAIN DYSFUNCTION IN ADOLESCENTS AND YOUNG ADULTS: DIAGNOSTIC AND THERAPEUTIC PERSPECTIVES

LOREN H. CRABTREE, JR.

A number of investigators have determined that minimal brain dysfunction (MBD) may persist into adolescence, young adulthood, and adulthood (Heussy, Metoyer, and Townsend 1974; Mann and Greenspan 1976; Mendelson, Johnson, and Stewart 1971; Menkes, Rowe, and Menkes 1967; Weiss, Minde, and Werry 1971; Wood, Reimherr, Wender, and Johnson 1976). Further, MBD has been identified as an underlying condition in a variety of delinquent populations (Hartacollis 1969; Morrison and Minkoff 1975; O'Neal and Robbins 1958; Quitkin and Klein 1969) and psychiatric populations (Cantwell 1978; Healy and Bronner 1936; Hill 1944; Offord, Sullivan, Allen and Abrams 1979). In previous studies, Horowitz (1981) and Crabtree, Gever, and Horowitz (1981) reported that approximately one-third of young psychiatric inpatients satisfied their criteria for the designation of MBD. For inclusion, they required a basic skill deficiency of greater than two years in language and/or math, a positive history of developmental lag, and current evidence on psychological testing of perceptual motor dysfunction or equivalent evidence of underlying organic interference. Frank brain damage and organic brain syndrome were excluded. In their studies, more hospitalized adolescent patients (38 percent) than hospitalized young adult patients (20 percent) had underlying MBD. Of the adolescent and young adult patients with MBD, almost one-half presented as an hyperactive-dyscontrol disorder which is the equivalent of the hyperactive child syndrome; about one-third as hypoactive diffuse developmental disorder which is the bizarre, awkward, social isolate—the school misfit who presents as borderline retarded or who academically overachieves at the expense of other developmental tasks; and about one-fourth as specific cognitive disorder which is a discrete attention and/or cognitive difficulty, well compartmentalized and commonly compensated for by significant ego constriction.

Although many of these patients presented, as expected, with behavior problems and delinquency, over one-half of the patients with MBD had a clinical psychosis, either transient, intermittent, or more enduring. Significantly more hypoactive-diffuse developmental disordered patients, whether adolescent or young adult, were psychotic and were commonly misdiagnosed as schizophrenic. Significantly more young adult patients with MBD than adolescent patients with MBD had concomitant psychoses.

These considerations strongly suggest that underlying organic brain dysfunction is not uncommon in hospitalized adolescent and young adult psychiatric patients. In many instances, this feature is not obvious to the examining psychiatrist and is, therefore, frequently overlooked. We were most commonly distracted from making this diagnosis when the patient was psychotic, when the patient presented as hypoactive and withdrawn, or when the patient had a well compartmentalized, specific deficit.

These findings compel the clinician to the question as to how underlying MBD, both undetected and properly diagnosed, impacts on the psychiatric treatment of such patients (individual and family psychotherapy, chemotherapy, milieu therapy, and aftercare). This presentation will focus on these treatment modalities for the adolescent and young adult patient with MBD.

Individual Therapy

The essence of the psychotherapeutic experience is the transmission of understanding to the patient and empathy for his unique experience of self as damaged, defective, and helpless to control the forces and interferences within. Though it may be argued that all psychiatric patients, particularly hospitalized patients, share in common the experience of wounded narcissism and helplessness, the patient with MBD has, in addition, the experience of a brain which will not consistently work for him, a brain which continues to occasion overwhelming frustration and humiliation in his relations to others and the unbearable pain of feeling incompetent. For those with the hyperactive picture, yearnings for peer acceptance combine with deficit-based impulsivity, explosivity, and poor judgment to propel them toward negative notoriety and delinquency. For those with the hypoactive picture, the sense of being a misfit commonly leads to withdrawal, school and work phobia, or overcompensatory enslavement to achievement and social isolation.

Significant involvement in the drug scene in adolescence and young adulthood is a common final pathway for a variety of dynamic, psychopathological, and sociocultural forces. In particular those MBD patients with an hyperactivity pattern seem to move into the drug scene—especially marijuana use. This attempt at adaptation and compensation—leading many to their first real sense of belonging to the peer group—constitutes another variable predisposing the young person with MBD to legal and/or psychiatric difficulty.

In my experience, empathetically appreciating the sense of defectiveness and helplessness to manage the inexorable pressure experienced toward interpersonal, social, and societal catastrophe has proven an essential component of the psychotherapeutic experience. Failure to diagnose underlying MBD clearly renders the therapist vulnerable to predictable countertransference problems, modeled, as they often are, after the response set of the patient's parents. Indulgence in these behaviors in response to the frequently frustrating, dyscontrol-ridden patient and his transferences to the therapist constitutes a transformation of the therapist in the parents' image (Nunberg 1951) and establishes a predictable and not uncommon therapeutic impasse.

In addition to the importance of proper diagnosis to the dimension of empathy and to the avoidance of therapeutic impasse, proper diagnosis is also crucial to make predictable and therefore more manageable a host of other clinical phenomena and specific treatment needs of the patient. These may be subsumed under the dimension of the specific need for structure, congruent with the patient's concrete thinking and lessened capacity for introspective work and insight. The therapist of the patient with MBD must use more than his usual deliberation about how he will handle the need for briefer length of sessions and greater frequency of sessions—especially early in the treatment relationship. He must attend to the patient's need for specific concrete focus, briefer structure, basic vocabulary, and repetition. He must assist the patient in learning problem-solving techniques—such as an approach to complex tasks by breaking a task down into several more concrete and therefore manageable parts and then integrating the separate solutions. The psychotherapist, unaware that he is working with a patient with underlying MBD, may fail to appreciate the enormous utility of working on those basic skills of daily living that we ordinarily take for granted. Unfortunately, the patient commonly cannot bring himself to ask for such help—again consistent with his dread of the experience of defectiveness and stupidity which asking for such help would bring him. His predilection remains to pretend not to care or not to be trying. "I'd rather be thought of as bad than stupid," seems to be his motto. Through the conveyance of understanding and willingness to work with basic concrete tasks with respect rather than with condescension, the therapist is in the position to teach the patient the importance of stating, "I don't understand." Asserting this will help the patient receive repetition and/or more basic explanation from the therapist and others, often what is needed for fuller comprehension and communication. In this and other ways, the patient is helped to take responsibility for his deficiency. This becomes the foundation for the experience of more adaptive ego mastery.

Chemotherapy

A previous study of 100 consecutive young adults used the Crabtree-Horsham Affective Trait Scale (CHATS), which consists of a variety of traits, clinical phenomena, and historical informations which are congruent with the diagnosis of affective illness and/or potential for lithium responsiveness (Crabtree 1981). Interrater reliability was established for the CHATS scale, for various treatment outcome measures, and for the determination of lithium responsiveness. It was established that a high score on the CHATS was a valid predictor of lithium responsiveness and of overall treatment outcome, independent of psychiatric diagnosis.

From the sample of 100 young adult patients, twenty MBD patients were selected for comparison with the remaining eight young adult patients. Eighty-five percent of the MBD patients were found to be in the category of high CHATS (defined at the mean), as compared with only 51 percent of the non-MBD patients. This is a statistically significant difference ($\chi^2 = 7.48, P < .01$).

In that study it was delineated that young adult patients in the high CHATS category who were given a trial of lithium carbonate had an 87 percent likelihood of being judged as lithium responsive (as compared with a 15 percent likelihood for patients in the low CHATS category who were given a trial of lithium carbonate). This finding supports the notion that there may be an important relationship between brain dysfunction and affective illness.

From the total sample of patients who received a trial of lithium carbonate, nine young adult patients with MBD who received a trial of lithium carbonate were selected. Since all nine were in the high CHATS category, lithium responsiveness was compared with the other twenty-two patients without MBD in the high CHATS category who received a trial of lithium. The project team judged that seven of the nine (78 percent) patients with MBD were lithium responsive, which is not significantly different from the comparison subgroup. This supports the notion that certain patients with underlying MBD may be lithium responsive.

Tricyclic medication was prescribed for six of the nine patients with MBD who were given a trial of lithium and one other patient with MBD who was not given lithium. In all seven instances, the tricyclic was judged to be useful in augmenting the stabilizing and modulating effect attributed to lithium or in establishing a stabilizing (as opposed to an antidepressant) effect when it was used alone. The desired effect occurred at lower dosage levels of tricyclic medications (50–100 mg daily) and more promptly (within two to three days), suggesting the need for an alternative explanation as to mode of action.

The ongoing use of phenothiazines was observed to constitute an added interference to functioning in the MBD patient, except during superimposed acute psychotic episodes. In the sample no young adult patient with specific cognitive disorder needed medications. Minor tranquilizers and sedation were not used since adolescents and young adults with MBD specifically and this age group in general are vulnerable to drug abuse and addiction.

EXAMPLE 1

Joan, an eighteen-year-old, single Caucasian, was referred for consultation preparatory to hospitalization for the recent emergence of an elaborate psychosis including hallucinations and delusions. During her childhood she had been diagnosed as having MBD, and she had been treated effectively during childhood and adolescence for this disability. However, she remained impulsive, explosive, irritable, and immature. She developed and was treated for a drinking problem and had bouts of depression of suicidal proportions. She was referred for inpatient care, however, when she revealed to her therapist that beneath her depression and her wish to die was a secret world filled with fantasy, unreality, and hallucinations. Psychological testing confirmed the persistence of perceptual motor dysfunction, impulsivity, cognitive concreteness, and splitting and delineated the psychosis which was overwhelming her.

She was hospitalized on the Adolescent Unit of Horsham Hospital. Lithium carbonate was prescribed for her which was dramatically effective. Her psychosis was shortlived. Her impulsivity and labile mood swings soon gave way to clearcut evidence of self-control and stabilization. However, following this dramatic recovery—and we found this to be the rule rather than the exception for hospitalized patients with MBD—she was beset with disabling personality problems.

Joan struggled with deep-seated insecurity and bad feelings about herself. This aspect was played out in clear focus as she attempted to climb the ladder of success on the Adolescent Unit within their level system. We were able to see that before each step up she would feel overwhelmed with self-doubt and insecurity. Each time she received a level increase, giving her more freedom and independence, she experienced greater tension, apprehension, and insecurity. She believed that she would feel only joy and happiness at these times of success. She learned, first, that increased tension at such times was predictable and, second, that she could overcome this surprising appearance of tension if she resisted using her past security operation, that is, withdrawal to the safety and security of lower-level functioning, and if she gave herself time to develop security and familiarity at the higher level of functioning and independence. Without this clear social system structure, her fear of change would not have been so evident to her and the staff, and she would have handled promotion regressively and self-defeatingly.

Joan illustrates the presentation of an enduring psychosis in a person with previous delinquent symptoms (impulsivity, explosivity, alcohol addiction) and affective symptoms (depression). Her story is not unusual for this form of MBD; hyperactive dyscontrol disorder including a concomitant psychosis, a more common form in the young adult than adolescent. She illustrates further importance of accurate diagnosis for chemotherapy and planning, for structuring understanding of her self, and for reducing the dysphoria and disorganization in the family.

The Family

In addition to the usual social and family history, and assessment of family dynamics for all families, the families of sixty of the 100 admissions in our study were specifically assessed for degree of family dysfunction using the Beavers-Timberlawn Evaluation Scale and the Family Global Health Pathology Scale (Lewis 1976). The families of hospitalized young adults in our study were found to cluster in the mild, mid-range, and chaotic range of family dysfunction. This trend correlated with severity of individual psychopathology in the index patient. Of sixty families studied, eleven families with a hospitalized young adult with MBD were compared with the remaining forty-nine families whose hospitalized young adult did not have MBD. Severity of individual psychopathology in the eleven patients with MBD correlated significantly with degree of family dysfunction ($r = +.615, P < .025$). All eleven families were rated as dysfunctional. Neither finding differs significantly from the findings for the families of the non-MBD young adults in our study (Crabtree and Cram 1981).

Young adult patients with a specific cognitive disorder tended to be rated as mildly dysfunctional and to come from mild to moderately dysfunctional families. Patients with hyperactive-dyscontrol disorder tended to be rated as moderately to severely impaired and to come from moderately to severely dysfunctional families. Patients with hypoactive diffuse developmental disorder were rated as the most severely impaired individually. Degree of dysfunction in their families, however, showed two trends: severely dysfunctional and chaotic family dysfunction was congruent with the severity of individual psychopathology and families with only a mild degree of dysfunction were incongruent with the severity of psychopathology in the index patient but were more characteristic of families of neurotic patients. This latter finding supports the notion that the severity of organic interference and constitutional genetic loading, along with the severity of family pathology, are important determinants in relation to ultimate individual psychopathologic outcome. These findings indicate a clear need for family work as part of an integrated treatment for the young adult with MBD.

Seventy percent of the patients and families in our sample either had never been aware of the presence of MBD or were woefully perplexed and bewildered if it had been diagnosed. The other 30 percent had been aware and were organized around its existence. The diagnosis of MBD, or an equivalent label conveying the presence of an organically based interference to learning and development, was commonly overlooked in our patients, at times because so many other features imposed themselves for attention. Helping the family to develop a workable, tenable perspective about MBD which is positive but realistic and does not set the patient and family up for unrealistic expectations, thereby perpetuating the vicious cycle of failure and recrimination, is crucial to effective work with the family of the young adult with MBD.

Milieu Therapy

The Young Adult Program of Horsham Clinic is a specialty program for hospitalized patients, age eighteen to twenty-five years old, whose average stay is three months and whose diagnostic spectrum includes the psychoses (approximately 50 percent) and the neurotic, characterologic, and self-abuse syndromes (approximately 50 percent). The young adult program consists of the full range of psychotherapies, chemotherapies, and a core program in training for independent living, career choice, and social skills.

In our setting we use a clearly defined, structured-level system for all patients to concretize and integrate the level of function with responsibilities, expectations, freedoms, and privileges. In our experience, this degree of structure is commonly not enough for the young adult patient with MBD. In fact, 60 percent of our MBD patients required a point sheet or a special concrete contract added to the level system structure in order to cope with the stimulation, ambiguities, and stresses of routine hospital life. The MBD patients with specific cognitive disorder, however, who tend to show less psychopathology, did not need a special program.

We rated the degree of peer group "belonging" in the young adult program. Unexpectedly, 60 percent of the young adult patients with MBD were rated as having good to adequate peer relations. Most with positive ratings were patients with specific cognitive disorder who tended to be achieving and accommodating and of the healthier hyperactive patients (without psychosis). However, most hypoactive patients and some of the more impaired psychotic hyperactive patients were rated poor, and two of these patients were significantly scapegoated in the milieu. Though much less profound a problem for out total group than we had anticipated, the scapegoating phenomenon surrounding the more dysfunctional MBD patients must be handled in an ongoing way. We attempt to clarify scapegoating to the MBD patient himself (that he is "setting this up") and to convey this perspective to the peer group, as well, rather than attempting to rescue and protect him. This allows the peer group to confront the usually provocative, scapegoated patient, providing sublimation for their aggression and for the habitual masochism of the vulnerable patients.

Further illustration of common features in the presentation and treatment of the young adult in-patient with MBD emerges from the following case example:

EXAMPLE 2

Bud is a nineteen-year-old, single Caucasian male whose psychiatric admission was his first, precipitated by acute depression and a suicide attempt. He had a chronic history of school failure and delinquency including drug abuse, petty larceny, and vandalism. He had had three years of psychoanalytically oriented outpatient psychotherapy.

Bud was an adopted child, hyperactive and bursting with energy from the start. He had disciplinary and learning problems throughout grammar school. He had been evaluated psychoeducationally during the fourth grade and was sent to a special school for learning-disabled children, where he performed better and was under control. He returned home to attend junior high school and since that time his behavior was reported to have been out of control.

He had been in constant trouble with authorities—those at school until he was expelled and then the law. He drifted into the drug scene where, though he had his first sense of belonging to a peer group, he became gradually poly-drug addicted. He wandered, robbed, and vandalized property. He was jailed on several occasions. He used what was described as poor judgment—at times bizarre—such as going out in the snow with one shoe on. He eventually attempted suicide, which led to hospitalization.

Psychological reevaluation in comparison with testing as a child confirmed the persistence of perceptual motor dysfunction, impulsivity, and mood lability, showed that he had regressed in overall cognitive function, and at times evidenced primitive thinking and paranoid features.

Bud's clinical presentation had two striking components: impulsivity, explosivity, manipulativeness, and delinquency alternating with a self-presentation that was good, righteous, God loving, and God fearing. His verbal productions and content at times were bizarre and idiosyncratic as he described himself as struggling to overcome Satan's influence.

Lithium and amitriptyline were used in combination and led to significant stabilization of his extreme impulsivity and affective dyscontrol and disappearance of bizarre and idiosyncratic psychotic thinking. Attempts to discontinue either medication were followed promptly by regression and decompensation. We did not use phenothiazines for the acute psychotic features because patients with MBD commonly experience the phenothiazines as noxious, especially patients with the hyperactive-dyscontrol disorder and the specific cognitive disorder.

This useful chemotherapeutic result, however, was hardly enough. Although the patient functioned with less glaring deficiency, he remained impulsive and mood dominated, and his sense of self, his identity, remained essentially unintegrated. Bud's approach toward life and treatment remained manipulative and delinquent, though controlled. With medication, vandalism gave way to angry outbursts, but he appeared less lost, more coherent, less unusual, and less grandiose.

He was in our structured-level system, but he could not mobilize to get off the first level (orientation level). He provoked much anger in the staff, who became divided over those who could accept him and those who could not. We introduced a structured point sheet with daily incentives and weekly accumulated incentives. His behavior pattern immediately changed. He attended, cooperated, and participated in all events. In fact, he had to be limited to five contributions per group, so enthusiastic did he become.

After two months, he and his family were able to understand and face that he had MBD as well as a borderline personality disorder. This made the apparent paradoxes and contradictions in his character somewhat understandable. Bud and his family were able to organize around the notion that his control problem was central and aftercare, therefore, would be at a rehabilitation center for at least six months.

Aftercare Needs

Our outcome study (Crabtree 1981) using three standardized outcome measures shows that most of the MBD patients, as is true of the entire hospitalized group of young adults, improve to some degree by the time of discharge. In fact, 57 percent of all young adult admissions are rated in the high improvement category on the Combined Treatment Outcome Measure. Sixty percent of the young adult patients with MBD are in the high improvement category. But the functional level which is attained through this improvement, in 55 percent of the cases of young adults with MBD, is below that which is considered necessary for out-patient, nonresidential functioning. In general, patients with specific cognitive disorder improve and attain adequate functional ratings by the time of discharge. They commonly return to independent living. Young adult patients in the hyperactive and hypoactive categories show significant improvement as well, but many attain below adequate to marginal levels of functioning. Accordingly, only one-third of the total group of MBD patients were discharged to independent living, work and/or school, and outpatient therapy. Most were transferred to a halfway house, transitional partial programs, drug and alcohol rehabilitation programs, and in one instance to another hospital. Many of our patients clearly need remediation for persistent basic skill deficiencies; rehabilitation efforts and training for independent learning, working, and living; and structured training for impulse control, affect control, and drug and alcohol abuse problems.

Conclusions

One hundred consecutive young adult admissions to Horsham Hospital were assessed to determine the incidence of MBD in this psychiatric population. Twenty of these patients satisfied the criteria for inclusion. Of these twenty patients, nearly one-half were categorized as hyperactive-dyscontrol disorder, about one-third as hypoactive-diffuse developmental disorder, and one-fourth as specific cognitive disorder. Over one-half had a concomitant psychotic picture.

Two case reports and data from our study of these one hundred young adult patients and their families illustrated that the physician must assess and diagnose, prescribe appropriate medications, educate the young adult patient with MBD as well as his family and the staff, and delineate existing disability to assure realistic treatment and aftercare planning. Diagnosis of underlying organic interference assists the therapist in appreciating the patient's core experience of defectiveness and powerlessness, and aid in transmission of empathy and understanding to the patient and to the avoidance of common countertransference problems and therapeutic impasse.

317

Psychotherapy must be tailored to the individual patient's needs—essentially for structure—utilizing greater specificity of focus, brevity, repetition, and concreteness of communication. Specific techniques to enhance interpersonal coping and problem solving are essential.

Hospitalized young adult patients with MBD tend to be rated high on the Crabtree-Horsham Affective Scale for affective traitedness. A significant number of these patients are lithium responders and tricyclic responders, alone or in combination. Phenothiazines may prove counterproductive except for the management of acute psychotic episodes. Minor tranquilizers and sedation are contraindicated because of the specific vulnerability of this population to drug abuse and addiction.

The families of hospitalized young adult patients with MBD were rated as dysfunctional and the degree of family dysfunction correlates with severity of individual psychopathology in the index patient, in most cases. Many young adult patients with MBD and their families are unaware of the existence of underlying organic interference or are bewildered about its nature and meaning.

Most young adult inpatients with MBD need more structure than is ordinarily provided in the psychiatric hospital setting. The sense of belonging to one's peer group is particularly important for these patients and may be a significant problem, especially for those with hypoactive syndrome, and may be associated with scapegoating. Aftercare for many young adult patients with MBD must include rehabilitation efforts for drug abuse, impulse control, remediation for persistent deficiencies in basic skills, and training for independent living.

NOTE

This work is an outgrowth of the MBD Project of the Horsham Clinic and the Institute of Pennsylvania Hospital. The Project Team consists of the author; Barbara H. Cram, Ph.D.; Benson Gever, Ph.D.; Harvey Horowitz, M.D.; Lisa Schell, M.S.; and Alan Zaur, M.D.

REFERENCES

Cantwell, D.P. 1978. Hyperactivity and antisocial behavior. *Journal of the American Academy of Child Psychiatry* 17:252–262.
Crabtree, L. 1981. The Crabtree-Horsham affective trait scale: a study

of the prediction of lithium responsiveness and treatment outcome. Unpublished.

Crabtree, L., and Cram, B. 1981. The family of hospitalized young adults: a study of patterns of dysfunction. Unpublished.

Crabtree, L.; Gever, B.; and Horowitz, H. 1981. Minimal brain dysfunction in adolescent and young adult inpatients. Unpublished.

Hartacollis, P. 1968. The syndrome of minimal brain dysfunction in young adult patients. *Bulletin of the Menninger Clinic* 32:102–114.

Healy, W., and Bronner, A.F. 1936. *New Light on Delinquency and Its Treatment*. New Haven, Conn.: Yale University Press.

Heussy, H.R.; Metoyer, M.; and Townsend, M. 1974. Eight to ten year follow-up of 84 children treated for behavioral disturbances in rural Vermont. *Acta Paedopsychiatrica* 40:230–235.

Hill, P. 1944. Amphetamines in psychopathic states. *British Journal of Addiction* 44:50–54.

Horowitz, H. 1981. Psychiatric casualties of minimal brain dysfunction in adolescents. *Adolescent Psychiatry* 9, this volume.

Lewis, J. 1976. *No Single Thread*. New York: Brunner-Mazel.

Mann, H.B., and Greenspan, S.I. 1976. The identification and treatment of adult brain dysfunction. *American Journal of Psychiatry* 133:1013–1017.

Mendelson, W.; Johnson, N.; and Stewart, M. 1971. Hyperactive children as teenagers: a follow-up study. *Journal of Nervous and Mental Diseases* 153:273–279.

Menkes, M.M.; Rowe, J.; and Menkes, J. 1967. A twenty-five year follow-up study of the child with minimal brain dysfunction. *Pediatrics* 39:393–399.

Morrison, J.R., and Minkoff, K. 1975. Explosive personality as a sequel to the hyperactive child syndrome. *Comprehensive Psychiatry* 16:343–348.

Nunberg, H. 1951. Transference and reality. *International Journal of Psycho-Analysis* 32:1–9.

Offord, D.R.; Sullivan, K.; Allen, N.; and Abrams, N. 1979. Delinquency and hyperactivity. *Journal of Nervous and Mental Diseases* 167:734–741.

O'Neal, P., and Robbins, L.N. 1958. The relation of childhood behavior problems to adult psychiatric status. *American Journal of Psychiatry* 114:961–969.

Quitkin, F., and Klein, D.F. 1969. Two behavioral syndromes related to possible minimal brain dysfunction. *Journal of Psychiatric Research* 7:131–142.

Weiss, G.; Minde, K.; Werry, J.S. 1971. Studies on the hyperactive child. VIII. Five-year follow-up. *Archives of General Psychiatry* 24:409–414.

Wood, D.R.; Reimherr, F.W.; Wender, P.H.; and Johnson, F.E. 1976. Diagnoses and treatment of minimal brain dysfunction in adults. *Archives of General Psychiatry* 33:1453–1460.

PART IV

ADOLESCENT SUICIDOLOGY

INTRODUCTION—ADOLESCENT SUICIDOLOGY

ARTHUR D. SOROSKY

It is a well-established fact that the adolescent therapist must possess exceptional capacities for empathic understanding. At the same time he must be capable of emotionally detaching and protecting himself from the ever-present danger of suicidal acting out in his young patients. It is a rare adolescent in psychotherapy who does not experience, at one time or another, symptoms along the presuicidal continuum of ideation, threats, and attempts. Furthermore, it is a rare adolescent therapist who will not have to experience the premature death by suicide of one of his troubled patients.

Suicidal fantasies and behavior are frequent sequelae of the pain of depression, the emptiness of the borderline syndrome, the despair of schizophrenia, and the confusion of drug and alcohol abuse. The ultimate act is more likely to occur when cries for help have gone unheeded and the patient's fears, frustrations, and feelings of helplessness have developed into feelings of isolation, panic, and hopelessness. Therefore, therapeutic intervention is necessary as early as possible in the suicidal process, as repeated attempts are typical and of graduated severity.

An understanding of the suicidal youngster requires a thorough understanding of adolescent psychodynamics. Adolescents are finding it increasingly difficult to disengage from family ties to enter into a world filled with pressures, competition, and social isolation. The fear of failure to succeed in the adult virtues of love and work have driven many a youngster to suicide.

In this part we present a series of chapters which illustrate some of the key issues in adolescent suicidology. It is not meant to provide a comprehensive overview but rather to contribute some new thoughts, approaches, and understanding to this very delicate aspect of adolescent psychotherapy.

Derek Miller believes that recent changes in society, disintegration of the nuclear and extended family, increase in divorce, breakdown in consistent social ties, and drug abuse have complicated adolescence and made young people increasingly vulnerable to suicidal behavior. He describes the psychodynamics of suicide as a defense against the true meaning of death; conflicts about omnipotence, helplessness, incomplete body-image formation, and time sense; failure to develop a capacity for ambivalence; and the lack of resolution of the oedipal complex. He discusses the environmental response to suicide as well as types of suicidal behavior: intentional, marginally intentional, and accidental. The evaluation of suicidal potential depends on direct inquiry and includes social and family determinants, biological factors, and psychological factors—all to be considered in a treatment plan.

Sue V. Petzel and Mary Riddle examine the psychosocial and cognitive aspects of adolescent suicide. They studied family adjustment, parent loss, family conflict, parent characteristics (personality and perceptions, family emotional and health problems, disciplinary techniques), school adjustment (performance, attendance, relationships, behavior, attitudes, stress and social relationships), loss and social characteristics, sexual adjustment, religious affiliation, situational factors, housing and economic factors, military service and war, climatic conditions, cultural factors, media and suggestibility, availability of means, availability of emotional help, cognitive functioning, death concept and attitudes, hopelessness and helplessness, individual characteristics (emotional adjustment, behavioral problems, mood disturbances, diagnostic groups, and general personality functioning), self-concept, and intent and motivation. Petzel and Riddle conclude that adolescents attempting suicide generally are of average intelligence, have a negative outlook, are emotionally reactive, probably are depressed and act out their feelings, and have experienced chronic family and social disruption. Adolescents completing suicide may be even more isolated and disturbed and less visible than those attempting suicide.

Norman Tabachnick considers the interrelatedness of adolescent psychology and suicidal dynamics and believes that these two are closely linked to create the unique features of adolescent suicide. He applies this idea to the psychotherapy of suicide in adolescents, emphasizing the special techniques demanded by this stage of life, and considers such issues as object loss, loneliness and alienation, hopelessness, and helplessness. Tabachnick finds that the metaphor of maternal deprivation is a key one in suicide and the resolution of this conflict through the replacement of old lost objects is the crucial goal of therapy.

Gabrielle A. Carlson differentiates primary affective disorder and secondary affective disorder in adolescents. Primary affective disorder (depression and manic-depressive illness) occurs without a preexisting psychiatric disorder and with a positive family history for affective disorder. Secondary affective disorder manifests similar symptoms but arises in those adolescents with a history of a prior nonaffective psychiatric disorder and a family history of characterological difficulties. These young people present more complicated treatment problems, are often more suicidal, and have more chaotic family situations which result from and then perpetuate the inherent psychopathology. Carlson believes that careful examination of children, adolescents, and their parents reveals symptoms of depression, and the so-called masking symptoms are actually well-documented symptoms of depression in adults.

Maurice J. Rosenthal examines sexual differences in the suicidal behavior of young people and discovers that more men than women commit suicide, more women than men attempt suicide without completing it, and that males tend to use more violent and more lethal methods than females. He hypothesizes that in males the impulse to suicide is less opposed by the wish to live and the dread of dying because it would be deemed cowardly, unmasculine, and self-contemptible. Women, on the other hand, face cultural pressures which foster the notion of personal helplessness and turning to others for rescue. Rosenthal believes these differences have therapeutic implications and outlines an approach to crisis intervention in suicidal adolescent patients.

Shelley Doctors discusses a form of suicidal gesture, delicate self-cutting, and compares this with wrist cutting in general. This phenomenon usually occurs in women with evidence of disturbances in early object relations and the sense of self, seems related to conflicts around the experience of the genitals and genital sensations, and is performed during a period of depersonalization. These girls, owing to developmental interferences, utilize action to express feelings of frustration, an example of which is delicate self-cutting. Self-cutting serves to express the violation of boundaries and to concretely demarcate disintegrating body boundaries. Doctors concludes that through this dramatic act the patient consolidates her cohesive sense of self by soothing herself in the face of the terror of feeling she is falling apart and protecting her relationships from the further ravages of her overwhelming anger.

Michael L. Peck identifies a suicidal subtype, the loner, a particularly isolated group of teenagers with no close relationships and an inability to communicate. This group, frequently diagnosed as manifesting borderline, schizoid, or depressive personality organization, requires early recognition and intensive psychotherapy of the individual and family.

Robert A. Caper describes severe depressive disorder in adolescence which manifested itself as delinquent, acting-out behavior. Caper in his psychoanalytic approach to drug abuse and depression in adolescent girls finds it important to deal with two aspects of his patients' personalities. The depressed infantile core must be recognized and relieved. Further, the struggle with parental imagoes using sadistic, triumphant aspects must be analyzed. The appearance of a capacity for genuine concern and empathy is good evidence that resolution of severe conflict is occurring and is illustrated by the intense transference-countertransference struggles that the therapists of severely depressed adolescents must tolerate. Caper believes a psychoanalytic approach can result in durable improvement in markedly disturbed adolescents.

Irving H. Berkovitz focuses on the powerlessness, helplessness, and hopelessness in late adolescents that leads to violent action. He believes that effective expression of anger during childhood and early adolescence helps achieve separateness and autonomy. When feelings of powerless depression and hostile attachment prevail, the stage is set for the unpredictable eruption of strong, occasionally violent, uncontrolled impulses that may lead to homicide or suicide. Eventually a reorganization of the vulnerable ego occurs as the sequel to reaching deeply repressed, murderous anger.

Thomas Mintz believes that suicidal thoughts are ubiquitous during adolescence and that suicidal problems evolve out of developmental issues. He discusses the clinical issues of frank and covert suicidal efforts. The therapist's countertransference is of great importance during crisis intervention with adolescents and their families.

22 ADOLESCENT SUICIDE: ETIOLOGY AND TREATMENT

DEREK MILLER

Adolescence is a period in which suicide is, statistically speaking, a highly significant cause of death. As a life stage it must be examined before the adolescent's vulnerability to suicide, real or attempted, can be understood. The psychological responses to the physiological changes of puberty are not the same as the psychological reactions of adolescence. Without puberty, however, adolescence is hollow, but pubertal change does not necessitate that the individual become adolescent (Miller 1978b).

Psychological reactions to puberty involve a struggle with a number of issues: in particular, the mastery of an insidious sense of helplessness, a profound sense of split-off omnipotence, and a preoccupation with the bodily self. In addition, thinking processes which in pre-adolescence may have become more formal (Piaget and Inhelder 1969) regress to less sophisticated cognitive modes, the capacity for empathy is impaired, a possible beginning of an ability to be ambivalent is temporarily lost, and a sense of the future and the past is attenuated.

Adolescence proper is a psychosocial process necessary to develop autonomy, awareness of a separate and independent self. Recent societal trends make adolescence, as a specific developmental period, almost impossibly complex. There has been a widespread disintegration of the nuclear family. Parental divorce is almost as common as marital divorce. Divorce almost invariably puts an end to shared parenting and provides little reality against which to resolve oedipal conflicts. Furthermore, there has been a breakdown of the extended family, and consistent social ties have disintegrated owing to vertical and horizontal social mobility. The easy availability and abuse of regressive drugs has made it difficult for young people to develop meaningful emotional involvements with others and to learn that toleration of frustration is part of mature adulthood.

At one time it was possible to divide adolescence into three separate if overlapping stages (Miller 1974). Early adolescence, lasting approximately three years, encompassed puberty and was associated with a high degree of internal turbulance. Middle adolescence, a stage of identity consolidation, lasted two to three years, during which an apparent conformity to adult norms appeared. Late adolescence, a time of coping, was a period in which the new sense of self was tested, experimented with, and enlarged upon.

Except for those young people who avoid significant drug abuse, who have an intact family, who have significant extrafamiliar relationships which are valued, and who participate in a broad educational experience which includes cognitive, creative, and imaginative stimulation, the traditional norms of adolescence hardly exist in some parts of Western society. Many young people have difficulty in developing an autonomous sense of self, becoming instead, "other-directed" adults (Riesman 1954). A feeling of one's self-worth comes to depend almost entirely on the approval of others, often perceived as an amorphous "they," with autonomy hardly present.

Incidence of Suicide

Young people who depend for a sense of worth on being valued by others are particularly vulnerable to psychological stress. Their internal world often appears devoid of conscious fantasy, and they depend for psychological stimulation on external forces, mainly peers, music, and drugs of abuse. When individuals are vulnerable to stress in a society which implicitly (and sometimes explicitly) devalues living, suicide becomes a common technique of conflict resolution (Miller 1980).

Suicide is currently the most common cause of death in the eighteen to twenty-four age group and the third most common in the age group of fifteen to nineteen. In the age group of ten to fourteen it causes as many deaths as appendicitis and diabetes (Weissman 1974). Many adolescent suicides are attributed to accidental deaths, because reliable statistics are unavailable (Petzel and Cline 1978).

Young people generally do not leave a farewell note, and the problem, like many adolescent difficulties, tends to be denied by society.

There are probably five times as many suicides as are actually reported and ten times as many suicidal attempts as completed acts.

The Act of Suicide

True suicide probably requires an accurate concept of the meaning of death. However, the regression and reworking of the adolescent developmental period means that many adolescents inappropriately maintain an early childhood attitude through chronological early adulthood: that of a profound conviction of their own omnipotence and immortality. Thus many adolescents may appear to be attempting suicide, but they do not really believe that death will occur. They seek the experience of death without dying, or they may wish to frighten others. Paradoxically a failed suicide attempt by a young person may reinforce the individual's sense of omnipotence. On the other hand, a conviction about the ease of the act and the probability of survival is reinforced. Many youngsters may then play chance games out of their own sense of omnipotence (Peterson, Awad, and Kendler 1973). By repeated attempts they seek a superman type of mastery to deal with their own helplessness.

Whether an adolescent is capable of understanding the concept of death depends on whether a significant, irrevocable loss of loved figures has been experienced and on the type of thinking of which the youngster is capable. Adolescents who cannot abstract are not totally able to understand death in conceptual terms. A concrete thinker perceives death as a deliberate going away, and even this awareness may depend on having irrevocably lost an important object, person, or thing. Furthermore, an understanding of death requires a sense of finite time. Since the span of today's adolescence has become so elongated, many chronologic young adults are still as much prisoners of the present as would be expected from an early adolescent in a more traditional developmental mode.

Most urban adolescents are no longer tested against natural forces. Contact sports that enhance an awareness of physical vulnerability are the preserve of the few. A false sense of personal power is given to adolescents who are allowed to drive automobiles at sixteen, an age when many have not yet developed a final sense of body image and still have poor reality testing. The perpetuation of a sense of omnipotence and a failure to develop a capacity for ambivalence, both of which are still present in many late adolescents, may mean that individuals who ought to be able to mourn an irrevocable loss are not able to do so.

329

When a loved individual does die, adolescents may deny the significance of death, feeling that the person they have lost is still alive inside themselves. It is as though they keep internal ghosts. These ghosts may be transformed into a type of transitional object (Winnicott 1953). A loved internal figure is talked to as, in the past, a child might have talked with a teddy bear. When life becomes difficult one might attempt to join these internal images of loved ones. Many young people report that they think frequently of dead friends, parents, and grandparents when they are under emotional stress.

When adolescents deal with object loss by internalizing the image of the dead loved one, they create further emotional deprivation. Involvement with an intrapsychic ghost can lead to emotional withdrawal from real people, with the adolescent becoming more isolated, deprived, and empty. The experience of stress is then even more likely to create a wish to join the lost loved one. Thus, a widespread social-system-induced vulnerability to stress ultimately affects personality development as significantly as do nurturing deficits or genetic sensitivity in a social system which otherwise reinforces growth and maturation.

Along with the difficulty of adolescents in developing a capacity to be ambivalent and to resolve oedipal conflicts, many more young people of today are thus vulnerable to suicidal acts. The significance of ambivalence is that if it cannot be developed without constant external support, an adolescent is likely to remain dependent on an archaic superego. Thus there exists a constant need to seek freedom from unbearable guilt from external sources (Fenichel 1945; Freud 1917; Menninger 1931). If mother is either loved or hated (inevitable before ambivalence becomes possible), a solution to unbearable hatred is to fuse with the attacking object (Zilboorg 1936). Because suicide is also a defense against unresolved oedipal conflicts (Glover 1955), vulnerability is further increased. Finally an adolescent with no sure sense of self is extraordinarily vulnerable to separation (Boyer and Giovacchini 1967), and suicide is often a defense against this painful experience.

The Environmental Response To Suicide Attempt

When an adolescent attempts suicide, the response aroused in parents and friends is that of anxiety and guilt. If the suicidal gesture is not successful, the initial anxiety and guilt may be followed by denial, rage, depression, and fear before there is an acceptance of the situation.

Anxiety and guilt in the parents of a suicidal adolescent need to be recognized, otherwise inevitable denial and rage will be ignored. Parents may then find themselves the unwitting reinforcers of a successful future attempt, as it is not unusual for an adolescent to make more than one suicidal attempt. Often when adolescents in treatment begin to insist prematurely that they are now recovered, parental denial may make it possible for them to believe their youngster and interrupt treatment.

Types of Suicidal Behavior

All problem behavior fulfills an economic function in the psyche. Suicidal behavior can be both an attempt to relieve intrapsychic tension as well as a source of such tension. The mere thought of suicide may protect the individual from its actual performance.

A sixteen-year-old girl had a two-year history of uncontrollable intrusive thoughts. These were either sexual or self-destructive and included visual hallucinations of throwing herself out of the window. Throughout this period she felt sure that she would not actually kill herself. Outpatient psychotherapy having failed, she was referred to an adolescent treatment center. She was placed in their special care unit and diagnosed as suffering from a schizophrenic reaction. She was given haloperidol, the intrusive thoughts disappeared, but for the following weeks she was acutely suicidal.

On the other hand, the thought may be the precursor of the act:

A sixteen-year-old boy was admitted to an adolescent treatment center with a history of repeated self-mutilation in which he had attempted to knife himself. Under stress he became acutely delusional and heard a voice telling him to kill himself. This was a precursor to suicidal behavior. He also used threats of killing himself as a way in which he could get his parents to grant his quite unreasonable wishes. For example, a desire to be married.

Adequate medication with phenothiazines ended the hallucinatory episodes. The resolution of the characterological problem in which he was threatening suicide was more difficult.

331

The severity of problem behavior in adolescents, apart from its possible consequences, is not necessarily indicative of its etiology or prognosis of the underlying illness. Suicidal behavior can thus be classified as intentional, marginally intentional, and accidental.

Intentional Suicidal Behavior

Intentional suicidal behavior is associated with efforts at self-destruction which appear deliberate to others, although that may not be the adolescent's real intent. The behavior is usually preceded by more or less subtle warnings which may not be conscious. If the warnings are ignored, such failure at communication may well reinforce the likelihood of the act occurring. Thus all suicidal threats should be taken seriously and skilled intervention should be sought. In this circumstance, the transient expression "I wish I were dead" is not the same as "I am going to kill myself."

The warning of intent is sometimes done by subtle throwaway lines, as illustrated by the following:

A seventeen-year-old boy committed suicide in a hospital chapel by placing a plastic bag over his face. He had been a patient on an adolescent medical ward and was about to be discharged to outpatient psychiatric care, as his physical symptoms did not have an organic basis. He appeared comfortable and accepting of this idea. His death was then even more shocking.

The only possible indication of intent took place on the previous day. He was out for a walk with a young female patient and in the midst of a rather long philosophical discussion he mentioned in passing that individuals should have control of their own destinies including their own life.

One reaction to such a death in the involved survivors, particularly those in the helping professions, is to wonder if the situation could have been averted. Nowhere is this more evident than in a hospital when a patient commits suicide.

One type of intentional suicide is associated with a cognitive, conscious decision to kill the self—a type of predatory aggression (Grey 1972). There may be no evidence that the aggression is directed against a bad introject (Zilboorg 1937). The suicidal decision may be secret, with no previous evidence of intent. A similar story occurs when an apparently well-adjusted adolescent who relates well to parents, teachers, or peers commits suicide. Such young people often do not have a history of psychiatric illness.

Some, retrospectively, have been withdrawn, isolated adolescents who have not made a significant emotional investment outside of themselves. They are individuals with many acquaintances but no true friends. Since conformity is highly valued in the educational system and nuclear family, these youngsters have not been perceived as having problems. Diagnostically, when seen after a failed attempt, they are found to be schizoid individuals whose suicidal attempt is either a despairing rejection of their profound feelings of emptiness or they may be overtly schizophrenic. Others have been depressed for years either on the basis of emotional deprivation or neuroendocrine vulnerability as manifested in endogenous unipolar or bipolar affective disorder.

Other suicidal adolescents have not been withdrawn and seem to have been the healthy offspring of a healthy family. The explanation for their deaths seems to be that some individuals under stress are genetically vulnerable to depression (Miller 1978a). Their pattern is to avoid psychic pain by seeking and conforming to environmental consistency. If the nuclear family has been consistent in its explicit and implicit messages, such young people may appear quite healthy. The unavoidable stress to be faced is the ultimate psychosocial demand for autonomy and separation which appears towards the end of adolescence. At this point acute depression may occur and suicide supervenes.

Some young people who abuse drugs and alcohol, apart from their psychological immaturity, appear to have a potential genetic neuroendocrine vulnerability. Impulsive suicide may occur when they are intoxicated. The stress which leads to such suicides may be psychological, biological, or both. These young people are ill prepared to meet the normative persecutory experiences that are a concomitant of helplessness or the recognition that one cannot be loved as one would wish. The suicidal adolescent may, from a dynamic viewpoint, be destroying a bad introject during the time when alcohol or drugs weaken superego controls. On the other hand, the genetically vulnerable adolescent may significantly affect his own brain biochemistry with drugs and alcohol.

The development of a sense of self requires the capacity to introject and then incorporate the perceived image of emotionally significant individuals and the interaction between them (Miller 1974). The development of a "bad" introject occurs when adolescents perceive themselves as being subjected to overt cruelty by their parents in their environment. To deal with the stress this creates, children and adolescents may identify with this destructive behavior either overtly or covertly (Miller and Looney 1976). Such young people may become intentionally suicidal, homicidal, or both. When homicidal, they may project the bad internalized object onto others; when suicidal, although they may make such a projection, they internalize the bad object. In its destruction they destroy themselves. Occasionally, after the individual onto whom a projection of a bad object was made has been destroyed, the adolescent suicides, thus killing both the introject and its projection.

Intentional suicide also takes place in association with acute emotional deprivation. The depriving figures are felt as deserving of punishment, and this may be associated with the wish to kill oneself to inflict revenge on others. Self-destruction is the ultimate punishment that can be inflicted on others by a boy or girl who may know that such individuals care for them but feel that they do not. Some adolescents may kill themselves in a narcissistic rage. The issue of being hurtful to others is irrelevant; at an emotional level others do not exist. This rage state is associated with an acute feeling that one cannot receive that to which one is entitled.

Another type of intentional adolescent suicide is associated with public self-immolation. Altruism and self-sacrifice are common phenomena in adolescents, perhaps representing an ascetic psychological defense against infantile greed and dependence. Vulnerable to social contagion, some young people may destroy themselves under group pressure. This pressure may be chronic or acute. Chronic contagious group pressure for self-destruction is transmitted by the media. Reports of monks burning themselves to death in Saigon produce imitators in Prague and elsewhere in the West. The suicide is symbolically designed to save the world or to convey to the world an awareness of its deficiencies.

Some adolescents who have no real sense of an autonomous self gain other-directed support by joining cults. If under acute stress a charismatic leader convinces a group that self-destruction is better than being destroyed from the outside, group suicide and homicide may become a preferred solution. This type of suicide has a long and revered history, particularly among minority groups who are, or see themselves, as being persecuted, such as the Israelites of Masada, the Jews of York in the thirteenth century, and more recently the followers of the Reverend James Jones in Guyana.

The etiology of intentional suicide behavior thus includes neuroen-docrine vulnerability; schizophrenia, unipolar and bipolar illness; as well as serious character disturbance. The latter particularly includes those who suffer from the borderline syndrome or pathological primary narcissism. The suicidal act requires an identification with a societal attitude which devalues the significance of human life. This may exist along with either an altruistic or revenge leitmotif, often existing in parallel.

Marginally Intentional Suicidal Behavior

This is usually chronic in nature and is typically seen in those indi-viduals who severely neglect the self; for example, those suffering from anorexia nervosa or those who are accident prone. Adolescents who are repeatedly involved in car accidents, motorcyclists who do not use protective clothing, and those who drive while intoxicated by alcohol, marijuana, or other drugs demonstrate marginally intentional suicidal behavior.

These activities, which are individually related to the regressive re-inforcement of omnipotence, requires societal collusion. Drug and alcohol abusers are particularly vulnerable to marginally intentional suicidal behavior. This group includes the middle-class youth who drives when intoxicated and the ghetto youngster, normally streetwise, who deliberately exposes himself on the turf of hostile gangs. Another example is the chronic heroin abuser who knows that the cut of the drug varies, yet continues to use unfamiliar sources.

On clinical examination these individuals are grandiose and narcis-sistic but they often suffer from a pervasive sense of low self-esteem. Sometimes these individuals enact suicide while hoping that they will be found and saved.

Accidental Suicidal Behavior

Some schizophrenic adolescents have no conscious intention to commit suicide but do so out of a wish to reconcile or fuse with another part of the self. This has been described in twin studies (Maen-chen 1968), but it can also occur in those schizophrenic adolescents who perceive themselves as having "living" introjects (Resnik 1972). Such deaths also can result from a symbolic self-castration, stemming from a desire to engage in a fantasied experience. For example, adolescents who tie themselves up in order to masturbate may accidentally hang themselves.

Accidental suicide may result from the failure of some young adolescent males to be aware of their own physical limitations. Many athletic boys brought up in urban areas and overprotected by their parents have little awareness of their physical limitations. They have been too well protected from natural hazards and so may have little or no sense of necessary physical constraints. Accidental deaths due to poor judgment occur in adolescents who are skating, swimming, or sailing. Such young people are like small boys climbing inappropriately large trees. In contrast, expert mountain climbers who get killed when they climb alone are probably marginal rather than accidental suicides; they know well the hazards of this activity.

The abuse of toxic drugs, particularly LSD and hallucinogens, often produces an acting out of an omnipotency wish. The relationship between the feeling that one can fly from high buildings and infantile fantasies is clear. Grandiosity can be reinforced by regressive drug abuse; under the influence of hallucinogens, fantasies become delusions which may be played out in reality.

Accidental suicide may occur in those social systems which reinforce adolescents' self-destructive behavior. For example, bodily mutilation in psychiatric hospitals is an institutional symptom. Self-mutilation in often highly eroticized and is apparently designed to project helplessness and rage into the environment, and, at the same time, to have the environment return negative attention. Typical behavior includes suicidal threats; cutting wrists, arms, abdomen, or thighs; and putting hands through glass. Although such behavior is rarely directly suicidal, it may lead to accidental suicide. In vulnerable individuals, who thus gain environmental permission for this type of symptomatic behavior, intentional suicide may follow. In a statistically significant way suicidal gestures may be followed by actual suicide (Patel 1974).

The Evaluation of Suicidal Potential in Clinical Practice

The initial interview with an adolescent helps to determine the likelihood of self-destructive behavior. Even if the adolescent has made a positively felt relationship with an interviewer, ideas of suicide are unlikely to be volunteered unless the youngster is acutely distressed. Even then the subject may only appear if the inquiry is made about suicidal thoughts or previous attempts. If the questions are not asked, the information is rarely volunteered.

In evaluating the likelihood of suicide a careful study of the potential social, biological, and psychological determinants of such behavior is necessary. In initial interviews treatability is assessed primarily on the basis of the adolescent's ability to relate to a therapist in such a way that problem behavior can be contained, the type of frustration that caused it can be determined, and the severity of the problem ascertained.

With behavior that is dangerous to the self or others, there is no room for symptomatic maneuverability. The behavior must be stopped. An issue is whether or not the adolescent is able to make the commitment that efforts at self-hurt will not be made without giving the therapist a chance to intervene. A therapist cannot function effectively with the persistent anxiety that a boy or girl in treatment is likely to attempt suicide. If such an assurance cannot be obtained, inpatient treatment is indicated, although this may be necessary for other reasons. It is my opinion that adolescents are almost always honest about suicidal impulses. If they are unable to agree not to kill themselves without first contacting the therapist and offering a chance for appropriate intervention, they will make this known.

Social and Family Determinants of Suicidal Behavior

Young people who are vulnerable to suicide often have a long history of social and psychological problems which may include antisocial behavior, particularly of a monosymptomatic type. A failure to make satisfactory interpersonal relationships and a pervasive feeling of emptiness are common findings. The youngster may come from a subculture in which life is especially devalued. Particularly vulnerable are certain minority groups.

A history of parental suicide makes the adolescent particularly vulnerable (Maxmen and Tucker 1973). The explicit and implicit message of this parental act is that such behavior is acceptable. Furthermore, mourning in children and adolescents for lost parents is almost always incomplete. The child who loses a parent of the same sex may have to attempt to replace that parent with the one who survives. After parental suicide, if the remaining parent remarries (another loss) the child may then become a greater suicidal risk as a result of what is felt as a final abandonment.

Apart from parental suicide, other parental patterns are common in the etiology of adolescent suicide. Parents may be significantly over-involved with their youngster. They may be highly intrusive, thus making it difficult for a boy or girl to develop a sense of autonomy. They may depersonalize their child by being overpermissive or over-restrictive. A history of significantly perceived parental rejection often precedes attempted suicide.

Biological Factors

Unipolar and bipolar illnesses and schizophrenia are still commonly misdiagnosed in children and adolescents because of their atypical pre-sentation. Adolescents who suffer from episodic dyscontrol syndromes are vulnerable to suicide because of the helplessness the syndrome engenders. Finally, those who do not develop a capacity for predatory violence as a defense against affective rage are more likely to be suici-dal risks.

Most adolescent depression is associated with behavioral disorders (Masterson 1970). Either passive compliance or focal anger directed towards objects or individuals who come to represent an externaliza-tion of the image of an unloving parent are commonly found. Depres-sion should be suspected if the behavioral disorder is initially monosymptomatic and occurs at apparently inexplicable intervals, if there is a history of mental illness in the family, if there is an eating or sleeping disorder, and if the world is felt as particularly persecutory in the morning.

Adolescents who suffer from epilepsy may be vulnerable to suicide (Gunn 1973), particularly those who suffer from the temporal lobe form. Pregnancy, menstruation, and physical illness are all of some significance in the etiology of suicidal behavior, depending on how well the adolescent masters the helplessness these syndromes produce.

Psychological Factors

Patients who seriously think of suicide generally have a pre-conceived plan. There is no evidence that direct questioning increases the chance of the plan being put into operation. It is important to check whether patients have the means to kill themselves. If they are known to have these, and the potential instruments are not withdrawn, the therapist is placed in a position of unwitting collusion, much in the same manner as the family members are involved.

A common pervasive feeling prior to suicide is that of extreme helplessness and a frantic need to act. It appears to the patient that the only effective way of changing the situation is self-destruction. Sometimes this helplessness is related to an overpowering feeling of rage.

In summary the diagnostic clues to potential suicide are as follows:

1. On inquiry, the patient will reveal that the idea of suicide has occurred. The reasons for not acting may be unsatisfactory: "I am afraid I will fail" or "I don't want to hurt myself." Depression is present either due to neuroendocrine dysfunction or deprivation. The act is associated with guilt, anger, or thoughts of revenge. Depression may be felt as an emptiness.
2. There is a history of previous attempts often associated with episodic dyscontrol as a stress response.
3. There may be a history of previous treatment and its failure. Sometimes the failure of treatment may be owing to a physical illness. Adolescents who are fearful of a recurrence of a serious illness, such as carcinoma, may attempt suicide.
4. There may be unresolved problems with separation and bereavement. Death tends to cause guilt in surviving children. Those who feel acutely guilty may attempt to kill themselves. This is also related to the fantasy wish of joining the loved ones.
5. Relatives have been told by patients that they are thinking of suicide, whereas the patient will not always indicate this to the physician. If this is not reported, the inaction of the relatives is taken as permission.
6. There may be a history of repeated accidents, especially in automobiles.
7. The basic personality structure prior to the attack is significant. Many patients who previously had a highly organized compulsive personality, may, when faced with overwhelming despair, attempt suicide. Immature personalities who make repeated attempts ultimately may be successful. These attempts should not be dismissed as merely attention-seeking behavior.

Treatment

Initially, an assessment must be made of the need of the patient for life protection. To some extent this need is assessed in terms of a review of the social, psychological, and biological systems which impinge upon the patient. If the suicidal crisis is a reaction to an overwhelming stress, it is clear that the patient needs emergency protection. This is a particularly relevant issue if divorce or death are the stress precipitants. When these occur, apart from the direct effect on the adolescent, the social system in which the patient lives is less supportive than it otherwise might be.

Sometimes the suicidal crisis is a representation of an internal decompensation, as described by Menninger (1962). The decompensation may not occur as the result of a reality stress; it may be related to the patient's internal perception. Under these circumstances the patient will almost certainly need ongoing protection.

Determining the need for hospitalization depends on the strength of a relationship that is made with the interviewer, on whether the therapist knows that he or she can offer continuity of care, and on whether other people in the patient's world are supportive.

Some adolescents are so emotionally bankrupt, particularly the chronic drug abusers or alcoholics, that they have no significant objects in their lives. This may be a particular issue when they have been involved in drug dealing, because drug dealers alienate others in their role as exploiter. In addition, their family and friends are often angry and alienated. Their survival then seems, to themselves, to be quite irrelevant to others. As a result, these individuals may become highly suicidal and will require hospitalization.

If the adolescent patient has to be hospitalized, the issue of appropriate suicidal precautions is relevant. Ultimately it is not possible to protect a patient who is determined, whatever the situation, to suicide. However, if suicidal precautions respect the dignity of the patient, overt self-destructive efforts within a hospital setting are less likely.

An essential attitude on the part of an adolescent program which looks after potentially suicidal individuals is an expectation that people will survive, that life is worth living.

If the patient is suffering from unipolar or bipolar illness, appropriate medication is called for. However, most antidepressant drugs do not have an immediate effect, and there is always the possibility that when they do begin to take effect the patient will become suicidal. In my opinion there is no indication for the use of electroconvulsive therapy in adolescents.

Insofar as family relationships are concerned, the family should be warned, as with adults, that the period of recovery from depression is when the patient is most vulnerable. If the underlying illness or character disorder is not susceptible to psychotherapy, the family should be told, as an essential part of the informed-consent procedure, that safety cannot be guaranteed.

Conclusions

Suicidal adolescents require every parameter of good therapy. Treatment procedures designed only to deal with acute crises, which encapsulate brief interventions, lead at best to chronic adult mental illness and at worst to the ultimate death of the adolescent.

REFERENCES

Boyer, L.B., and Giovacchini, P.L. 1967. *Psychoanalytic Treatment of Schizophrenic and Characterological Disorders*. New York: Aronson.

Fenichel, O. 1945. *The Psycho-Analytic Theory of Neurosis*. New York: Norton.

Freud, S. 1917. Mourning and melancholia. *Standard Edition* 14:237–258. London: Hogarth, 1957.

Glover, E. 1955. *The Technique of Psychoanalysis*. New York: International Universities Press.

Grey, J.S. 1972. The structure of emotions and the limbic system. *Ciba Symposium* 8:92–93.

Gunn, J. 1973. Affective and suicidal symptoms in epileptic patients. *Psychological Medicine* 3:108–114.

Maenchen, A. 1968. Object cathexis in a borderline twin. *Psychoanalytic Study of the Child* 23:438–456.

Masterson, J. 1970. Depression in adolescent character disorders. *Proceedings of the American Psychological Association* 59:242–257.

Maxmen, J.S., and Tucker, G.J. 1973. No exit: the persistently suicidal patient. *Comprehensive Psychiatry* 14:71–79.

Menninger, K.A. 1931. Psycho-analytic aspects of suicide. *Archives of Neurology and Psychiatry* 25:1369–1391.

Menninger, K.A. 1962. *The Vital Balance*. New York: Viking.

Miller, D. 1974. *Adolescence: Its Psychology, Psychopathology and Psychotherapy*. New York: Aronson.

Miller, D. 1978a. Affective disorders in adolescence: mood disorders and the differential diagnosis of violent behavior. In F.J. Ayd, ed.

Depression: The World's Major Public Health Problem. Baltimore: Ayd.

Miller, D. 1978b. Early adolescence: its psychology, psychopathology and implications for therapy. *Adolescent Psychiatry* 6:434–447.

Miller, D. 1980. The treatment of severely disturbed adolescents. *Adolescent Psychiatry* 8:469–481.

Miller, D., and Looney, J. 1976. Determinants of homicide in adolescents. *Adolescent Psychiatry* 4:231–252.

Patel, N.S. 1974. A study of suicide. *Medicine, Science and the Law* 14:129–136.

Peterson, A.M.; Awad, G.A.; and Kendler, A.C. 1973. Epidemiological differences between white and non-white suicide attempts. *American Journal of Psychiatry* 130:1071–1076.

Petzel, S.V., and Cline, D.W. 1978. Adolescent suicide: epidemiological and biological aspects. *Adolescent Psychiatry* 6:239–266.

Piaget, J., and Inhelder, B. 1969. *The Psychology of the Child*. New York: Basic.

Resnik, H.L.P. 1972. Erotized repetitive hanging: a form of self-destructive behavior. *American Journal of Psychotherapy* 26:4–21.

Riesman, D. 1954. *The Lonely Crowd*. New York: Anchor.

Weissman, M.M. 1974. The epidemiology of suicide attempts: 1960–1971. *Archives of General Psychiatry* 30:737–746.

Winnicott, D.W. 1953. Transitional objects and transitional phenomena: a study of the first not-me possession. *International Journal of Psycho-Analysis* 34:89–97.

Zilboorg, G. 1936. Differential diagnostic types of suicide. *Archives of Neurology and Psychiatry* 35:270–291.

Zilboorg, G. 1937. Considerations of suicide with particular reference to the young. *American Journal of Orthopsychiatry* 7:15–31.

23 ADOLESCENT SUICIDE: PSYCHOSOCIAL AND COGNITIVE ASPECTS

SUE V. PETZEL AND MARY RIDDLE

Adolescent suicide is an increasing problem. The current (1975) rate, 11.8 per 100,000[1] for fifteen- to twenty-four-year-olds, is the highest rate ever recorded in the United States for this age group and is closer to the total population rate (12.7) than it has been throughout this century (U.S. Department of Health, Education, and Welfare 1956, 1963–1979, 1967). While suicide represents the ninth leading cause of death for persons of all ages, it represents the third leading cause of death for fifteen- to twenty-four-year-olds, preceded only by accidents (60.3) and homicide (13.7) for this youth group (U.S. Department of Health, Education, and Welfare 1979). Although such statistics help to dramatize the problem of suicide for adolescents, they do not contribute to better understanding. It is through greater understanding of the epidemiological and biological aspects (Petzel and Cline 1978) as well as the psychosocial and cognitive factors that more effective prevention and intervention strategies may be developed.

Studies of Social Determinants

FAMILY ADJUSTMENT

For the suicidal adolescent, the organization of the family and the interactions within it have been major areas of study. These studies suggest that suicidal youths experience greater family disorganization than nonsuicidal youths and that continued youthful suicidal behavior may be associated with an inability to achieve adequate family relationships. Elements of family disorganization have included parent loss and family conflict, and a variety of parent characteristics such as emotional problems, health problems, and negative attitudes that characterize parent-child relationships. Parent disciplinary techniques also have been considered in relationship to adolescent suicide. Data regarding families and adolescent suicide tend to be based on demographic research, clinical observations, and case studies rather than empirical studies even though methods of direct, experimental study of the family as a unit have developed in recent years.

PARENT LOSS

Studies with adults suggest that a childhood characterized by parental discord and the intentional separation of parent from child is associated with attempted suicide in adult life, while a childhood characterized by the loss of a parent through natural causes appears unrelated (Crook and Raskin 1975). Many studies also have examined the effect of parent loss on subsequent youthful suicidal behavior. Loss of a parent or other loved one probably stimulates suicidal activity in adolescents in different ways, including an effort to copy the parent's example and self-blame for the loss and desired reunion with the lost one (Seiden 1969). Theories of Zilboorg (1936) and Bowlby (1961), as well as studies with adults (Dorpat, Jackson, and Ripley 1965; Maletsky 1973; Ropschitz and Ovenstone 1968), suggest that parent loss in childhood predisposes to depression and suicidal behavior later in life. Parent loss also may be associated with continued suicidal behavior in adolescents (Barter et al. 1968).

Recent studies of adolescents attempting suicide indicate an incidence of actual or threatened parent loss by divorce, separation, desertion, and/or death ranging from 25 to 84 percent (Barter et al. 1968; Crumley 1979; Haider 1968; McIntire and Angle 1970, 1971a, 1971b; Margolin and Teicher 1968; Sabbath 1971; Schrut 1968; Senseman 1969; Teicher 1970; Whitlock and Edwards 1968). Most studies have not used control groups. However, when the same indices of loss have been used for suicidal and nonsuicidal adolescents, studies have found (Dizmang et al. 1974; Jacobs 1971) and failed to find (Mattsson, Seese, and Hawkins 1969; Peck and Schrut 1971; Stanley & Barter 1970; Stevenson, Hudgens, Held, Meredith, Hendrix, and Carr 1972) a greater incidence of parent loss in suicidal compared with nonsuicidal adolescents. In studies documenting a positive correlation between parent loss and the development of suicidal behavior, loss has been part of a pattern of family and social disruption. No significant difference in the nature of parent loss (e.g., death, divorce, separation, adoption, other) has been suggested in recent studies (Adam, Lohrenz, and Harper 1973). However, a greater percentage of parent losses occurring before age twelve for suicidal compared with psychiatrically disturbed–nonsuicidal controls has been reported (Stanley and Barter 1970). A greater incidence of parents divorcing, separating, and/or remarrying during the onset of adolescence also has been reported for suicidal compared with nonsuicidal adolescents (Jacobs 1971). When the incidence of suicidal fantasy for individuals who have and have not experienced childhood parental losses has been studied, a significant correlation between early parent loss (i.e., loss of parent before child was sixteen) and suicidal ideation has been reported, while no correlation was found between development of suicidal ideas and the specific age of the child when the parent was lost. Such results suggest that the presence of both parents throughout childhood protects the child from suicidal thoughts and that suicidal thoughts are not universal in the adolescent period (Adam et al. 1973).

FAMILY CONFLICT

Family conflict, characterized by anger, ambivalence, rejection, and/or communication difficulties, is frequently present in families in which adolescent suicidal behavior occurs. Marital and parent-child conflict, especially chronic conflict, are not unique to families of suicidal adolescents but have been reported within families of suicidal individuals of all ages (Roberts and Hooper 1969; Ropschitz and Ovenstone 1968; Rosenbaum and Richman 1970; Spalt and Weishbuch 1972).

Children and adolescents attempting suicide tend to view their family conflict as extreme and long standing (Sabbath 1969, 1971; Teicher 1970). Parents particularly are seen as major sources of anger and as unable to be depended upon for support (Cantor 1976). The conflict-filled home environment of adolescents who attempt suicide includes frequent quarreling leading to emotional disorganization (Haider 1968); strife, distrust, and resentment of parent(s)/stepparent(s) (Jacobs 1971); and decreasing communication (Mattsson et al. 1969; Schrut 1968). Disturbed relations with parents have been described as the "most important extrinsic factor in the emotional disturbances" of adolescents attempting suicide (Lukianowicz 1968). A climate of family discord and unhappiness, including major communication problems, also has been reported by parents of adolescents who successfully complete suicide (Bagley and Greer 1972; Sanborn, Sanborn, and Cimbolic 1973). Additional documentation of family conflict has been provided by Williams and Lyons (1976), who compared twelve individually matched, intact family tetrads, six normal and six containing an adolescent female who had exhibited suicidal behavior. This represents the most direct study of family interactions and adolescent suicidal behavior. The families of suicidal girls, compared with families of normal girls, contained higher rates of conflict and negative reinforcement. Suicidal adolescent girls engaged in conflict with either or both parents but displayed little conflict with their siblings.

Hendin (1969) studied young adult blacks attempting suicide (ages nineteen to thirty-five) and noted a relationship between black suicide, rage, and violence. Although Hendin included few adolescents in his study, description of family background during childhood and adolescence for his suicidal sample indicates chronic dislike of family, aggression and abuse within the family, lack of understanding and rejection by parents, violent death within the family, and rage, especially toward the mother. Other reports of violence and aggression within families of suicidal adolescents have included descriptions of paternal aggression associated with alcohol abuse and directed at the suicidal adolescent (Sabbath 1971) and family chaos in which violence served as a model (Maletsky 1973).

Family conflict has been reported not only as part of the family background of suicidal adolescents but also as one of the experiences occurring at the time of the adolescent's suicidal behavior. Acute conflict between child and parental figures has been described as the most common event triggering childhood and adolescent emergency psychiatric referrals, many of which were associated with suicidal attempts or threats (Mattsson et al. 1969). For adolescents, a "poor" relationship with parents has been described as the most frequent reason given for attempted suicide (Senseman 1969), and family problems appear to be one of the significant stresses occurring at the time of self-poisoning (McIntire and Angle 1970, 1971a, 1971b).

In families of suicidal adolescents, conflict within the family may involve the suicidal adolescent directly, as in parent-child conflict, or, as with marital discord, may be part of the family environment. For suicidal adolescents, conflict between their parents may be inferred when parent loss is the result of divorce and, frequently, separation.

For adolescents attempting suicide, conflict between parents also frequently has been identified explicitly (Barter et al. 1968; Senseman 1969). A detailed statistical study of parental discord has not been reported, but disappointment (Sabbath 1971), "sadomasochistic interaction" (Cazzullo, Balestri, and Generali 1968) and quarreling (Haider 1968; Jacobs 1971; Schrut 1968; Stanley and Barter 1970) have been identified. Stanley and Barter (1970) studying adolescent attempted suicide reported "family conflict," defined as marital discord, did not differ in amount between experimental and control (psychiatrically disturbed–nonsuicidal) groups. However, threats of divorce or separation were significantly more frequent than fighting/quarreling or alcohol abuse among parents of adolescents attempting suicide compared with parents of controls. Therefore, it may be the specific nature of the discord and not the extent of conflict that is significant.

Rejection of the adolescent by the family represents another dimension of family conflict characterizing family relationships of suicidal adolescents. Family rejection also may characterize suicidal individuals of all ages (Ropschitz and Ovenstone 1968; Rosenbaum and Richman 1970). Studies have emphasized the intensely ambivalent nature of the parent-child relationship, especially the mother-child relationship, in suicidal adolescents (Friedman, Glasser, Laufer, Laufer, and Wohl 1972; Hendin 1969; Margolin and Teicher 1968). In addition, paternal and parental abandonment (Resnik and Dizmang 1971; Sabbath 1969, 1971) and parental indifference and denial in response to problems of their suicidal children repeatedly have been described (Cazzullo et al. 1968; Yusin, Sinay, and Nihira 1972). Sabbath, in particular, has proposed the concept of the "expendable child." In cases of attempted and completed suicide, Sabbath described chronic problems in the parent-child relationship. During adolescence, suicidal teenagers felt abandoned and complied with a parental wish, explicitly or tacitly conveyed, to be rid of them. Rosenbaum and Richman (1970) interviewed family groups of nonsuicidal and suicidal individuals (all ages). They found family conflicts in both family groups. However, the suicidal person was the object of aggression, was not able or permitted to respond, and was seen as able to save the family by removing himself.

Rejection in a different direction also has been suggested. Jacobs (1971), looking at parental remarriage, reports 40 percent of adolescent suicide attempters had stepparents. In every case, the stepparent was seen by the adolescent as unwanted. Similarly, Teicher (1970) reports that among adolescents attempting suicide who have stepparents, 84 percent felt the stepparent was unwanted.

Family conflict and parent loss often are described as indices of family disorganization. Other indices of family stress and disorganization have been reported to be associated with adolescent suicidal behavior. These include a high incidence of multiple primary caretakers (Dizmang et al. 1974); an inability to achieve an adequate family relationship, including an inability to live at home (Barter et al. 1968); frequent residential changes (Jacobs 1971; Schrut 1968; Teicher 1970); and problem-making environmental changes, for example, sibling leaving home, foster home placement, parents remarrying, death in family (Teicher 1970).

PARENT CHARACTERISTICS

Since families, and especially parents, have been implicated as contributing to adolescent suicide, it is relevant to identify what qualities may typify parents of suicidal adolescents and how suicidal adolescents perceive their parents. The roles, contributions, and perceptions of parents probably differ with their gender and may vary with the gender of the suicidal adolescent. The psychological and physical health of parents also may have contributing effects in the etiology of adolescent suicide.

PERSONALITY AND PERCEPTIONS OF PARENTS

Adolescents attempting suicide have characterized their fathers as helpful and friendly but insignificant in their lives (Friedman et al. 1972) and have allowed them to escape criticism or anger even when they had been totally rejected by their fathers (Hendin 1969). Lack of a meaningful relationship with a male during early development has been reported in adolescent males attempting suicide. Early maternal deprivation, role reversal with the mother or parents (Margolin and Teicher 1968; Teicher 1970), and a negative relationship with both parents also have been reported for suicidal adolescents. Mothers frequently were seen as rejecting and hostile or domineering and fathers as alcoholic and noncommunicative (Senseman 1969). An inability to please parents and unjust isolation within the family have been described by adolescent girls attempting suicide, who often feel guilty for being a burden to

348

their mothers who raised them as single parents. Other repetitive themes described by adolescent girls attempting suicide included maternal (*a*) depreciation of femininity, (*b*) disparagement of men and sexuality, (*c*) expectation of abandonment by men, and (*d*) covert support for the daughter's promiscuity (Schrut 1968).

Several studies have used control groups to identify characteristics of parents of suicidal adolescents. Peck and Schrut (1971) studied suicidal and nonsuicidal college students. Students rated early parent-child experiences as highly contributory to suicidal predispositions, with the mother first and then the father judged as contributing. In the committed suicide group, parents had greater overt striving for success for themselves and their children and lacked acceptance of their children. Parents of attempt and ideation groups were more passive, had few goals for their children, and responded with little support or enthusiasm to their children's success or failure. Peck and Schrut suggest suicide attempt and ideation students realize they cannot please or get a response from parents and, under stress, turn to suicidal behavior to be heard.

Marks and Haller (1977) compared adolescents who attempted suicide with emotionally disturbed nonsuicidal adolescents. Suicidal boys, in contrast with other emotionally disturbed male adolescents, had mothers who drank alcohol excessively and were not close to their fathers during childhood. Suicidal girls, in contrast with other emotionally disturbed adolescent females, viewed both parents as passive while they were young. Fathers were viewed as cold, fearful, critical, and capricious and mothers as more predictable. During adolescence, alienation from fathers continued. Thus, suicidal adolescent girls in particular experienced estrangement from parents.

Other family studies suggest families of adolescent girls attempting suicide represent a malfunctioning system, differing from families of normal girls by their less effective productivity, impaired interaction, ineffective communication, and higher rates of negative reinforcement (Williams and Lyons 1976). In addition, parents of suicidal adolescents, compared with parents of other adolescents in crisis (aggressive, psychotic, psychotic-drug groups), have demonstrated less reaction (i.e., anger, worry, fear, or confusion) to the crisis and have been perceived by the adolescents as less concerned about socially acceptable behaviors (Yusin et al. 1972). These parents disapproved of behavior by silence and withdrawal and were less likely to use physical punishment, to expect obedience, or to want improved communication with their children. They also were not likely to contact a psychiatric facility about the suicidal crisis.

Psychopathology in families of adolescents demonstrating suicidal behavior has been identified in many studies. Dimensions associated with parental problems have included parent (*a*) suicide and suicide preoccupation, (*b*) depression, (*c*) alcoholism, and (*d*) vague, more general categories, such as "unresolved problems" or "mental history."

Reports of parental or family suicidal behavior for adolescents attempting or completing suicide vary from 10 to 15 percent (Crumley 1979; Margolin and Teicher 1968; Sanborn et al. 1973; Schrut 1968; Teicher 1970, 1975). In approximately 2 percent of completed suicides for persons of all ages and 10 percent of adolescent completed suicides (ages ten to nineteen), a family history of suicide has been reported (Patel 1974). Studies using control groups have found (Jacobs 1971; Spalt and Weisbuch 1972) and failed to find (Peck and Schrut 1971; Stevenson et al. 1972) a greater history of parental/family suicide for suicidal compared with nonsuicidal adolescents. In a study of college students and basic trainees, 59 percent had had experience with suicidal behavior in others and 13 percent who had experienced suicidal behavior in relatives were the most likely to have had a serious suicidal crisis themselves (Leonard and Flinn 1972). For the persistently suicidal, 50 percent of the suicidal teenagers, while only 38 percent of the suicidal young adults, had a family history of suicide attempts (Maxmen and Tucker 1973). All persistently suicidal teenagers with a family history of suicide were females having a sister who also had made an attempt. The study of attempted suicide in social networks (ages fifteen to sixty-five) similarly has indicated that more younger than older individuals attempting suicide have positive contact with relatives and friends who also have attempted suicide and the age effect is particularly important for women (Kreitman, Smith, and Tan 1969).

To understand the impact of parental suicide on children, Shepherd and Barraclough (1976) followed thirty-six children who between the ages of two and seventeen had experienced the suicide of a parent. Interviews with the surviving parent five to seven years after the suicide indicated the children demonstrated some increased vulnerability for psychological problems, especially delinquency, but most "had enough resources to weather the crisis." No incidence of suicidal behavior/ideation for the children was documented. The children functioning less well were those whose parents had had marital separations, trouble with the police, and abnormal personalities. Approximately half of the children were assessed as functioning adequately, half as not. These two groups of children showed no difference in age, sex, social class, family size, or sex of parent lost; however, only children tended to be doing better. No direct clinical assessment was made of the children, so it is difficult to evaluate the data. However, in assessing the children's response to parent suicide, Shepherd and Barraclough conclude that the quality of life prior to the parent suicide was important.

A positive psychiatric history in the family of suicidal adolescents has been found in 20 to 54 percent of cases (Sanborn et al. 1973; Senseman 1969). Peck and Schrut (1972), however, reported no significant difference in occurrence of a positive psychiatric history among parents of suicidal compared with those of nonsuicidal older adolescents. Stevenson et al. (1972) also reported that suicide attempts in suicidal compared with nonsuicidal psychiatric adolescents were not significantly affected by family history of psychiatric illness or suicide. According to Peck and Schrut (1971), whenever a psychiatric or suicidal problem did occur, regardless of which group, the mother was more likely to be identified as experiencing the problem.

In addition to general descriptions such as "suicide" and "psychiatric" problems, other nonspecific problems reported for parent(s) or family members of suicidal adolescents have included "an abnormal parental personality" (Lukianowicz 1968) and "parents' unresolved problems," including those associated with their own sexual and aggressive drives and their own parental relationships (Sabbath 1969, 1971). More specific parent problems have included depression in female relatives of male adolescents who have attempted suicide (Margolin and Teicher 1968) or who have a high incidence of suicidal ideation or behavior (Maletsky 1973); paternal depression (Sabbath 1969); violence and aggression by male relatives (Duncan 1977; Hendin 1969; Maletsky 1973; Margolin and Teicher 1968; Sabbath 1969, 1971); high use/abuse of alcohol by parent(s) (11–50 percent: Anastassopoulos and Kokkini 1969; Haider 1968; Jacobs 1971; Margolin and Teicher 1968; Marks and Haller 1977; Sabbath 1969, 1971; Senseman 1969; Stanley and Barter 1970; Teicher 1970); and maternal withdrawal prior to and after pregnancy (Margolin and Teicher 1968). Evidence of alcohol abuse by parents has not differentiated between adolescents attempting suicide and psychiatrically disturbed adolescents (Stanley and Barter 1970) but has been reported to be greater in suicidal than in nonsuicidal-nonpsychiatrically disturbed adolescents (Jacobs 1971). Reports also have suggested that long-standing family psychopathology is found within families of children seen on an emergency basis whether or not the emergent condition was suicidal behavior (Mattsson et al. 1969).

In addition to psychiatric problems, there may be a higher incidence of serious physical health problems for parents or other family members of suicidal (attempt, threat, ideation) compared with non- or successfully suicidal adolescents (Jacobs 1971; Peck and Schrut 1971). Descriptions of chronic problems for suicidal adolescents have included frequent family illness leading to the adolescent's assumption of a parental role, for example, caring for sick or younger siblings and taking charge of the household or family business (Teicher 1970).

DISCIPLINARY TECHNIQUES

Discipline has not been a factor widely studied for suicidal adolescents. However, disciplinary action by parents of suicidal adolescents relates to relevant family issues, including family conflict, handling aggression within families, feelings of rejection experienced by adolescents within their families, and the adolescent's perception of the parent.

Adolescents attempting suicide perceive their parents' discipline as unfair and as rejection (Jacobs 1971; Lester 1968a; Teicher 1970). Parents of suicidal adolescents, meanwhile, view their disciplinary efforts as leading to increased frustration (Jacobs 1971). Suicidal adolescents report nagging (Teicher 1970) and withholding privileges and withdrawal (Yusin et al. 1972) as primary methods of parental disapproval for their behavior. As viewed by the adolescent, parents of suicidal adolescents, compared with parents of disturbed-nonsuicidal adolescents, demonstrated the lowest incidence of a reaction (i.e., anger, worry, fear, or confusion) to crisis behavior demonstrated by the adolescent (Yusin et al. 1972). Teicher (1970) suggests that the parents' failure to discourage behavior that the suicidal adolescent considers bad is taken by the adolescent as a sign of rejection. In at least one case study, "harsh physical punishment" by parents of an adolescent girl who attempted and later committed suicide has been reported (Duncan

1977). However, using a control group, no difference was found between suicidal and nonsuicidal college students in their experience of physical or psychological techniques of punishment (Lester 1968a).

In general, reports suggest that parents of suicidal adolescents underreact to misbehavior, or, at least, fail actively and explicitly to communicate their reaction, concern, and disapproval, resorting instead to ignoring, withholding, and withdrawal.

SCHOOL ADJUSTMENT

School is the second major social system in which adolescents are involved. However, little attention has been directed to the influence of school on adolescent suicidal behavior. Not all suicidal adolescents have problems at school. However, for many suicidal students, problems associated with school performance, attendance, relationships, behavior, and stress have been described. The limited attention directed to school in relation to adolescent suicide underestimates contributions of the school system to earlier identification, prevention, and intervention services for students at risk for suicidal behavior.

SCHOOL PERFORMANCE

School performance consists of academic performance and of participation in nonacademic but school-related or sponsored activities. Difficulty with academic performance has been the most frequently reported school factor associated with adolescent suicide. Such difficulties have varied from poor and deteriorating performance to underfunctioning and underachievement (Connell 1972; Finch and Poznanski 1971; Sabbath 1971; Sanborn et al. 1973; Schrut 1968; Senseman 1969; Suicide among American Blackfeet Indians 1970). Pressure by parents for better school performance, especially in the adolescent with limited intellectual abilities, may be a stress leading to suicidal behavior (Glaser 1971). Unsatisfactory academic performance and associated suicidal behavior have been viewed as signs of depression (Connell 1972; Mattsson et al. 1969). Although school failure for adolescents has been described as one precipitant of suicide attempts and emergency psychiatric referrals, adolescents continuing to make suicide attempts following psychiatric hospitalization do not have a higher rate of school failure than those discontinuing such attempts (Barter et al. 1968).

Control groups have been used infrequently in studies evaluating school performance of suicidal adolescents. Peck and Schrut (1971), comparing college students committing, attempting, and threatening suicide with nonsuicidal students, found more nonsuicidal than suicidal students had above-average grades in high school and college. However, only 8 percent of suicidal students were failing. Stanley and Barter (1970) reported 79 percent of suicidal adolescents attempting suicide were receiving passing grades, while only 68 percent of psychiatrically disturbed–nonsuicidal adolescents were passing; these differences were not statistically significant. These results suggest only a small percentage of suicidal adolescents in school may actually be failing; the majority are passing, although they may be achieving below expectation for their level of abilities. Thus, academic performance of suicidal students may be similar to that of other students having emotional but not specifically suicidal problems.

College students, having chosen to continue in school, may represent a different situation than younger students, required to attend school. Several authors have described a relationship between suicidal behavior and high achievement or high academic standards among college students (Fox 1971; Lester and Lester 1971; Ross 1969; Seiden 1969). The relationship between student suicide and academic achievement varies from university to university, but students at more prestigious universities, where standards are the highest, exhibit unusually high rates of suicidal behavior.

Participation in nonacademic activities represents the second major component of overall school performance. Minimal effort has been made to identify such participation or lack of participation for suicidal adolescents. However, Marks and Haller (1977) reported that male adolescents attempting and threatening suicide are involved in a greater number of school activities than emotionally disturbed nonsuicidal male adolescents.

SCHOOL ATTENDANCE

Variables associated with school attendance for suicidal adolescents have included the incidence of nonattendance, number of schools attended, and attendance at special schools.

Reasons for suicidal adolescents not attending school have included expulsion and suspension, truancy, dropping out, school refusal, and health and emotional problems. As high as 36 percent of adolescents attempting suicide may not be enrolled in school at the time of the attempt (Teicher 1970), and adolescents with lifelong school difficulties particularly may have dropped out of school by the time of their attempt (Barter et al. 1968). Suicidal adolescent girls are reported to drop out of school more often than suicidal boys or other emotionally disturbed girls (Marks and Haller 1977). Suicidal adolescents, as well as other emotionally disturbed adolescents in crisis, are reported to have done nothing about getting back into school at the time of their attempt/crisis (Yusin et al. 1972).

Unsatisfactory scholarship has not been the primary reason for school nonattendance for suicidal adolescents. For example, Teicher (1970) reported in a study of adolescents attempting suicide that 89 percent had reasons other than poor scholarship for not attending school, reasons which contributed to the suicide attempt itself. These included illness, pregnancy, prior suicide attempts, and behavioral problems. Other studies also have reported that the reason for suicidal adolescents not attending school, such as fear of school, is directly related to the attempt itself (Lukianowicz 1968).

Suicidal adolescents have been reported to attend a large number of different schools, possibly changing schools frequently in the five years or less preceding the attempt (Jacobs 1971; Lukianowicz 1968). In a follow-up study of children who had had a parent commit suicide when the child was five to seven years of age, those children who attended more than two schools following their parent's suicide were less likely to be functioning well; however, the incidence of suicide attempts by these children was not documented (Shepherd and Barraclough 1976).

School attendance, rather than nonattendance, has been identified as a particular problem for suicidal American Indian youths. Attendance at schools where teachers and classmates are predominantly white contributes to emotional problems—including suicidal behavior—for American Indian youths. Indian youths frequently are sent to boarding schools geographically distant from their home, further contributing to isolation from families and to possible suicide behavior. Another contributing factor to higher rates of suicidal behavior among boarding school students may be that high-risk students, such as those from broken or disorganized families, frequently are selected for admission (Shore 1975). Resnik and Dizmang (1971) suggest the alienation of the Indian child within the school system contributes to suicidal behavior during adolescence and may be a pattern that applies to other minority children.

SCHOOL RELATIONSHIPS

The extent to which suicidal adolescents have difficulty relating to teachers and classmates is unknown. Clashes with other students, conflict with teachers, and lack of friends at school have been reported for suicidal adolescents. However, conflicting results indicate that male adolescents attempting and threatening suicide, compared with other emotionally disturbed adolescent males, have fewer problems with relationships at school and that teachers were influential to them. At the same time, suicidal adolescent girls, in contrast with other emotionally disturbed girls, were less likely to have a favorable attitude toward teachers (Marks and Haller 1977).

School personnel may not be aware that a suicidal student is experiencing stress. This may reflect the personnel's lack of information about cues related to suicide, the difficulty predicting suicide despite adequate information, and/or relative social isolation of the student within the school. Sanborn et al. (1973) reported that of eight adolescent students committing suicide, only four schools reported having noticed anything in the adolescents' behavior indicative of stress. Sartore (1976) points out that discussion of suicide in schools is "virtually ignored" and that students as well as school personnel need information about suicide.

SCHOOL BEHAVIOR, ATTITUDES, AND STRESS

School difficulties for adolescents attempting and threatening suicide have included disciplinary and behavior problems, lack of interest, dislike of school, boredom, and fear. Labeling a student a failure when he is having school difficulties also may be a stress contributing to suicidal behavior (Sartore 1976). Suicidal adolescent girls are reported as less likely to have behaved well in school than suicidal boys or than other emotionally disturbed girls (Marks and Haller 1977) and more frequently have school adjustment difficulties (e.g., poor grades, truancy, and disciplinary problems) (Barter et al. 1968). Additional sources of stress associated with school for adolescents committing suicide include attendance at competitive schools and parents' high expectations and criticism regarding school.

356

SOCIAL RELATIONSHIPS

Information regarding social relationships of suicidal adolescents is extremely limited. Most frequently described factors include the effect of loss, descriptive characteristics of their social behavior, the role of sexual adjustment, and the influence of religious affiliation.

LOSS AND SOCIAL CHARACTERISTICS

Loss or threatened loss of a boyfriend, girl friend, or parent and intense reactions to loss are common precipitants to adolescent suicidal behavior. Interpersonal conflict also commonly precipitates crisis behavior for adolescents, including suicidal behavior. Suicidal adolescents have been described as demonstrating a pattern of unstable and intense interpersonal relationships and having problems tolerating being alone (Crumley 1979). Frequently suicidal adolescents are described as socially isolated, withdrawn, alienated, lonely, and rejected. Loneliness also has been described as playing a prominent role in precipitating suicidal behavior for older age groups (Ropschitz and Ovenstone 1968). For suicidal adolescents, increasing withdrawal and asocial behavior particularly may occur immediately prior to a suicide attempt, while social difficulties for other suicidal adolescents appear long standing (Jacobs 1971; Lukianowicz 1968; Schrut 1968). The pattern of social withdrawal, rejection, and suicidal behavior has been described as part of a picture of depression for adolescents. However, withdrawal by the suicidal adolescent also has been viewed as an adaptive technique which, as part of the suicidal process, precedes the suicidal behavior and contributes to progressive social isolation (Jacobs 1971).

Several studies have included control groups in the effort to characterize social relationships of suicidal adolescents. Peck and Schrut (1971) compared college students committing, attempting, and threatening suicide with nonsuicidal students. Sixty-one percent of the suicidal, compared with 31 percent of the nonsuicidal, students "spent considerable spare time in solitary activities" before high school. Nonsuicidal students dated more frequently in high school and college than suicidal. Those students who committed suicide were more isolated and less likely to send out communication signals for help. Similarly, Barter et al. (1968), in a follow-up study of adolescents attempting suicide after hospital discharge, reported that those adolescents not

357

making posthospital attempts more often had an active social life than those continuing such attempts. Marks and Haller (1977) suggest suicidal adolescent females more closely fit the picture of social isolation than males. Their results indicate that adolescent males attempting suicide, in contrast with other emotionally disturbed male adolescents, associated more with older girls and less with boys their own age during childhood; as adolescents, they continue to lack close relationships with male peers. In contrast, suicidal girls, compared with other emotionally disturbed females, had few or no friends during childhood, could talk about their personal problems with no one, and, during adolescence, did not value friendships. Cantor (1976) reported that youthful female suicide attemptors (ages eighteen to twenty-five) have high affiliative, succorant, and nurturant needs. More specifically, high succorant needs, interacting with an inability to reach significant others, distinguished young women who attempted suicide from those who frequently thought about suicide.

Contrasting results regarding social adjustment have been described. Stanley and Barter (1970) reported adolescents attempting suicide do not differ in social adjustment (i.e., poor relationships, withdrawn, number of outside activities) from other emotionally disturbed adolescents. However, continued suicide behavior was associated with inadequate peer relationships. Yusin et al. (1972) compared four groups of adolescents engaging in crisis behaviors (i.e., suicidal, aggressive, psychotic, and psychotic-drug). The suicidal group had more friends of the same age than the other groups but were the least interested in becoming leaders in peer groups.

One of the few efforts to examine the nature of relationships established by suicidal youths is represented in Lester's (1969) study of resentment and dependency. He reported that suicidal college students and other emotionally disturbed individuals had a smaller dispersion of dependencies than those who were nonsuicidal-nondisturbed, suicidal individuals had more ambivalence toward those whom they knew, and suicidal individuals demonstrated excessive dependency upon those whom they resented.

SEXUAL ADJUSTMENT

Suicidal adolescents occasionally have been described as experiencing problems related to sexuality. Based primarily on case studies, such problems have included sexual inhibition (Finch and Poznanski

358

1971), conflicts associated with homosexuality (Finch and Poznanski 1971; McIntire and Angle 1970, 1971b; McIntire, Angle, Wikoff, and Schlicht 1977; Mattsson et al. 1969; Peck and Schrut 1971), use of sex in exchange for lack of closeness (Bernstein 1972), paternal sexual assault (Lukianowicz 1968), pregnancy (McIntire and Angle 1970, 1971a, 1971b; McIntire et al. 1977; Petzel and Cline 1978), promiscuity (Mattsson et al. 1969; Roberts and Hooper 1969; Sabbath 1971; Schrut 1968), sexual conflicts (Mattsson et al. 1969), confusion over sexual identity (Sabbath 1969), and maternal disparagement of men and sexuality (Schrut 1968). Senseman (1969) reported that guilt over sexual activity is one of the common reasons given for adolescents' suicide threats/attempts. Roberts and Hooper (1969) identified six life styles characteristic of suicide attempters of all ages. One of these, the "sexualized" style, includes many of the sexual characteristics noted in case studies of suicidal adolescents and is characterized by promiscuity, multiple, premature, or precipitous marriage, and homosexuality.

Few studies have used controls in describing the sexual adjustment of suicidal adolescents. Peck and Schrut (1971) compared college students attempting, threatening, and committing suicide with nonsuicidal controls. Of the suicidal students, 43 percent had not had sexual intercourse, only 18 percent of nonsuicidal students had not had intercourse; 56 percent of suicidal students and 47 percent of nonsuicidal students were males. There was a tendency for those committing suicide (90 percent male) to have less sexual experience than the other suicidal groups (40 percent male). These results suggest suicidal adolescents have less sexual experience than expected for their age and gender. However, Stanley and Barter (1970) reported that suicidal and nonsuicidal emotionally disturbed adolescents did not differ in sexual adjustment. Therefore, suicidal adolescents may be similar to other emotionally disturbed adolescents in terms of the adequacy of their sexual adjustment. Whitlock and Edwards (1968) compared young women attempting suicide who were and were not pregnant. Pregnant suicide attempters had difficulty establishing stable sexual and personal relationships; control for emotional adjustment was not included. Marks and Haller (1977) reported that reasons for referral for treatment of suicidal girls in contrast with other emotionally disturbed girls/boys or suicidal boys included sex difficulties.

From a perspective entirely different than a focus on sexual problems, Lester (1970) studied the influence of sexual mores upon youthful suicide in nonliterate cultures, hypothesizing that the adolescent suicide rate would be higher among cultures in which premarital sexual expression was severely punished. There were statistically non-significant trends in the expected direction, and it was concluded that the proportion of suicides committed by adolescents within each of the seventeen societies examined was not related to measures of sexual permissiveness. However, differences across cultures in the adult suicide rates could have obscured significant findings since only the ratio of adolescent to adult suicides was examined.

RELIGIOUS AFFILIATION

The role of religion, another dimension of social affiliation, has received limited attention for the suicidal adolescent. Efforts have been primarily demographic. No significant relationship between religious affiliation or belief in an afterlife and attempted, threatened, and committed suicide has been reported for children and adolescents. However, nonsuicidal, compared with older suicidal, adolescents attend religious services less often (Peck and Schrut 1971), adolescent girls attempting suicide, compared with other emotionally disturbed girls, seldom attend church (Marks and Haller 1977), and those committing suicide more frequently express belief in an afterlife than other suicidal groups (Peck and Schrut 1971). In addition, an increase in self-poisoning for late teenage Jewish males has been reported (McIntire and Angle 1971b).

Recent reports suggest a relatively high percentage (20–22) of people of all ages, including adolescents, attempting/threatening suicide are Catholic. Gabrielson, Klerman, Currie, Tyler, and Jekel (1970) studied a population pregnant as teenagers who by the time of their suicide attempt ranged in age from seventeen to twenty-five. A higher percentage of these young women who threatened/attempted suicide were single, Catholic, and not living at a poverty level, compared with non-suicidal women who also had borne children in their teens. Results are interpreted to suggest that the acceptability, or relative lack of acceptability, of the pregnancy in the women's social group might be a contributing factor, especially given the attitudes of the Catholic religion. The relative high percentage of attempts among Catholics particularly is interesting in view of earlier expectations, based primarily on demographic information from Catholic and Protestant countries, that suicide will be relatively lower among Catholics than among other religious groups. The effect of religion upon the behavior of adolescents is undoubtedly more complicated than a simple denominational breakdown, and other dimensions merit consideration. Strength of religious conviction, for example, may be relevant (Ross 1969).

Studies of Situational Factors

Components of the general social climate, such as customs, values, and economic conditions, as well as inanimate factors such as weather have been explored as indirect influences upon the incidence of suicide. However, few efforts have been made to investigate relationships between these factors and adolescent suicide.

HOUSING AND ECONOMIC FACTORS

Although residential mobility appears to be associated with higher rates of attempted and completed youthful suicide, it is not clear whether residential location is significant. A higher rate of suicidal behavior among urban dwellers has been suggested (Bakwin 1957; Finch and Poznanski 1971), but this expectation was not confirmed in a study of adolescent suicide attempts in the Denver area (Stanley and Barter 1970). Poor housing as a factor among black suicide attempters who were young, but not solely adolescents (mean age, 20.2), and medium-to-low family income (Jacobziner 1960; Teicher 1970) among urban adolescent suicide attempters have been reported. Unemployment and/or debt (Bagley and Greer 1972; Seiden 1969; Smith and Davison 1971), particularly among youthful males, and overcrowded living conditions as factors in youthful suicide also have been described. A higher proportion of pregnant adolescent attempters, on the other hand, have been reported to come from nonpoverty than from poverty areas (Gabrielson et al. 1970). There is no recent sufficient information to challenge Seiden's (1969) conclusion, in his earlier review of youthful suicide, that there is no evidence that suicide is more frequent among rich or poor. However, as with other factors, it is not financial status by itself that is a significant component in adolescent suicide but the interaction between income status and other factors, such as gender, living conditions, and work conditions.

The effect of fluctuations in the economy on youthful suicide is unclear. Seiden (1969) states youthful suicides are highest during periods of economic depression, as is observed among adults, while

Yacoubian and Lourie (1969) suggest high suicide rates observed during depressions do not hold for adolescents. Neither author provides data to support his conclusions nor have more recent studies or relevant data been published.

MILITARY SERVICE AND WAR

Fear of induction into the military service may precipitate youthful suicide attempts (Senseman 1969). Suicidal behavior has been reported to be most prevalent for young men in a military setting during basic combat training at the beginning of military service when the novelty of military life wears thin and the reality of combat becomes apparent (Russell, Conroy, and Weiner 1971). Anxiety over exposure to firing weapons, loss of identity, unfamiliar living conditions, and growing, poorly directed anger at the army may contribute to increased stress during this period. Stress is relieved as familiarity with the routine increases. Similar findings indicating the majority of suicide attempts occurred during basic training also have been reported in a study which included a more diverse group of military personnel (Sawyer 1969). This group included women and stockade prisoners, each of whom had higher rates of attempted suicide than young male trainees. During the period of the study, there were nine completed suicides, only one of whom previously had attempted suicide. At least seven of these nine were absent or had just returned from an absence at the time of their death, suggesting a relationship between completed suicide and recent absence with or without leave from the military base.

The effect of war upon youthful suicide may be different from its effect on adult suicide (Choron 1972; Finch and Poznanski 1971; Yacoubian and Lourie 1969). The adult suicide rate decreases during wartime, while the adolescent rate increases. The increase is apparently accounted for by youthful males, since the rate for youthful females remains relatively constant.

CLIMATIC CONDITIONS

Seasonal variations in the suicide rate appear to be relatively independent of age. For adolescents as well as adults, spring is the most common time for attempted and completed suicides to occur, with May as the peak month. Lester (1971) found a secondary peak in October but did not look at adolescents as a separate group, while Haider (1968) found half of his young subjects (ages six to nine) attempted suicide in the fall. There does not appear to be a relationship between seasonal variability in the suicide rate and weather; for example, rates are independent of temperature and precipitation.

CULTURAL FACTORS

Population base rates for suicide among different countries have been compared as a means of examining cultural influences upon youthful suicide. Such comparisons assume cultural differences account for some of the variability. Using data from the early 1950s, Japan had the highest adolescent suicide rate. A common explanation of this high rate is that suicide has been considered honorable in Japan. The proportion of total suicides in Japan committed by adolescents also is unusually high, although in general there is a significant positive relationship between youthful suicide rates and those of adults across nations. Bakwin (1957) also reported high rates of youthful suicide in eastern Europe and France around the turn of the century, concluding that the "Prussian way of life," with strict, rigid, punitive child-rearing practices, appears to have been a major factor.

Recently in Japan the adolescent suicide rate and the rate for the population as a whole has decreased (Suicide—International Comparisons 1972; U.S. Department of Health, Education, and Welfare 1974). This decrease parallels dramatic social change in Japan brought about by the rapid adoption of westernized customs and values. If the change in the adolescent suicide rate is related to cultural factors, it might be expected that older Japanese, who had lived in a different social climate, would retain the former high rate of suicide. In fact, the rate of suicide among Japanese aged sixty-five years and above is still one of the highest in the world for this age group.

MEDIA AND SUGGESTIBILITY

Suicide epidemics have been described, some of which are mass suicides, such as in Jonestown, Guyana. Often the epidemics appear to stem from suggestibility. In a study of young suicide attempters, ages three to fourteen years, suggestion appeared to play a role (Lourie 1966). The methods of suicide selected by these youngsters resembled methods from television and movies or overheard in conversation.

While there are appeals from time to time to suppress reporting of

363

suicides in the media, under the assumption that these reports may trigger more suicides, previous literature reviews generally have concluded that the media have little effect on the suicide rate. Three studies have directly addressed the question of media influence, comparing completed suicide rates before and after newspaper strikes (Blumenthal and Bergner 1973; Motto 1967, 1970). Only two of these compared age- and sex-specific rates, but all concluded there was no overall decrease in the suicide rates during periods in which newspapers were scarce. However, suicide rates for youthful women decreased during the period of the strike. While Blumenthal and Bergner's (1973) findings failed to reach significance, Motto's (1970) decrease for women under thirty-five was significant at the .01 level. These findings are not conclusive but suggest the possible influence of newspapers on the suicidal tendencies of youthful women. However, no attempt was made to relate this influence specifically to newspaper reports of suicide.

AVAILABILITY OF MEANS

The availability of a relatively convenient means of committing suicide may affect the incidence of suicidal behavior. Studies suggest an increase in suicidal behavior coinciding with an increase in the availability of specific, potentially lethal, prescription medications and possibly associated with the ready availability of handguns. Furthermore, the proportion of suicidal behavior involving medications, as opposed to other methods, has increased with their increased availability. While studies have not analyzed medication use among adolescents as a separate group, increased rates of suicidal behavior among adolescents parallel increases among older-aged groups. The most dramatic increase in the rate of suicidal behavior was seen among young males ages fifteen to twenty-five years and among men and women ages twenty-five to fifty-four years (Aitken, Buglass, and Kreitman 1969). It is premature to assume that people attempt suicide merely because the means are at hand. However, Oliver and Hetzel (1973) made a careful attempt to exclude alternative explanations in their study of completed suicide and reported it was likely that the pattern they found represented "a changing proportion of persons at risk who, through ready availability of a lethal dose of sedative drugs, achieved the fatal outcome of an act performed without strong suicidal intent." Smith (1972), too, seems to accept a causal relationship between changing prescription rates and changing patterns of hospital admissions for self-poisoning.

The availability of firearms, the leading method of suicide for youths aged ten to twenty-four (U.S. Department of Health, Education, and Welfare 1963–1976), merits increased attention. Browning (1974) reported that the firearms used in suicides for persons of all ages appeared easily available. Moreover, these guns, primarily handguns, were responsible for three of the four teenage suicides in his study but only 43 percent of all suicides (i.e., all ages) and were obtained for the purpose of suicide or, originally, for self-protection. Browning suggests that if such findings are indicative of the national pattern of firearm use in suicides, there are considerable ramifications of such easy availability of a highly lethal means, and the removal of at least the handgun from general availability may be the only way to test the hypothesis that the suicide rate might be lowered.

AVAILABILITY OF EMOTIONAL HELP

In recent years there has been a dramatic growth of suicide prevention centers providing a telephone answering service, available at all hours, for people in crisis. Studies have suggested these services have (Fox 1971; Senseman 1969) and have not had (Suicide: a world problem 1971) a significant impact on overall suicide rates. Either way, the effect on adolescent suicide, specifically, is not clear, and critics claim these centers do not reach the most seriously suicidal people (Klagsburn 1976). On the other hand, increased availability of emotional help provided by social workers introduced into dormitories has been associated with decreased suicide attempts among youthful Indian and Eskimo boarding school students (Harvey, Gazay, and Samuels 1976).

Studies of Cognitive Functioning

A neglected area of study is the contribution of cognitive functioning to adolescent suicidal behavior. Studies with adults (Yufit, Benzies, Fonte, and Fawcett 1970) and studies which have included adolescents (Melges and Weisz 1971) suggest that suicidal persons have less focus on the future and a less elaborate concept of future time. Motivation for suicide for adolescent suicide attempters includes escape from pessimistically distorted future expectations (Hynes 1976). Suicidal adolescents also are reported to have diminished problem-solving capacity (Levenson and Neuringer 1971) and to have fewer responses besides suicide available to them under stress (Maxmen and Tucker 1973). Suicidal adolescent girls have been described as having extremely poor judgment and deviant ideation (Marks and Haller 1977). Overall intellectual abilities for suicidal adolescents appear to be average to high average (Dudley, Mason, and Rhoton 1973; Maxmen and Tucker 1973), with superior abilities second and a retarded level of intellectual functioning uncommon (Senseman 1969). For younger adolescents, intellectual abilities for suicide attempters are higher than for adolescent psychiatric patients in general (Dudley et al. 1973). Death concept, attitudes about death, and negative outlook have received more attention as possible cognitive factors influencing adolescent suicide.

DEATH CONCEPT AND ATTITUDES

The concept of death for the developing child has been studied for a number of years. The emphasis in most studies has been on children rather than adolescents and on clinical or case material rather than on more controlled observations. Studies suggest that children connect death with deprivation and aggression (Schilder and Wechsler 1934) and children and adolescents demonstrate increased emotional response to the concept of death (Alexander and Adlerstein 1958). The child's concept of death has been viewed as developing over time. From a developmental perspective, children are described as perceiving death early as reversible and later as a cessation of bodily activities (Nagy 1959). More recently, the emphasis on age and development as important influences in determining a child's concept of death has been challenged. Bluebond-Langner (1977), working with terminally ill children, has suggested that children's views of death reflect their experiences, concerns, circumstances, and self-concept rather than their specific chronological age.

The effect of the child or adolescent's concept of death on their tendency toward suicidal behavior is unknown. Rather prematurely, Glaser (1971) warns that seriously disturbed children may be at greater risk for suicide since they may act on their age-appropriate comprehension of death as incomplete and reversible. McIntire and Angle (1971b) interviewed children and adolescents following self-poisoning. Their results support a developmental view of the concept of death but do not support a correlation between suicide and this developing concept. In contrast, Lourie (1966) emphasizes the importance of early patterns of thinking which result in suicidal thinking later in life. Using case studies of suicidal children (ages three to fourteen), he suggests that when a child's early ideas of death relate to experiences of separation from parents and the child's perception of inflicting hurt on the parent, later thoughts may occur such as, "I'll hurt you (or symbolically kill you off) by removing myself."

It is difficult to separate attitudes and concepts about death. Various attitudes possibly related to suicidal or self-destructive behavior have been identified. Cash and Kooker (1970) administered an attitude-toward-death scale to nonsuicidal college students, suicidal psychiatric patients, and nonsuicidal psychiatric patients (ages fourteen to fifty). More suicidal individuals demonstrated inconsistent attitudes, suggesting suicidal individuals experience an approach-avoidance conflict toward death. Frederick, Resnik, and Wittlin (1973) constructed a Morbidity Attitude Survey Scale to obtain information about the relationship between drug abuse, addiction, and self-destructive behavior. Addicts demonstrated more aberrant attitudes toward life and death and were more self-destructive than nonaddicts. Results suggest that the risk-taking behavior in which addicts engage, including suicidal behavior, is consistent with a more deviant attitude toward life and death than is normal. In an effort to better understand motivation behind suicide and attitudes toward death, Edland and Duncan (1973) categorized suicide notes into seven psychodynamic constellations proposed by Hendin (1963) (age range not specified). Edland and Duncan make no statement regarding the developmental appropriateness or relative deviancy associated with the categories. However, constellations used, such as a view of death as punishment for society, might relate to dimensions explored in other studies, such as relative conceptual deviancy or developmental adequacy.

HOPELESSNESS AND HELPLESSNESS

Studies indicate a correlation between suicidal behavior and negative outlook. Melges and Weisz (1971) reported that suicidal ideation was associated with a negative outlook or hopelessness and with a feeling of less personal control over outcomes (helplessness). Other studies also have reported a significant correlation between negative expectations or hopelessness and seriousness of intent of suicide attempters. In addition, seriousness of intent of attempters has been found to be more closely related to hopelessness than to the syndrome of depression in general (Minkoff, Bergman, Beck, and Beck 1973). Marks and Haller (1977) reported a gender difference, describing feelings of hopelessness as characteristic of adolescent suicidal girls in contrast to other emotionally disturbed girls/boys or suicidal boys. Administration of a projective test (Thematic Apperception Test) to three groups of adolescents (suicidal, psychiatrically disturbed–nonsuicidal, normal) indicated that the self-destructive adolescent did not see the world as more overpowering and overwhelming than did other adolescents. However, the ability of adolescent suicide attempters to handle oppressiveness may differ. Thus, the suicidal adolescent may feel helpless not because he feels phenomenally overwhelmed but because he cannot cope with his environment due to possible cognitive deficiencies (Levenson and Neuringer 1972).

Studies of Individual Characteristics

Identification of individual characteristics of suicidal adolescents— what loosely might be defined as personality characteristics—have included dimensions of emotional adjustment, self-concept, and motivation. Research efforts primarily have been descriptive with relative inattention to characteristics of general adolescent development that might play a role in the suicidal process.

EMOTIONAL ADJUSTMENT

If there are qualities specifically characteristic of suicidal adolescents, it is necessary, by definition, that these characteristics distinguish the suicidal adolescent from the average, well-adjusted youth as well as from other adolescents experiencing psychosocial problems. In other words, if suicidal behavior is not normative in adolescence, is such behavior simply part of an overall picture of emotional maladjustment?

There are many ways to assess the level of an adolescent's emotional adjustment. These include evaluating the presence of specific problems, such as behavioral, drug, or affective difficulties; formal diagnostic classification; and assessing the level of general personality functioning. The results of evaluating suicidal adolescents in all of these ways indicate that suicidal behavior, and probably suicidal ideation as well, are not normative during adolescence. However, it is a more complex endeavor to separate suicidal behavior from a general picture of psychosocial maladjustment. In particular, the reoccurring issue of possible depression and efforts to identify its presence in studies of suicidal adolescents have been complicated by practical and theoretical issues.

BEHAVIORAL PROBLEMS

Descriptions of behavioral problems for suicidal adolescents have included references to their impulsivity, acting out, and rebelliousness. However, the inconsistency with which such behaviors have been defined is a major obstacle in comparing findings.

Contradictory results regarding adolescent suicide have attributed youthful suicide threats and attempts to impulsiveness as well as to rational decision making. Several studies have suggested that impulsiveness may be a long-standing, deeply ingrained personality trait among suicidal adolescents (Crumley 1979; Haider 1968; Toolan 1962). However, the evidence is less compelling when control groups are used (Mattsson et al. 1969; Stanley and Barter 1970). Impulsivity, or a history of acting out suggesting impulsivity, appears to be a common trait among emotionally disturbed youths whether or not they are suicidal. These controlled studies report no significant differences in characterological impulsivity or history of delinquency between adolescent suicide attempters and nonsuicidal, emotionally disturbed controls.

Additional inconsistent findings have occurred in studies of behavior problems in suicidal adolescents. Jacobs (1971) found no difference for suicidal youths, compared with a matched nonsuicidal control group, in behavior problems associated with rebelliousness. While rebelliousness may include a component of impulsivity, Jacobs did not specifically identify impulsivity in his study. However, suicidal adolescents generally displayed more behavioral problems than controls, with significant behavioral differences associated with mood, avoidance of stimulation, and escape. Mattsson et al. (1969), on the other hand, controlled for impulsivity and found no difference between adolescent suicide attempters and psychiatric controls in "autoplastic pathology," a category of behavior which shares some features with the dimensions along which Jacobs's suicidal adolescents differed from controls. Since "autoplastic pathology," defined as withdrawal, fears, and somatic complaints, is not identical with Jacobs's description of "behavioral problems," it is not surprising that the results of the two studies differed. Unfortunately, the well-designed, controlled study by Stanley and Barter (1970) did not examine behavior problems of the type associated with suicidal behavior in Jacobs's study.

Consideration of multiple factors, such as gender and time variables, in relation to specific, objective indices of behavioral problems, may clarify the association between behavioral problems and adolescent suicide. For example, Marks and Haller (1977) compared adolescents exhibiting suicidal behavior (thoughts, threats, and attempts) with emotionally disturbed, nonsuicidal adolescents. Comparisons based upon ratings by adolescents or their psychotherapists of 1,250 variables indicated suicidal adolescent boys, but not girls, were more often rated as impulsive and as having a history of running away than were controls. Suicidal girls, compared with controls, were rated as having more childhood behavior problems. In a retrospective study, Dizmang et al. (1974) compared youthful American Indians who completed suicide with a matched control group. Although few objective variables were included in the study, comparison of arrest records indicated no difference in total number of arrests between the two groups. However, important differences emerge in comparing the time at which the arrests occurred. Indians who committed suicide were significantly younger at the time of their first arrest and had a significantly greater number of arrests in the year immediately preceding their suicide. Factors such as sequence of events over time are consistent with Jacobs's (1971) findings that it is characteristic of suicidal adolescents to have a long history of behavior problems and that these problems escalate in the weeks or months preceding the suicide attempt.

Investigations of behavioral problems of suicidal adolescents have been complicated by several factors. Results vary with use of a control group, the type of behavior problem investigated, gender of the adolescents studied, and the time period during which the adolescents' lives were considered. The most productive approach to future study of the role of impulsivity and behavior problems in adolescent suicide would include investigation of genders separately; study of specific behaviors separately; an attempt to gain a historical perspective of the changing pattern of behavior problems; and use of a matched, nonsuicidal control group. Of the studies reviewed, Marks and Haller's (1977) comes closest to meeting these criteria.

DRUG USE

Few studies have investigated the relationship between drug use and suicide among adolescents. In a review article, Seiden (1969) suggested "mind altering" effects of LSD might increase suicide potential for youths by increasing the likelihood of delusions that self-destructive behavior is not dangerous; by enhancing previously present suicide proneness; as the result of an LSD-induced fantasy of the necessity of death for altruistic reasons; and in association with flashbacks. In spite of the intuitive appeal of these scenarios, Seiden concludes there is scanty evidence of a direct causal connection between drug usage and suicide. Ross (1969), in another review, also concluded studies have "revealed little or no connection between" LSD usage and suicide for college students.

The relationship between drug use and suicide was investigated by Dolkart, Hughes, Jaffe, and Zaks (1971) for thirteen- to nineteen-year-old "yippies" during a political convention, a group in which drug use was very high. A measure of degree of drug involvement, based upon frequency and number of different types of drugs used, had a low, statistically significant positive correlation with suicidal preoccupation.

Some studies have focused upon the relative frequency of suicidal behavior among adolescents and young adults who use drugs. This appears to be a highly vulnerable group. Frederick et al. (1973) found a significantly higher rate of previous suicide attempts reported by youthful heroin addicts than by delinquent and normal controls. Twenty-one percent of addicts and 8 percent of controls reported attempting suicide at some time in the past. Although the majority of addicts in this study were black, and a very high suicide attempt rate was reported for a black control group (20 percent), the data supported "the influence of addiction over race."

Although no control group was used, Hassal (1969) reported an even higher suicide attempt rate among young (under thirty) male alcoholics. Forty-five percent reported having attempted suicide at some time in their lives, while 80 percent reported suicidal thoughts or impulses. This is a remarkably high rate for any group.

At least two studies have suggested that the relationship between drug use and suicide is more complex than simple differences in overall rates of use. Peck and Schrut (1971) found no difference in nonprescription drug use when suicide attempters and threateners were com-

371

pared with controls, but suicidal subjects were significantly more likely to use barbiturates and sedatives in a nonprescribed manner. A group of youths who had committed suicide, also part of this study, used all types of drugs less often than did other suicidal groups or controls. McIntire et al. (1977), in a study of adolescents with a history of self-destructive but not necessarily suicidal behavior, reported adolescents at low risk for repeated self-destructive behavior of low lethality had significant alcohol problems, while those at high risk for gestures of increasing lethality did not necessarily have such problems.

Available studies indicate adolescents who are seriously addicted to drugs are far more likely to attempt suicide than adolescents who are not addicted. However, addicted adolescents apparently do not constitute a very large proportion of adolescent suicide attempters. Methodological inconsistencies across studies prevent identification of drug use patterns among suicidal adolescents. Careful definition of terms, study of specific types of drugs separately, and appropriate use of control groups will be important in future research in this area.

MOOD DISTURBANCES

Widely differing views exist regarding the role of mood disturbances in adolescent suicidal behavior. Depression is the most frequently discussed affective component of a possible mood disturbance for suicidal youths, but anger and rage (McIntire and Angle 1971b) and irritability (Lester 1968b) also have been described as characteristic of suicidal adolescents. Depressive tendencies may be far less prominant in suicidal adolescents than in suicidal adults (Balser and Masterson 1959; Seiden 1969). However, the controversy regarding the nature of depression during adolescence suggests that teenagers, especially younger teenagers, manifest depression primarily through a number of nontraditional expressions that may interfere with recognizing depressive symptoms for youths whether or not they also are suicidal (Toolan 1962; Weiner 1970). Despite such controversies, quantitative estimates of the prevalence of depression reported for suicidal adolescents range from 40 percent (Mattsson et al. 1969) to 80 percent (Crumley 1979; Marks and Haller 1977), while estimates for control groups of disturbed, nonsuicidal adolescents range from 13 percent (Mattsson et al. 1969) to 46 percent (Marks and Haller 1977). In two studies investigating mood disturbance among suicidal adolescents compared with control groups of disturbed, nonsuicidal youths, rates of depression were significantly higher among the suicidal groups (Marks and Haller 1977; Mattsson et al. 1969). For adolescents previously hospitalized for self-destructive behavior, those at low risk for repeated self-destructive behavior of low lethality have been described as not significantly depressed but as having high ratings for hostility; a prediction of high risk for recurrent self-destructive behavior correlated with high ratings of depression or depression-hostility (McIntire et al. 1977).

It has been suggested that depression appears to lift just before the suicidal act occurs (Seiden 1969). Such an apparent improvement in mood may be in response to the sense of relief brought about by having decided to end one's life. However, considering the lack of empirical knowledge about youthful suicide, including its relationship to cognitive variables such as decision making as well as the uncertainty regarding the nature of mood factors, the presence of decreased depression prior to youthful suicide remains hypothetical.

DIAGNOSTIC GROUPS

No consistent trends are seen in studies classifying adolescent suicide attempters into formal diagnostic categories. In four of nine studies using discrete psychiatric diagnoses, schizophrenia was the most frequently diagnosed category. In three studies, personality disturbances predominated, while no psychiatric disturbance occurred with equal frequency in one of the three. In the two remaining studies, neuroses predominated in one and adjustment reactions in the other. While schizophrenia was most frequently diagnosed in four of the nine studies, this diagnosis was made for less than 10 percent of the subjects in another four of the studies. In the two of the nine studies using control groups, there was no difference in diagnosis between suicidal subjects and controls in one (Mattsson et al. 1969) and, in the second, the diagnoses appear very similar between the two groups but no test of significance was reported (Sanborn et al. 1971). The findings in the nine studies are summarized in table 1.

Diagnoses do not appear to vary systematically with the year of each study, with the descriptions provided of settings, or with subject characteristics. However, formal diagnostic labels have limitations and are open to criticism. For example, when subjects have been studied in more depth, depression emerges as a prevalent factor (Crumley 1979; Mattsson et al. 1969). In addition, the use of the diagnosis of "adjust-

TABLE 1
PROPORTIONAL FREQUENCY (%) OF SUBJECTS BY DIAGNOSTIC GROUP

Source	Description of Subjects	Subjects (N)	Age Range (Years)	Percent of Subjects by Diagnostic Group								
				Schizophrenia	Major Affective Disorder	Unspecified Psychosis	Anxiety/Depressive Neurosis	Personality Disorder	Adjustment Reaction	Retardation/ Brain Damage	No Psychiatric Diagnosis	Other
Balser and Masterson (1959)	Hospital in-, outpatients, private practice patients; attempted suicides	37	13–19	62	...	...	...	...	...	...	...	38
Toolan (1962)	Admissions to hospital children's service; suicidal threats/ attempts	102	5–16	44	...	...	16	34	2	4	...	...
Lawler, Nakielny, and Wright (1963)	Children seen at a hospital after suicide attempt	22	8–15	18	14	...	41	23	...	...	...	5

Study	Description	N	Age								
Haider (1968)	Hospital in-, outpatients referred after suicide attempt	64	7–18	3	…	44	45	8	…	…	5
Leese (1969)	Hospital inpatients (?) seen after suicidal behavior	20	12–17	…	…	20	70	…	5	…	5
Mattsson, Seese, and Hawkins (1969)	Children seen in emergency room for psychiatric problems, 75 suicidal, 95 nonsuicidal; data grouped	170	14–17	9	…	27	16	45	…	…	3
Senseman (1969)	Psychiatric admissions with history of suicide attempt/threat	73	12–21	33	1	26	5	27	5	…	4
McIntire and Angle (1971b)	Admissions to poison control centers, accidental and intentional poisoning	1103	6–18	…	2	4	31	3	31	…	29
Sanborn, Casey, and Niswander (1971)	Hospitalized male drug abusers; nonsuicidal	12	18–25	33	0	25	25	17	8	…	17
Sanborn et al. (1971)	Hospitalized non-drug-abusing males; suicide attempts	12	18–25	50	8	25	17	…	17	0	0
Crumley (1979)*	Private practice; suicide attempts	40	12–19	15	68	18	62	5	…	…	155

* Many subjects received several diagnoses, but no information is given regarding the overlap.

ment reaction" among suicidal and nonsuicidal youths has been described as "indiscriminate," as a reflection of psychiatric trainees' inexperience, and as indicative of supervisors' reluctance to view childhood disturbances as indicators of neurotic and personality disorders (Mattsson et al. 1969). A further complication reported in formal diagnosing is that depression may appear diminished immediately after a suicide attempt. This apparent decrease may be the result of a "defensive denial of illness, as well as a temporary lessening of depression following a suicide attempt" (Crumley 1979). There also has been speculation that depression appears to lift immediately prior to the suicidal act (Seiden 1969). Thus, the time interval between attempt and diagnosis, as well as the experience and skill of the diagnostician, can have a marked effect upon the final diagnosis. However, studies provide little information about these variables.

If there is an association between psychiatric diagnosis and the probability of attempting suicide among adolescents, it remains unclear. As Stevenson et al. (1972) concluded in their comparison of psychiatrically disturbed adolescents who attempt suicide or communicate suicidal intent and adolescents who do not, ". . . in this age group type and duration of the psychiatric illness are not the essential determinants of such behavior, although severity of the illness may be a determinant."

GENERAL PERSONALITY FUNCTIONING

Diagnostic classification has been of little use in distinguishing suicidal adolescents from other youths, emotionally disturbed or not. Many studies, however, have provided personality descriptions independent of diagnostic categories.

Several studies describing personality characteristics of adolescent suicide attempters in which no control group has been used present the suicidal adolescent as a vulnerable, poorly defended individual for whom depression is a significant factor, but this depression is expressed differently from typical expressions seen with adults (Crumley 1979; Haider 1968; Toolan 1962). The suicidal adolescent is described as particularly vulnerable to loss or threatened loss, as reacting strongly to minor stresses, as experiencing poorly controlled rage attacks, and as almost frantically struggling to escape inactivity or boredom. This need to escape, combined with resentment over environmental pressures, often results in acting out. Toolan (1962) attributes the restlessness, boredom, compulsive hyperactivity, and acting-out behaviors specifically to depression as manifested during adolescence. The suicide attempt is an ultimate desperate effort to solve an intolerable situation. Teicher (1970) and Jacobs (1971) emphasized the role of situational factors in the developmental history of these suicidal adolescents, depicting a chain of events resulting in a history of unreliable interpersonal support that escalates just prior to the attempt.

Balser and Masterson's (1959) perspective of the suicidal adolescent's personality, also obtained from a study in which no control group was used, differs considerably. The suicidal adolescent, based on their data, is delusional, withdrawn, fantasizes extensively, has few somatic complaints, and constructs a picture of supposed wrongs done to him. Additional characteristics include little overt anxiety, undisturbed sleep and appetite, and possible, but not necessarily probable, complaints of depression. This picture contrasts with the depressive reaction ordinarily seen in the adult who makes a suicide attempt and with previous descriptions in which suicidal adolescents were not focused inwardly upon themselves but appeared determined to avoid their own depressive thoughts by any means available. It is plausible that Balser and Masterson selected their suicidal sample from an atypical adolescent population. Perhaps use of a control group from the same atypical population would result in revealing differences between suicidal and control groups in the direction predicted by the other uncontrolled studies, that is, a picture which would include for suicidal adolescents the expression of depression indirectly through behavioral manifestations.

In general, controlled studies of the emotional adjustment of adolescent suicide attempters focus on very narrow, specific aspects of adjustment and do not attempt to arrive at a description of personality as a whole. The study by Marks and Haller (1977) is exceptional and represents a controlled, cross-validated study in which ratings on 1,250 variables were examined. A small sample of adolescents who threatened but did not attempt suicide did not differ from the large group of suicide attempters on ratings, while both differed from the control group in similar ways. Suicidal adolescents were sad, depressed, intropunitive, and described themselves as emotional. Suicidal males were tense, jumpy, high strung, perfectionistic, prone to worry and suspiciousness, and had exaggerated needs for affection but few relationships with male peers; distress was channeled into projection, depression, and somatization. Suicidal males were generally less resentful than controls and often were referred for treatment because of impulsive behavior. Suicidal females were tearful, despondent, resentful, weak, unstable, and unpredictable. Weak defenses, poor judgment, deviant ideation, marginal control, flat affect, subjective feelings of depression, few or no friends, and sex difficulties also characterized suicidal adolescent females. Although they were not lazy, fearful, or hysteroid, they were seen as extremely disturbed.

Marks and Haller's (1977) findings generally are consistent with results reported in studies not using control groups. Marks and Haller, however, do not include ratings of variables such as reaction to loss or minimal stress, rage experiences, ability to communicate problems, reliability of social support, or tolerance to boredom, but it is unclear whether these variables were examined. The 1,000 or so ratings from which there were no significant differences between suicidal and nonsuicidal groups were not discussed and no systematic attempt was reported comparing findings with those of previous studies. The only variable describing suicidal adolescents in the studies not using controls for which Marks and Haller reported different results is "resentment." Resentment was characteristic of their female suicidal adolescents but notably uncharacteristic of suicidal males.

The single other controlled study by Lester (1968b), specifically investigating "resentment," included adolescents threatening as well as attempting suicide. Marks and Haller's study suggests these two groups are actually similar; therefore, it is possible the findings of the two studies can be compared. Lester reported slightly greater resentment for suicidal youths compared with nonsuicidal controls, but it was related to degree of neuroticism, which also was greater in the suicidal group. When neuroticism was controlled, resentment was not associated with suicidal behavior. No effort was made to investigate possible gender differences, such as reported by Marks and Haller.

Controlled studies also have indicated greater irritability among suicidal youths regardless of degree of neuroticism (Lester 1968b); perception of environmental presses independent of suicidality (Levenson and Neuringer 1972); thought disturbance independent of suicidality (McIntire et al. 1977); and increased history of emotional disturbance for suicidal youths (Peck and Schrut 1971). Yusin et al. (1972), comparing suicide attempters with adolescents displaying other forms of crisis behavior, described suicidal youths as "an unhappy, uninvolved group of adolescents who wanted human relationships, yet did not seem to have a sufficient number of them."

378

The findings reported in these controlled studies are consistent with the general description of adolescent suicide attempters presented in studies not using control groups. Adolescents attempting suicide appear to be depressed, poorly defended, emotionally reactive, uncomfortable, socially isolated youths who do at times act out their frustrations in unacceptable ways. Features that may be characteristic of this group but need further substantiation include susceptability to rage attacks, overreaction to loss or threatened loss, and an intolerance of boredom or inactivity resulting in the need to frantically seek out stimulation or distraction.

Suicide attempters rather than those successfully completing suicide have been the focus of efforts to piece together factors that lead to suicide. Individuals who attempt suicide are available for study after their group membership has been established. Adolescents who commit suicide, on the other hand, are an elusive group. Some efforts have been made to construct retrospectively a picture of these successfully suicidal adolescents on the basis of available records and interviews with family, friends, and associates. In a study of ten consecutive completed adolescent suicides, with no control group, Sanborn et al. (1973) concluded that while four subjects were noticed to be under stress by school personnel and the majority demonstrated academic or emotional difficulty adjusting to the school environment, with the exception of an explicit suicide threat, "it was almost impossible to distinguish the suicidal adolescent from the 'normal' adolescent."

Peck and Schrut (1971), on the other hand, found committed suicide youths differed from three control groups (suicide attempters, suicide threateners, and normal volunteers) and had a greater frequency of psychiatric hospitalizations, a higher rating of emotional disturbance, and fewer prior suicide attempts than other suicidal groups. Loss or threatened loss of a loved one actually occurred less often in the completion group than in the other suicidal groups, but this may have been an artifact of other factors (e.g., the committed group tended not to have a loved one to begin with). In general, sources of overt stress seemed lower, as if the suicide completers were so vulnerable that less impetus was required in order for them to act. The other suicidal groups communicated their distress and intentions more openly.

Based on the evidence available, adolescents who commit suicide may be even more isolated, more disturbed, but less visible than adolescents who attempt suicide. Suicide completers are a difficult group to study and findings to date are only suggestive.

379

SELF-CONCEPT

A variety of descriptive terms associated with self-concept, as well as with related qualities of self-esteem and self-blame, have been reported for suicidal adolescents. However, the few studies investigating dimensions of self-concept of suicidal adolescents have reached no consensus.

Feelings of low self-esteem have been attributed to youthful suicide attempters in studies by Senseman (1969) and Toolan (1962). However, in neither study were control groups used nor was there an attempt made to rule out the effects of youth or general emotional disturbance upon self-concept. According to Senseman (1969), suicidal youths expressed their low self-image with words such as "unloved, alone, inadequate, failure, inferior, unworthy, unattractive, difficult, no good, bad, a nobody, nothing but a burden" and many other negative descriptions. Similarly, Toolan (1962) reported the adolescent suicide attempter is convinced of his "bad, evil and unacceptable" qualities. In a study of recurrent adolescent suicidal behavior, McIntire et al. (1977) reported adolescents at low risk for continued suicidal behavior had relatively high ratings for self-esteem as well as hostility; high risk was associated with low self-esteem, hostility, and depression.

The controlled study of suicide attempters by Marks and Haller (1977) included responses to a personal data questionnaire and an adjective checklist. Suicidal males, compared with nonsuicidal emotionally disturbed adolescent males, saw themselves as taking things too seriously and as fearful of the future. Male and female suicidal adolescents described themselves as "emotional" significantly more often than did controls. The suicidal females described themselves more often as "artistic," "defensive," and "self-punishing" but less often as "cheerful" or "loud" than did controls. Psychotherapist ratings confirmed the suicidal girls' self-view as more intropunitive than controls. The suicidal boys also were rated by their psychotherapists as more intropunitive than controls, although the male adolescents did not share this view.

Additional attempts to explore the concept of intropunitiveness or self-blame among suicidal youths have produced discrepant findings. Levenson and Neuringer (1970) looked for evidence of intropunitiveness in responses to the Rosenzweig Picture Frustration Test in a controlled study comparing suicidal adolescents with nonsuicidal psychiatrically disturbed adolescents and with normal adolescents. Significant differences across groups indicated female adolescents were more intropunitive than male adolescents. There were no significant differences between suicidal groups and control groups nor was there a significant sex by group interaction. Weinberg (1970) examined the closely related concept of self-blame as revealed in Thematic Apperception stories in a study of suicide attempters and one successful suicide. No control group was used. Male suicidal adolescents were more prone to blame themselves for their difficulties, while females were likely to blame others.

The studies by Marks and Haller, Levenson and Neuringer, and Weinberg appear to have explored the same basic concept: self-punishment or self-blame. Their inconsistent findings may be attributable to the difference among settings—medical versus psychiatric—and the methods of data collection. One study found a gender difference in self-descriptions but no difference in ratings by others and significantly more self-punishment associated with suicidality (Marks and Haller 1977). Another found a similar gender difference, by means of ratings by others, and no significant association between self-punishment and suicidality (Levenson and Neuringer 1970). Finally, a gender difference in the opposite direction was reported in the third study (Weinberg 1970). It may be concluded that the relationship between intropunitiveness and suicidality is unclear, with or without an attempt to examine the effects of gender differences.

INTENT AND MOTIVATION

The identification of self-destructive intent as suicidal is complex. For many individuals, whether or not their behavior is classified as suicidal or nonsuicidal is a matter of interpretation. However, it is after self-destructive behavior has been identified as suicidal that consideration of motives behind such behavior generally occurs. For possibly suicidal adolescents, therefore, it is relevant to determine what is the intended action, or intent, of their self-destructive behavior as well as what factor(s), or motive(s), moves them to such intent.

Self-destructive behavior simplistically represents a behavioral continuum ranging from destructive behavior without intent to die to destructive behavior with intent to die. However, even when intent to die, or suicidal intent, is specifically defined as "the deliberate attempt to kill oneself," it can be difficult to distinguish "accidental" behavior without suicidal intent from destructive behavior with definite suicidal aim. There are many situations where an individual's intent to die is not definite but ambiguous and, therefore, his intention plays a partial, covert, or unconscious role, as in drug abuse, eroticized repetitive hangings, wrist cutting, and disregard for essential medical care. In many cases of apparent accident, such as self-poisoning, traffic accidents, and accidents with firearms, suicidal intent particularly is a possibility. For example, according to McIntire and Angle (1971a), ingesting a toxic substance by an older child is rarely accidental. Thus, considering the possible ambiguity of intent, what someone is able to say directly about their self-destructive intentions may be vague and incomplete. Interpretation of patterns of events, feelings, and behavior may lend additional understanding to intent and, for the completed suicide, such indirect, inferential information gathering may be the only means of assessing intent.

Once destructive behavior for adolescents has been classified as suicidal, it is most often further classified along the traditional continuum represented by the categories of threatened, attempted, and completed suicide; suicidal ideation and gestures may be part of this continuum. There have been efforts to conceptualize destructive behavior in alternative ways, including use of the concept of "lethality" (Shneidman 1968) and identification of particular self-destructive syndromes. For suicidal adolescents, the few efforts that have been made to incorporate lethality into understanding their suicidal behavior have been inconclusive (Weismann and Worden 1972) or have suggested that risk for continued suicidal behavior may be reliably predicted by considering lethality of intent along with other psychosocial variables (McIntire et al. 1977). Two particular self-destructive syndromes specifically including adolescents have been relatively newly described, eroticized repetitive hangings and the wrist-cutting phenomenon. Both are examples of self-destructive behavior which may appear to be suicide attempts but in which the intent, rather than to die, may be an effort—in the former—to deny fear of separation (Resnik 1972) and—in the latter—to avoid depersonalization or psychosis (Rinzler and Shapiro 1968).

The majority of studies with suicidal adolescents have interpreted from available anecdotal data both intent and motivation and have focused upon those youths attempting suicide; less frequently, studies have included independently or as a suicidal group, adolescents who have made attempts, gestures, and/or threats. Few studies have included adolescents who have committed suicide. Some studies have reported differences in a variety of characteristics between adolescents threatening and attempting suicide (Flinn and Leonard 1972), while others suggest there is little difference between teenagers who attempt suicide and those who think about it or threaten it (Marks and Haller 1977; Peck and Schrut 1971). Characteristics of adolescents completing suicide and their similarities or dissimilarities to other suicidal adolescents are little known.

Regardless of the specific suicidal adolescent group included, studies have revealed that suicidal intent for adolescents is unlikely to result from a single motive and occurs within the context of long-standing problems. Several common motives have emerged, with self-destructive action actually precipitated by such motivational factors or by other trivial factors. For adolescents, commonly reported motives have included loss, interpersonal difficulties, especially conflict, anger, manipulation, signal of distress, psychotic disintegration, wish to escape an intensely discomforting/intolerable situation, school difficulties, pregnancy or anxiety about sexual activity, and a variety of miscellaneous factors, such as a desire to join a dead relative, self-depreciation, and flirtation with death.

Physical illness represents an experience for some suicidal adolescents which may not be a common motive but which has been reported with sufficient frequency to merit further study. Marks and Haller (1977) reported that suicidal adolescent males, in contrast with other emotionally disturbed male adolescents, manifested gastrointestinal and nervous system somatic involvement and sometimes were physically handicapped. Thus, physical illness was reported as a correlate of adolescent suicidal behavior for boys but not girls. Weinberg (1970) reported that physical illness seemed to influence suicidal preoccupation in adolescent boys when illness was experienced as an obstacle to achieving competencies associated with masculine identity. Adolescent girls, on the other hand, tolerated physical illness to the extent that it elicited care and support but suicidal intent seemed to increase when illness was experienced as the cause of rejection. In addition, visible and disfiguring symptoms of physical illness for adolescents particularly appeared crucial factors in their suicidal intent. Stevenson et al. (1972) concluded that for the psychiatrically disturbed adolescent who has communicated suicidal intent and is hospitalized on a nonpsychiatric service, the duration and severity of the medical disorder may influence the suicidal symptoms. Jacobs (1971) reported a greater number of suicidal adolescents, compared with nonsuicidal controls, were likely to have experienced serious physical illness or injury in the years between onset of adolescence and their attempt, while the incidence of such problems did not differ appreciably prior to adolescence. Thus, physical illness in combination with other psychosocial factors, especially gender, sex roles, emotional disturbance, and time sequence may become a motivating factor for suicidal adolescents.

Despite many commonly identified motives in the lives of suicidal adolescents, there is conflicting evidence about the specific role such motives play in the etiology of suicidal behavior, especially when suicidal adolescents are compared with other emotionally disturbed youths. For example, when the precipitating event of psychiatric hospitalization has been compared for suicide-attempting adolescents and other emotionally disturbed adolescents, the precipitating event has not differed significantly (Stanley and Barter 1970). Mattsson et al. (1969) also reported that the most common situation triggering emergency behavior for suicidal and nonsuicidal children (ages four to eighteen) was acute conflict with parents. In this study, while many other common precipitating factors leading to emergency behavior for suicidal adolescents typically reported in other studies were less frequent among nonsuicidal disturbed than among suicidal children, the statistical significance of the differences is unclear. Yusin et al. (1972) reported that crisis behavior for adolescents in a suicidal group, compared with three other groups (aggressive, psychotic, and psychotic-drug), was frequently associated with loss which apparently, although not entirely clear from the study, was not related to crisis behavior in the other three groups. Thus, many motives associated with suicidal behavior may represent motives associated with the behavior of adolescents which brings them to the attention of health or mental health care providers. Once again, when carefully matched controls are used, the distinguishing characteristics of suicide attempters, including the motives associated with their behavior that attracts professional attention, probably are fewer than might be expected from casual reading of the literature.

Measurement

The most frequent methods of data collection reported in studies of adolescent suicide have been interviews, review of charts, anecdotal observations and recollections, and case studies. The use of objective measurements and adequately standardized tests has been minimal. The infrequent use of tests and other more objective approaches may reflect general skepticism and lack of information about such procedures and a relatively limited interest by psychologists in the study of adolescents and suicide. The limited number of standardized tests currently available assessing social, family, and psychological characteristics of the adolescent also interferes with the use of psychometric methods. Other possible contributions to the infrequent use of objective techniques in the adolescent suicide literature includes the nature of the subjects. Requesting an individual in a life-threatening or high-risk situation to complete a standardized test raises issues of sensitivity. For completed youthful suicides, only prospective studies can utilize measurement devices directly with the adolescent and prospective studies are rare. The necessity of parental approval for research with adolescents may evoke concerns by parents that researchers will intrude into private areas of their lives. While consent for an interview might be given reluctantly by parents, more formal and probably more time-consuming measurement methods may be viewed less receptively.

The most frequently employed method weakly increasing the objectivity of information gathered about adolescent suicide has been the use of a variety of questionnaires constructed to fit the design of a particular study (e.g., see Flinn and Leonard 1972; McIntire and Angle 1971a, 1971b). Rarely have issues of reliability and validity been addressed in the use of such questionnaires and infrequently has the same instrument been used in another published study. In addition to general questionnaires, standardized psychological tests and specifically devised tests occasionally have been used to study the psychosocial and cognitive aspects of adolescent suicide.

Formal measurement techniques have been inadequately utilized in the study of adolescent suicide. It particularly has been a rare study which has incorporated formal psychometric techniques in the study of the younger suicidal youth. Considering the relative absence of rigor in many studies, increased use of appropriate measurement approaches is likely to increase the meaningfulness of information, improve the ease with which studies can be replicated and contribute to clarifying distinguishing affective and personality characteristics of suicidal, compared with nonsuicidal, youths.

Discussion

Review of psychological and social determinants in the etiology of adolescent suicide reveals considerable attention directed to the role of the family and relative inattention to other social relationships or systems or to the contribution of cognitive and personality factors. Studies suggest that a pattern of family and social disruption characterizes the background of suicidal adolescents. Particular family or social experiences, such as loss of a significant other or problem-making environmental changes, affect an adolescent's disposition toward suicidal behavior as part of this pattern. Studies further indicate that suicidal adolescents are more solitary than nonsuicidal but not than other emotionally disturbed adolescents. Sexual adjustment may be somewhat less adequate for suicidal adolescents than adolescents in general but not less adequate than other emotionally disturbed adolescents. However, the infrequency with which sexual problems have been assessed may lead to underestimating sexuality as a problem for suicidal adolescents. Clear correlation between suicidal behavior for adolescents and school performance, relationships, or stresses does not exist and relevant research is lacking. Descriptively, suicidal adolescents appear to be of at least average intelligence, have a negative outlook, be emotionally reactive, and at times act out their frustrations.

Difficulty comparing and evaluating studies emphasizing psychosocial variables and adolescent suicide include the differences in age groups considered (e.g., ages ten to twenty-one, fifteen to twenty-four, fourteen to fifty-two), limited empirical studies, limited use of control groups, and use of clinical populations as experimental and control groups. The imprecision with which social and psychological factors have been defined and documented also makes it difficult to evaluate their role. Frequently, dependent variables have been vaguely described or too broadly defined. In addition, most studies have used adolescents attempting/threatening rather than completing suicide, and it is not valid to generalize results from one group to the other. Therefore, understanding about adolescent suicide reflects the study of adolescents who attempt or threaten suicide; there are indications that those adolescents who complete suicide are even more isolated, less visible, and more disturbed than those attempting suicide.

Despite methodological difficulties and limited availability of empirical data, additional and more specific trends regarding youthful suicide are apparent:

1. Family conflict repeatedly and consistently has been identified in the background of suicidal adolescents and as a leading precipitant to their suicidal behavior; it may be particularly the nature rather than extent of such conflict that is significant.

2. Parent gender/roles probably differentially affect suicidal adolescents, with the role of the mother particularly appearing to be significant, at least from the view of the adolescent.

3. The suicidal adolescent girl particularly appears to be estranged from parent(s).

4. The impact of suicide within families in increasing suicidal risk for family members, especially for the young, merits continued study and preventive mental health attention.

5. The age of the child at the time of parent loss may be more important than the nature of the loss in its impact on subsequent suicidal behavior during adolescence.

6. Suicidal thoughts are not necessarily universal during adolescence.

7. Difficulties at school appear more often to be a problem for suicidal girls than boys and for suicidal adolescents who continue making attempts.

8. Relative social isolation particularly applies to suicidal girls and to those adolescents making repeated attempts and/or successfully completing suicide.

9. Adolescents addicted to drugs are at higher risk for suicide attempts than those who are nonaddicted, but addicted adolescents do not constitute a large proportion of youthful suicide attempters.

10. No clear effect of residential location, employment opportunities, or economic conditions upon adolescent suicidal behavior has been found, but increased geographic mobility is associated with a greater frequency of suicidal behavior in this age group.

11. In general, there is no clear evidence of media influence upon suicidal behavior, although some studies have suggested a decrease in the completed suicide rates for youthful females when newspapers are scarce.

12. There appears to be an increased risk of completed suicide among youthful males during wartime.

13. Depression during adolescence probably is associated with increased risk for suicidal behavior and particularly for recurrent suicidal

behavior; however, identification of the role of depression in youthful suicide has been complicated by the controversy over the nature of adolescent depression.

14. There are no consistent trends found in formal diagnostic categories for suicidal adolescents.

15. For adolescents, the interaction of physical illness with additional factors, such as gender, sex roles, emotional disturbance, time sequence, and visibility of symptoms can become a motivating factor for suicidal behavior.

16. The contribution of cognitive factors to adolescent suicide, or, more generally, the role of learning in the development of adolescent suicidal behavior has been overlooked.

17. Many school, family, social, and psychological problems, as well as motivating factors, may be characteristic of emotionally disturbed adolescents rather than specifically related to suicidal behavior.

18. There are sufficient gender differences to recommend that male and female suicidal adolescents be considered separately.

19. Closer attention to the effects of school on suicidal adolescents and incorporating suicide as a topic in teacher training and in secondary education are recommended.

20. Increased use of psychometric techniques in the study of adolescent suicide is likely to improve the identification of personality and affective characteristics distinguishing suicidal youths.

21. As a public health approach to suicide, it is relevant to direct increased attention to the easy availability of highly lethal means of death, especially to specific prescribed medications and to handguns.

22. Identification of psychosocial factors associated with the etiology of adolescent suicidal behavior is likely to be more productive if increased consideration is given to the influence and interrelationship of multiple factors, such as gender, sequence of events over time, lethality of self-destructive behavior, and overall emotional adjustment.

From both a practical and theoretical view, Jacobs's (1971) description and integration of the multiple diverse factors contributing to suicidal behavior during adolescence continues to be the most complete. Jacobs specifically has described the adolescent suicide attempt as part of a process which includes long-standing problems, escalation of problems during adolescence, increasing failure of adaptive techniques, progressive isolation, relatively acute dissolution of residual relationships, a conceptual justification of suicide, and, finally, the attempt. The extent to which learning variables and cognitive factors interact within such a pattern essentially has not been elaborated and the extent to which many specific social difficulties and individual characteristics are associated or interact as part of this suicidal process needs further clarification. Nevertheless, Jacobs's model provides a framework to which additional elements can be added.

Suicide behavior as learned behavior has received little attention. However, Frederick and Resnik (1971) have made an effort to place suicidal behaviors from a theoretical view in the context of learning theory irrespective of age variables. The inattention to the role of learned behavior and cognitive factors by Jacobs and others specifically with suicidal adolescents underestimates the potential use of intervention techniques based on learning theory. For example, anxiety associated with threatened loss or fear associated with environmental stress might be reduced by use of desensitization and relaxation procedures (Wolpe 1958). Feelings of hopelessness, helplessness, or limited time perspective might be changed by challenging negative and distorted expectations for the future and/or negative and irrational self-concepts on which they are based. Having the suicidal adolescent develop or learn problem-solving skills also might be important. Recent interest in rational-emotive theory and counseling for youths (Tosi 1974) and cognitive controls and cognitive control therapy for children (Santostefano 1978) particularly may be useful but unexplored models to better understand and change adolescent suicidal behavior. Since cognitive functions in general undergo considerable transition during adolescence (Piaget and Inhelder 1958), it continues to be essential that the effects of age and normal development neither be overlooked nor overemphasized in studies directed at the role of cognitive factors in adolescent suicide.

In general, research into adolescent suicide has provided the basis for asking many relevant questions but has produced little substantive information. As Haim (1974) summarized with respect to research into adolescent suicide, "confronted by so many questions, one can only express astonishment once more that research has been so scanty."

Conclusions

Review of social, situational, cognitive, and individual variables contributing to youthful suicide indicates that adolescents attempting suicide generally are of average intelligence, have a negative outlook, are emotionally reactive, probably are depressed and act out their feelings, and have experienced chronic family and social disruption. Adolescents completing suicide, a relatively unknown group, may be even more isolated and disturbed and less visible than those attempting suicide. Factors such as gender, sex roles, emotional disturbance, sequence of events over time, and physical illness appear to play important roles in the development of suicidal behavior for this age group but need further clarification. The importance of learned behavior and cognitive factors for the suicidal adolescent and the use of formal measurement techniques in research into youthful suicide behavior have been overlooked. Interpretation of adolescent suicide as a process which includes multiple psychosocial factors is discussed. Closer attention to the interaction of multiple etiological factors over time and clearer distinction between those psychosocial factors that may distinguish suicidal adolescents from other emotionally disturbed youths are recommended.

NOTE

1. Rates expressed per 100,000 population per year in specified age group.

REFERENCES

Adam, K. S.; Lohrenz, J. G.; and Harper, D. 1973. Suicidal ideation and parental loss: a preliminary research report. *Canadian Psychiatric Association Journal* 18:95–100.

Aitken, R. C. B.; Buglass, D.; and Kreitman, N. 1969. The changing pattern of attempted suicide in Edinburgh, 1962–67. *British Journal of Preventive and Social Medicine* 23:111–115.

Alexander, I. E., and Adlerstein, A. M. 1958. Affective responses to the concept of death in a population of children and early adolescents. *Journal of Genetic Psychology* 93:167–177.

Anastassopoulos, G., and Kokkini, D. 1969. Suicidal attempts in psychomotor epilepsy. *Behavioral Neuropsychiatry* 1:12–16.

Bagley, C., and Greer, S. 1972. "Black suicide"—a report of 25 English cases and controls. *Journal of Social Psychology* 86:175–179.

Bakwin, H. 1957. Suicide in children and adolescents. *Journal of Pediatrics* 50:749–769.

Balser, B. H., and Masterson, J. F. 1959. Suicide in adolescents. *American Journal of Psychiatry* 116:400–404.

Barter, J. T.; Swaback, D. O.; and Todd, D. 1968. Adolescent suicide attempts: a follow-up study of hospitalized patients. *Archives of General Psychiatry* 19:523–527.

Bernstein, D. M. 1972. The distressed adolescent—pregnancy vs. suicide. In N. Morris, ed. *Psychosomatic Medicine in Obstetrics and Gynecology*. Basel: Karger.

Bluebond-Langner, M. 1977. Meanings of death to children. In H. Feifel, ed. *New Meanings of Death*. New York: McGraw-Hill.

Blumenthal, S., and Bergner, L. 1973. Suicide and newspapers: a replicated study. *American Journal of Psychiatry* 130:468–471.

Bowlby, J. 1961. Childhood mourning and its implications for psychiatry. *American Journal of Psychiatry* 118:481–498.

Browning, C. H. 1974. Epidemiology of suicide: firearms. *Comprehensive Psychiatry* 15:549–553.

Cantor, P. C. 1976. Personality characteristics found among youthful female suicide attempters. *Journal of Abnormal Psychology* 85:324–329.

Cash, L. M., and Kooker, E. W. 1970. Attitudes toward death of NP patients who have attempted suicide. *Psychological Reports* 26:879–882.

Cazzullo, C. L.; Balestri, L.; and Generali, L. 1968. Some remarks on the attempted suicide in the period of adolescence. *Acta Paedopsychiatrica* 35:373–375.

Choron, J. 1972. *Suicide*. New York: Scribner's.

Connell, H. M. 1972. Depression in childhood. *Child Psychiatry and Human Development* 4:71–85.

Crook, T., and Raskin, A. 1975. Association of childhood parental loss with attempted suicide and depression. *Journal of Consulting and Clinical Psychology* 43:277.

Crumley, F. E. 1979. Adolescent suicide attempts. *Journal of the American Medical Association* 241:2404–2407.

Dizmang, L. H.; Watson, J.; May, P. A.; and Bopp, J. 1974. Adolescent suicide at an Indian reservation. *American Journal of Orthopsychiatry* 44:43–49.

Dolkart, M. B.; Hughes, P.; Jaffe, J.; and Zaks, M. S. 1971. Suicide preoccupations in young affluent American drug users: a study of yippies at the Democratic convention. *Bulletin of Suicidology* 8:70–73.

Dorpat, T. L.; Jackson, J. K.; and Ripley, H. S. 1965. Broken homes and attempted and completed suicide. *Archives of General Psychiatry* 12:213–216.

Dudley, H. K., Jr.; Mason, M.; and Rhoton, G. 1973. Relationship of beta IQ scores to young state hospital patients. *Journal of Clinical Psychology* 29:197–203.

Duncan, J. W. 1977. The immediate management of suicide attempts in children and adolescents: psychological aspects. *Journal of Family Practice* 4:77–90.

Edland, J. F., and Duncan, C. E. 1973. Suicide notes in Monroe County: a 23 year look (1950–1972). *Journal of Forensic Sciences* 18:364–369.

Finch, S. M., and Poznanski, E. O. 1971. *Adolescent Suicide*. Springfield, Ill.: Thomas.

Flinn, D. E., and Leonard, C. V. 1972. Prevalence of suicidal ideation and behavior among basic trainees and college students. *Military Medicine* 137:317–320.

Fox, R. 1971. Today's students. Suicide among students and its prevention. *Royal Society of Health Journal* 91:181–185.

Frederick, C. J., and Resnik, H. L. P. 1971. How suicidal behaviors are learned. *American Journal of Psychotherapy* 25:37–55.

Frederick, C. J.; Resnik, H. L. P.; and Wittlin, B. J. 1973. *Archives of General Psychiatry* 28:579–585.

Friedman, M.; Glasser, M.; Laufer, E.; Laufer, M.; and Wohl, M. 1972. Attempted suicide and self-mutilation in adolescence: some observations from a psychoanalytic research project. *International Journal of Psychoanalysis* 53:179–183.

Gabrielson, I. W.; Klerman, L. V.; Currie, J. B.; Tyler, N. C.; and Jekel, J. F. 1970. Suicide attempts in a population of pregnant teenagers. *American Journal of Public Health* 60:2289–2301.

Glaser, K. 1971. Suicidal children—management. *American Journal of Psychotherapy* 25:27–36.

Haider, I. 1968. Suicidal attempts in children and adolescents. *British Journal of Psychiatry* 114:1113–1134.

Haim, A. 1974. *Adolescent Suicide*. New York: International Universities Press.

Harvey, E. B.; Gazay, L.; and Samuels, B. 1976. Utilization of a psychiatric-social work team in an Alaskan native secondary boarding school. *American Academy of Child Psychiatry Journal* 15:558–574.

Hassal, C. 1969. Development of alcoholic addiction in young men. *British Journal of Preventive and Social Medicine* 23:40–44.

Hendin, H. 1963. The psychodynamics of suicide. *Journal of Nervous and Mental Diseases* 136:236–244.

Hendin, H. 1969. Black suicide. *Archives of General Psychiatry* 21:407–422.

Hynes, J. J. 1976. An exploratory study of the affective future time perspective of adolescent suicide attempters: its characteristics, relationship to clinical identification and lethality, and its implications for postvention. *Dissertation Abstracts International* 37:1404–1405.

Jacobs, J. 1971. *Adolescent Suicide*. New York: Wiley-Interscience.

Jacobziner, H. 1960. Attempted suicides in children. *Journal of Pediatrics* 56:519–525.

Klagsburn, F. 1976. *Too Young to Die*. Boston: Houghton Mifflin.

Kreitman, N.; Smith, P.; and Tan, E. 1969. Attempted suicide in social networks. *British Journal of Preventive and Social Medicine* 23:116–123.

Lawler, R. H.; Nakielny, W.; and Wright, N. A. 1963. Suicide attempts in children. *Canadian Medical Association Journal* 89:751–754.

Leese, S. M. 1969. Suicide behavior in twenty adolescents. *British Journal of Psychiatry* 115:479–480.

Leonard, C. V., and Flinn, D. E. 1972. Suicidal ideation and behavior in youthful nonpsychiatric populations. *Journal of Consulting and Clinical Psychology* 38:366–371.

Lester, D. 1968a. Punishment experiences and suicidal preoccupation. *Journal of Genetic Psychology* 113:89–94.

Lester, D. 1968b. Suicide as an aggressive act: a replication with a control for neuroticism. *Journal of General Psychology* 79:83–86.

Lester, D. 1969. Resentment and dependency in the suicidal individual. *Journal of General Psychology* 81:137–145.

Lester, D. 1970. Attempts to predict suicidal risk using psychological tests. *Psychological Bulletin* 74:1–17.

Lester, D. 1971. Seasonal variation in suicidal deaths. *British Journal of Psychiatry* 118:627–628.

Lester, G., and Lester, D. 1971. *Suicide: The Gamble with Death*. Englewood Cliffs, N.J.: Prentice-Hall.

Levenson, M., and Neuringer, C. 1970. Intropunitiveness in suicidal adolescents. *Journal of Projective Techniques and Personality Assessment* 34:409–411.

Levenson, M., and Neuringer, C. 1971. Problem-solving behavior in suicidal adolescents. *Journal of Consulting and Clinical Psychology* 37:433–436.

Levenson, M., and Neuringer, C. 1972. Phenomenal environmental oppressiveness in suicidal adolescents. *Journal of Genetic Psychology* 120:253–256.

Lourie, R. S. 1966. Clinical studies of attempted suicide in childhood. *Clinical Proceedings of Children's Hospital of the District of Columbia* 22:163–173.

Lukianowicz, N. 1968. Attempted suicide in children. *Acta Psychiatrica Scandinavica* 44:415–435.

McIntire, M. S., and Angle, C. R. 1970. The taxonomy of suicide as seen in poison control centers. *Pediatric Clinics of North America* 17:697–706.

McIntire, M. S., and Angle, C. R. 1971a. Is the poisoning accidental? an ever-present question beyond the early childhood years. *Clinical Pediatrics* 10:414–417.

McIntire, M. S., and Angle, C. R. 1971b. "Suicide" as seen in poison control centers. *Pediatrics* 6:914–922.

McIntire, M. S.; Angle, C. R.; Wikoff, R. L.; and Schlicht, M. L. 1977. Recurrent adolescent suicidal behavior. *Pediatrics* 60:605–608.

Maletsky, B. M. 1973. The episodic dyscontrol syndrome. *Diseases of the Nervous System* 36:178–185.

Margolin, N. L., and Teicher, J. D. 1968. Thirteen adolescent male suicide attempts. *Journal of the American Academy of Child Psychiatry* 7:296–315.

Marks, P. A., and Haller, D. L. 1977. Now I lay me down for keeps: a study of adolescent suicide attempts. *Journal of Clinical Psychology* 33:390–400.

Mattsson, A.; Seese, L. R.; and Hawkins, J. W. 1969. Suicidal behavior as a child psychiatric emergency. *Archives of General Psychiatry* 20:100–109.

Maxmen, J.S., and Tucker, G. J. 1973. No exit: the persistently suicidal patient. *Comprehensive Psychiatry* 14:71–79.

Melges, F. T., and Weisz, A. E. 1971. The personal future and suicidal ideation. *Journal of Nervous and Mental Disease* 153:244–250.

Motto, J. A. 1967. Suicide and suggestibility—the role of the press. *American Journal of Psychiatry* 124:252–256.

Motto, J. A. 1970. Newspaper influence on suicide. *Archives of General Psychiatry* 23:143–148.

Nagy, M. H. 1959. The child's view of death. In H. Feifel, ed. *The Meaning of Death*. New York: McGraw-Hill.

Oliver, R. G., and Hetzel, B. S. 1973. An analysis of recent trends in suicide rates in Australia. *International Journal of Epidemiology* 2:19–101.

Patel, N. S. 1974. A study of suicide. *Medicine, Science and Law* 14:129–136.

Peck, M. L., and Schrut, A. 1971. Suicidal behavior among college students. *HSMHA Health Reports* 86:149–156.

Petzel, S. V., and Cline, D. 1978. Adolescent suicide: epidemiological and biological aspects. *Adolescent Psychiatry* 6:239–266.

Piaget, J., and Inhelder, B. 1958. *The Growth of Logical Thinking from Childhood to Adolescence.* New York: Basic.

Resnik, H. L. P. 1972. Erotized repetitive hangings: a form of self-destructive behavior. *American Journal of Psychotherapy* 26:4–21.

Resnik, H. L. P., and Dizmang, L. H. 1971. Observations on suicidal behavior among American Indians. *American Journal of Psychiatry* 127:58–63.

Rinzler, C., and Shapiro, D. A. 1968. Wrist-cutting and suicide. *Journal of Mount Sinai Hospital New York* 25:485–488.

Roberts, J., and Hooper, D. 1969. The natural history of attempted suicide in Bristol. *British Journal of Medical Psychology* 42:303–312.

Ropschitz, D. H., and Ovenstone, I. M. 1968. A two year's survey on self aggressive acts, suicides, and suicidal threats in the Halifax district. *International Journal of Social Psychiatry* 14:165–187.

Rosenbaum, M., and Richman, J. 1970. Suicide: the role of hostility and death wishes from the family and significant others. *American Journal of Psychiatry* 126:1652–1655.

Ross, M. 1969. Suicide among college students. *American Journal of Psychiatry* 126:220–225.

Russell, H. E.; Conroy, R. W.; and Weiner, J. J. 1971. A study of suicidal behavior in the military setting. *Military Medicine* 136:549–552.

Sabbath, J. C. 1969. The suicidal adolescent—the expendable child. *Journal of American Academy of Child Psychiatry* 8:272–285.

Sabbath, J. C. 1971. The role of the parents in adolescent suicidal behavior. *Acta Paedopsychiatria* 38:211–220.

Sanborn, D. E.; Casey, T. M.; and Niswander, G. D. 1971. Drug abusers, suicide attempters, and the MMPI. *Diseases of the Nervous System* 32:183–187.

Sanborn, D. E.; Sanborn, C. J.; and Cimbolic, P. 1973. Two years of suicide: a study of adolescent suicide in New Hampshire. *Child Psychiatry and Human Development* 3:234–242.

Santostefano, S. 1978. *A Bio-developmental Approach to Clinical Child Psychology.* New York: Wiley.

Sartore, R. L. 1976. Students and suicide: an interpersonal tragedy. *Theory into Practice* 15:337–339.

Sawyer, J. B. 1969. An incidence study of military personnel engaging in suicidal behavior. *Military Medicine* 134:1440–1444.

Schilder, P., and Wechsler, D. 1934. The attitudes of children toward death. *Journal of Genetic Psychology* 45:406–451.

Schrut, A. 1968. Some typical patterns in the behavior and background of adolescent girls who attempt suicide. *American Journal of Psychiatry* 125:107–112.

Seiden, R. H. 1969. Suicide among youth. *Bulletin of Suicidology* (suppl.) Washington, D. C.: National Institute of Mental Health.

Senseman, L. A. 1969. Attempted suicide in adolescents: a suicide prevention center in Rhode Island is in urgent need. *Rhode Island Medical Journal* 52:449–451.

Shaw, C. R., and Schelkun, R. F. 1965. Suicidal behavior in children. *Psychiatry* 28:157–168.

Shepherd, D. M., and Barraclough, B. M. 1976. The aftermath of parental suicide for children. *British Journal of Psychiatry* 129:267–276.

Shneidman, E. S. 1968. Orientation toward cessation: a reexamination of current modes of death. *Journal of Forensic Science* 13:33–45.

Shore, J. H. 1975. American Indian suicide—fact and fantasy. *Psychiatry* 38:86–91.

Smith, A. J. 1972. Self-poisoning with drugs, a worsening situation. *British Medical Journal* 4:157–159.

Smith, J. S., and Davison, K. 1971. Changes in the pattern of admissions for attempted suicide in Newcastle-upon-Tyne during the 1960's. *British Journal of Medicine* 4:412–415.

Spalt, L., and Weishbuch, J. B. 1972. Suicide: an epidemiologic study. *Diseases of the Nervous System* 33:23–29.

Stanley, E. J., and Barter, J. T. 1970. Adolescent suicidal behavior. *American Journal of Orthopsychiatry* 40:87–95.

Stevenson, E. K.; Hudgens, R. W.; Held, C. P.; Meredith, C. H.; Hendrix, M. E.; and Carr, D. L. 1972. Suicidal communication by adolescents: study of two matched groups of 60 teenagers. *Diseases of the Nervous System* 33:112–122.

Suicide among American Blackfeet Indians. 1970. *Bulletin of Suicidology* 7:42–43.

Suicide: a world problem. 1971. *Lancet* 2:1411.

Suicide—international comparisons. 1972. *Metropolitan Life Insurance Company Statistical Bulletin* 23:2–5.

Teicher, J. D. 1970. Children and adolescents who attempt suicide. *Pediatric Clinics of North America* 17:687–696.

Teicher, J. D. 1975. Children who choose death. *Emergency Medicine* 7:136–142.

Toolan, J. M. 1962. Suicide and suicidal attempts in children and adolescents. *American Journal of Psychiatry* 118:719–724.

Tosi, D. J. 1974. *Youth: Toward Personal Growth: A Rational-emotive Approach.* Columbus, Ohio: Merrill.

U.S. Department of Health, Education, and Welfare, Public Health Service, National Vital Statistics. 1974. *Mortality Trends for Leading Causes of Death, United States, 1950–1969.* DHEW Publication no. (HRA)74-1853, series 20, no. 16 (March): 44–46.

U. S. Department of Health, Education, and Welfare, Public Health Service, National Office of Vital Statistics. 1956. *Death Rates by Age, Race, Sex, United States, 1900–1953: Suicide.* Vital Statistics Special Report 43, no. 30 (August 22): 463–477.

U. S. Department of Health, Education, and Welfare. 1963–1979. *Vital Statistics of the United States, 1960–1975.* Washington, D. C.: Government Printing Office.

U. S. Department of Health, Education, and Welfare, Public Health Service, National Office of Vital Statistics. 1967. *Suicides in the United States, 1950–1964.* Public Health Service Publication no. 1000, series 20, no. 5 (August), pp. 15–17, 32–33.

Weinberg, S. 1970. Suicidal intent in adolescence: a hypothesis about the role of physical illness. *Pediatrics* 77:579–586.

Weiner, I. 1970. *Psychological Disturbance in Adolescence.* New York: Wiley-Interscience.

Weismann, A. D., and Worden, J. W. 1972. Risk-rescue rating in suicide assessment. *Archives of General Psychiatry* 26:553–560.

Whitlock, F. A., and Edwards, J. E. 1968. Pregnancy and attempted suicide. *Comprehensive Psychiatry* 9:1–12.

Williams, C., and Lyons, C. 1976. Family interaction and adolescent suicidal behaviour: a preliminary investigation. *Australian and New Zealand Journal of Psychiatry* 10:243–252.

Wolpe, J. 1958. *Psychotherapy by Reciprocal Inhibition.* Stanford, Calif.: Stanford University Press.

Yacoubian, J. H., and Lourie, R. 1969. Suicide and attempted suicide in children and adolescents. *Clinical Proceedings of Children's Hospital* 25:325–344.

Yufit, R. I.; Benzies, B.; Fonte, M. E.; and Fawcett, J. A. 1970.

Suicide potential and time perspective. *Archives of General Psychiatry* 23:158–163.

Yusin, A.; Sinay, R.; and Nihira, K. 1972. Adolescents in crisis: evaluation of a questionnaire. *American Journal of Psychiatry* 129:574–577.

Zilboorg, G. 1936. Suicide among primitive and civilized races. *American Journal of Psychiatry* 92:1346–1369.

24 THE INTERLOCKING PSYCHOLOGIES OF
SUICIDE AND ADOLESCENCE

NORMAN TABACHNICK

The purpose of this chapter is to delineate certain aspects of the psychology of suicide and certain aspects of the psychology of adolescence which interrelate to create the unique features of adolescent suicide. When one considers the psychologies of these two situations, there is an immediate impression that they are closely linked. Indeed, one might come to feel that in certain ways suicidal psychology is an essential part of adolescent psychology. The problems of the adolescent and his special ways of dealing with them make suicide very attractive. In most cases the situation will not go beyond the point of thinking about suicide, but suicide attempts and suicidal deaths do occur.

Although suicidal rumination may be an essential and perhaps normal part of adolescence, suicide itself is something that we are seriously concerned about. That life-affirming parental attitude suggests the second focus of this discussion which is an understanding of suicidal and adolescent psychology from the standpoint of psychotherapy. Although the psychotherapy of suicide revolves around principles which are important for all suicidal individuals, adolescence calls for special psychotherapeutic techniques and approaches.

The adolescent is a sensitive individual who no longer is a child but is afraid to acknowledge that he often still wants to be a child. This is because his inner development, his wishes, and the society that he lives in are all pushing him toward adulthood and expecting him to achieve it. But he often fears that he will not make it; that he *cannot* make it. Between his desires for adulthood and his fear of failure, between his secret longing for childhood and his conscious wish to no longer be a child, the adolescent is in limbo and a very painful limbo at that. And, here we see the first relationship to suicide. Suicidal concern typically arises in individuals who have doubts about their appropriate place in developmental life cycles. It also arises in persons who are concerned about social sanction and approval. The adolescent is vulnerable in both areas.

The discussion in this chapter is based mainly on the author's clinical training experience. It is affected by a theoretical background in psychoanalysis, but it does not exclude other data and theorizations about suicide and adolescence. There have been many years of work with adolescents at the Los Angeles Suicide Prevention Center, as well as data from other outpatient clinics. In addition, many suicidal adolescents have been treated in a private practice setting.

It is important to emphasize that these are the subject populations, because they do not encompass all suicidal adolescent situations. For example, a great deal of suicide occurs among adolescent delinquents and drug takers. These young people often are not seen in clinics or by private psychotherapists. The focus of this article is on general psychological principles which are basic to therapy with suicidal adolescents. Little attention is paid to the utilization of certain ancillary features such as medication or hospitalization.

Even when death does not result, the presence of suicidal thinking in an adolescent is a serious indication for paying attention and trying to help. When we speak about suicide, we envision a whole group of feelings and situations. They have to do with depression, loss, and feelings of hopelessness. Although any person thinking about suicide has an increased possibility of making a suicide attempt or killing himself or herself by suicide, those individuals who just think about suicide are certainly troubled and need attention.

Features of Suicidal Psychology

OBJECT LOSS

Most people in suicidal states are concerned with the loss of something very important to them. From a psychoanalytic standpoint we speak of object loss. In that framework we mean more than something external, something that is real, or something that an outsider could easily see as being important to the individual. Although object loss from a psychoanalytic standpoint may include such external losses, what the term means more essentially is that within the individual something crucial is felt to be gone. Thus, there may be times when to an outsider object loss would be difficult to appreciate. For example, a lover might say a few slighting words or indicate that he might not be available at a particular time to the suicidal individual. To the latter this may be experienced as a strong rejection or as if he has lost the object.

In most cases the lost object is an individual, a relative, a lover, or a dear friend. However, the objects may be nonhuman. For example, they may include one's good health, financial fortune, or status in society. Examples run the gamut of all things in which human beings place importance.

LONELINESS

In addition to a feeling of being distant from special important objects, suicidal people often describe a feeling of loneliness, or a sense of being alienated from the whole world. This is especially extreme in schizophrenic alienation. But, in those suicidal people who are not psychotic, one can see it in such symbolic manifestations as dreams of being alone at sea or wandering over a desert. Those dreams which show one to be isolated in a vast and horizonless environment are metaphors for suicidal isolation.

HOPELESSNESS

Associated with suicidal states are episodes of hopelessness. These are periods in which an individual attaches no special meanings to his life or when the meanings seem to be uncertain. One moment he may think that a change of occupation would make him feel better, but the next moment he reverts and tells himself, "No, I don't really think that that occupation or any occupation could make me feel that life is worthwhile." This uncertainty often exists in other areas, for example, personal relationships and philosophical values. Often a lack of hope is associated with an inner feeling of emptiness. There are questions about the central goals of one's life. Some suicidal individuals have a very good idea of what they would like to be; however, they feel that there is no chance. They frequently feel, for example, that they are too old to accomplish or to continue accomplishing certain important goals.

HELPLESSNESS

Close to hopelessness, but more specifically connected with one's own abilities, are feelings of impotence. These are not only related to sexuality but can also be tied to work ability, the attraction of friends, and indeed to any life goal.

A CASE OF ADOLESCENT SUICIDAL RUMINATION

Bob was an eighteen-year-old student who during the last months of his second semester at college was having a "catastrophic crash." He had looked forward to school, had had ambitions to do well, to have a good time, and to learn a lot. He was not too sure of how those wishes would be fulfilled, but when he started school he had confidence that he would find ways to realize his hopes. At the beginning, things had gone well. However, as time went on he became lonely, felt isolated from his friends, and began to miss his parents and his hometown 200 miles away. He became depressed, started to think about suicide, but didn't know what to do about it. He had kept contact with his parents. His mother, who implemented the important family decisions, brought him home. She called the therapist, alerting him of Bob's return, and set up an appointment. Bob was seen shortly after he returned to the city.

He was depressed and ashamed of himself. He felt that he had failed. Even more than that, he felt that the failure was an indication of inner deficiencies. What were they? Old ideas about not being a man came to the fore. He found himself attracted to boys and men. He wondered if he was homosexual. In addition, things were working out very poorly at school. He had hoped that he would be attracted and fascinated by many or all of his subjects and that the only problem with choice would be picking one of the many life goals which seemed attractive. Things had not gone that way. Much of the schoolwork was tedious and there were many things he could not understand. Some of the teachers were less than the inspirational ideals he had fantasized. And, in the face of all these external difficulties, he was also missing the inner enthusiasm which he had assumed would express itself.

Then, there was the problem of friends. He had expected a group of enthusiastic, fun-loving, intellectually alert students. He had assumed that he would make many friends; that they would form a joyous band who would participate in activities together. On the contrary, there were not too many people who had that brilliant attractiveness. Of the small number who did, none seemed to be interested in him. He felt isolated and became deeply depressed.

Bob had many features of the typical suicidal person. There were many object losses. Old ones included being away from the usual and important supports of home and especially being away from his mother. He had always been dimly aware of his mother's value to him but had not thought of himself as overly dependent. Actually, he thought his mother was dominating and had predicted that he would be glad to get away from her. Even though it was hard for him to acknowledge his feeling adrift without her, it was clear that this was the case.

There were new losses as well. He had looked forward to finding a stimulating environment at school, with new ideals (teachers) whom he could emulate and feel close to and new friends. Even in anticipation, these had become important objects to him. But, he was disappointed when he was unable to find significant replacements at school. Furthermore, since he began to feel that these problems had to do with inner deficiencies, he became discouraged about finding and developing relationships with new people or new activities that might have started to fulfill some of his ambitions.

He felt hopeless. The plan about his life and its purpose, and about the individual, who would be activating that plan and in turn being formed by it, was falling apart. He did not know what to do and he was uncertain if he should continue in school. But, he also felt a sense of failure in leaving. When his mother said, "You must come home and get into therapy," he was relieved. Even though he was ashamed at his own inaction, at least, and at last, something was being done.

Finally, he felt impotent. He did not know what to do and he doubted whether he had the strength or the essential core to do anything. He felt that he was not what was very important for him to be at that time, a "man," someone who was capable of actualizing personal and societal goals.

Bob's mother was a crucial figure, both for the onset of the suicidal problems and, as it turned out, in helping to resolve them. Feelings of suicide are not infrequently connected with the image of a nurturing mother. Very often these feelings are elicited by the mother who could nurture but does not want to, is not available, or who cannot be turned to even if she is available. She is the first important object and is the one who supplies those essential elements which make life worthwhile, transforming one into a living human being with a personal identity.

Although suicidal situations develop in the face of all kinds of losses, concerns about being adequately mothered probably are always present in suicidal individuals. Of course, in most cases the mother that is missing turns out to be the mother that we must be to ourselves. However, the metaphor of maternal deprivation is a key one in suicide (Tabachnick 1957, 1973).

The corollary to this is that the metaphor of maternal sufficiency is related to the overcoming of suicidal situations. The latter are resolved in different ways. Sometimes life situations bring back the old objects or bring new ones which take their place. Sometimes the therapist is the new object. Sometimes an individual summons from within himself new hope and thus, new objects. But, all of these share the conviction that a new good mother is discovered.

Features of Adolescent Psychology

Many features of adolescence cluster around the same key concepts which are prominent in suicide. They include:

OBJECT LOSS

There are real and fantasied object losses in adolescence, just as in suicide. The real ones have to do with the giving up by the adolescent and the taking away by society of many of the supports and caretaking relationships which have existed in earlier epochs of life. Object losses, however, must be seen in terms of the internal fantasy of the adolescent as well as the actual dissolution of real relationships. The adolescent is in a period of transition. By necessity he must leave old supports and move toward new responsibilities. Moving into self-reliance is a cherished goal, but its shadowy, often unconscious, underside is terror. The terror is often projected onto others and is manifested in vague anxieties, depression, and nightmares.

LONELINESS AND ALIENATION

As the adolescent makes transitions and tries new modes, loneliness occurs. The adolescent who as a child has had many strong and supportive contacts with adults, now finds that, increasingly, life must be lived alone. And again, just as in the suicidal, those dreams of being "at sea" and "deserted" are not uncommon.

404

HOPELESSNESS

And, following from these problems, there is grave questioning as to how much one can do. There is doubt over one's possession of the essential spark of vitality which makes for competence. The youngster wonders if he will amount to anything or will instead be a hopeless cripple, a defect, a homosexual. At such times, the adolescent often thinks he might be better off dead.

In essence, there is a feeling of hopelessness associated with an uncertain identity. Identity and hope are related to a secure knowledge of what one wants to do and a sense of having the competence to do it.

HELPLESSNESS

Because the previously supportive parental figures are no longer available and because the adolescent has tremendous inexperience in the new modes of living, there is a feeling of being helpless to deal with life's problems. Of course, that is not the entire picture. There are the newly discovered pleasures that come from work, intimacy, and sexuality. Thus, there is a to and fro oscillation. One moment the youngster is happy, pleased, and exulted; the next he is in despair.

During adolescence there is typically much frustration and anger. These feelings are understandable and normal, but society tells the adolescent to repress them. Of course society is unable to tell him precisely how much to repress and when to repress. Generally the adolescent manages to muddle through, to find ways of expressing and repressing which eventually lead to positive adaptations. But often he fails. It would appear that too often the adolescent represses too much. This dynamic may lead to suicide.

Adolescence is one of those developmental nodal points in which drive conflicts and self-problems are intertwined. Drive issues are very important in adolescence. They include concerns about assertion, intimacy, sexuality, and competitiveness. They are the subject matter of the main concerns. But beyond them is a highly important need—the stability and the strength of the individual's self. In adolescence, the self, which is the organ of integration and synthesis of the total human personality, undergoes crucial and significant development. One cannot say that either issue is more important than the other. Both are present and must be dealt with in an interrelated way.

One is struck by the similarity of suicidal psychology to adolescent psychology. We can see how suicide and suicidal concerns are a normal mode in adolescence. In a sense, any adolescent not showing some suicidal concern might be suspected of being insensitive to, or dishonest about, all that is going on in his life.

Psychotherapy of Suicidal Adolescents

The psychotherapy of suicidal patients has been studied in depth (Mintz 1966; Tabachnick 1970). Some of the key points in suicidal psychotherapy are related to the issues mentioned earlier as fundamental to the psychology of suicide and adolescence. They are object loss, loneliness and alienation, hopelessness, and helplessness. Let us examine the way in which those issues are dealt with in the general treatment of suicide and then note the modifications necessary in working with adolescents.

OBJECT LOSS

To replace the lost object is a principle of suicidal treatment. Indeed, if that does not occur, one must doubt that the treatment has been sufficient. In adults that object is replaced by one or more people. One of them is usually the therapist; the other one is either an old object with whom the patient is reunited or a new one, brought in because an older one is not available. It is typical of suicidal patients to move into very close relationships with these new objects. An adult patient who had lost her mother said to her therapist after several sessions, "I think of you a lot. Sometimes when something is troubling me and I'm not sure as to what I should do, I think of our discussions and see if they apply. I try to think of what you would tell me to do. It's like you are with me."

Adolescents, however, have difficulty in maintaining such intense relationships. Bob, the patient presented earlier, found a young woman friend after three months of therapy, but the relationship was tempestuous. There were many breakups and reconciliations; many feelings that the relationship was not worthwhile. He wondered if he should tie himself to just one person. The same issues were present in his therapy. Although he felt that therapy was helpful, he wondered if he needed more of it, whether the therapist was doing enough for him, and whether it might not be better for him to take care of things on his own, in other words—"to be a man."

In therapy the adolescent is trying out new ways of dealing with the mother, played out through her surrogate, the therapist. Previously he had to hold back most of the anger he felt toward his mother. He thought of her as essentially good. This is not to say that adolescents don't experience many dissatisfactions with their mothers. Of course they do, but it is only during adolescence that they seriously consider that it is important to become independent of mother. They begin to see her as an equal, someone with whom they can have a relationship, even a special relationship, but upon whom they are no longer dependent. The issue of simultaneously needing mother but changing the relative balance of need and independence is the key point here.

Also important are the feelings of the therapist in this situation. He must deal with a tempestuous, erratic patient who is considering leaving (rejecting) him. All therapists working with adolescents must deal with this problem. (Adolescents are always thinking of leaving.) But, in suicidal patients our general acceptance of adolescent independence is diminished. We are concerned that the patient's rejection of us, and thus, the patient's rejection of therapy, may lead to suicide. This makes us more anxious and may make us more rigid in treating the suicidal adolescent. This concern may mask the therapist's difficulty in accepting rejection by the patient.

LONELINESS AND ALIENATION

Loneliness is bewildering and loathsome. The therapist's task is to help the adolescent appreciate the positive value of loneliness. True it is unpleasant and difficult to handle. But that is not the worst of it for the adolescent. The crucial problem is the relationship of loneliness to personal inadequacy. The therapist has to help the patient to see that loneliness is related to being human and to being able to bear the anxiety of independence, so that he can have an opportunity to make a life and character that is his own.

HOPELESSNESS AND LOSS OF IDENTITY

Here, the problems are similar to those of loneliness and alienation. Hopelessness entails leaving behind the old certainties and finding oneself in a period of trial and error. One has to muddle around for a while before a new confidence develops. During that period one may have trouble holding on and feeling hopeful. In dealing with this issue the therapist must act as a "good enough" mother surrogate. Through his belief that the patient has the potential which will lead to learning and good adaptation, he provides him with a sustaining environment.

HELPLESSNESS

Again, helplessness is a way of giving a negative cast to an experiential state essential for human development. That state is produced by the ability to renounce old supports and to bear the resulting feelings of weakness. When that renunciation is possible, the adolescent can accept new objects, new friends, and new supports. These he finds in his day-to-day contacts and in his relationship with the therapist. But, it is important for him not to fall into the idea that his friends and his therapist will take care of him in the same way his mother did when he was a baby—because he no longer is a baby. The price for this realization and responsibility creates a feeling of helplessness. The goal is to be able to bear the feeling.

With all of this, one can expect a good deal of acting out on the part of the patient. This does not necessarily mean that he will make suicide attempts. In various ways he will defy the therapist. He will forget about or not show up for his appointments, often without even phoning. When the matter is discussed, he will retort, "I had other things to do. It was important for me to be with my friend at a particular event. It was important for me to study. You know there are other important things to life besides therapy." What can one say in response to this? There are other important things besides therapy and one does have to learn how to decide what is most important.

The therapist may feel that nothing could be more important than for his patient to be at the appointment at the time that the therapist has scheduled to see him. That, no doubt, is a very understandable feeling for the therapist. However, it is not necessarily a healthy attitude for the patient. He should be feeling (just as he said) that there are other important issues in his life. Just as the patient may have to learn to bear feelings of helplessness, the therapist must also learn to accept the acting out of his suicidal patient. Actually, it is common for adolescent suicidal patients to leave therapy by engaging in a struggle, dealing with their dependency towards the therapist. It would be unwise to deal with this struggle by interpreting unconscious hostility. In the first place, the interpretation is inaccurate because the irritation is often quite conscious. Second, it is quite appropriate for the patient to struggle with the therapist. The patient is dealing with the image of an engulfing mother who wants the patient to be dependent on her. The patient has to struggle, and to say finally, "It is my decision to be different than you, and to leave you even though you may not think that this is the best time for my leaving." It is up to the therapist to accept and perhaps even to encourage this by saying, "You know, you may be right. I am not sure that it is not a good time for you to leave. Even though I have some questions about it, I may be wrong."

When the therapist can say that, then he has mastered the problems of this developmental epoch, and when the patient can defy the therapist, he has in part mastered his problem. They can part with some irritation between them. The legacy will be a patient actively involved in the process of becoming a stronger adult.

Conclusions

There are a number of striking similarities in the psychology of adolescence and in the psychology of suicide. Four important issues which are significant in both groups are object loss, loneliness, hopelessness, and helplessness. These key issues are fundamental to the psychotherapy of suicide. Although much psychotherapy of suicide is similar for adults and adolescents, there are some special criteria which should be kept in mind in treating suicidal situations in adolescence. Thus although adolescents are concerned about object loss, they also have strong needs to become independent of objects. Loneliness, helplessness, and hopelessness in adolescents are connected to their efforts to achieve adult, as distinguished from childhood, identities. Thus the suicidal adolescent must not only overcome the anguish of those states but must also learn that to bear such anguish is important. The therapist, in terms of the distortions and working through of the transferences ascribed to him, will have to be different in working with suicidal adolescents than with suicidal adults.

REFERENCES

Mintz, S. 1966. Some practical procedures in the management of suicidal persons. *American Journal of Orthopsychiatry* 5:896–903.
Tabachnick, N. 1957. Observations on attempted suicide. In E. S.

Shneidman and N. L. Farberow, eds. *Clues to Suicide*. New York: McGraw-Hill.

Tabachnick, N. 1970. The crisis treatment of suicide. *California Medicine* 112:1–8.

Tabachnick, N. 1973. Creative suicidal crisis. *Archives of General Psychiatry* 29:258–263.

25 THE PHENOMENOLOGY OF
ADOLESCENT DEPRESSION

GABRIELLE A. CARLSON

As we have become more conversant with the clinical manifestations, natural history, dynamics, and treatment of affective disorders in adults, clinicians seeing children and adolescents are reexamining some of their previously held notions about depression and manic-depression in this age group.

Large epidemiologic studies of adolescents admitted to psychiatric hospitals record rates of depression from a negligible (Weiner and Del Gaudio 1976) 2.7 percent in state and county facilities to 19 percent in private general hospitals (U.S. Department of Health, Education, and Welfare 1977a). Psychoneurotic depression is the most frequent depression diagnosis, though this is greatly exceeded by diagnoses of schizophrenia and adjustment reaction. Where specific ages are noted, the incidence of depression increases with chronologic age such that depression in early adolescence is much less common than in late adolescence (U.S. Department of Health, Education, and Welfare 1977b). Where systematic and detailed examinations of adolescents have been performed, however, the diagnosis of affective disorder in hospitalized teenagers is much higher, between 20 and 40 percent (Hudgens 1974; King and Pittman 1969). Until the recent longitudinal studies by Masterson (1967), Offer (1967), and Rutter, Grahan, Chadwick, and Yule (1976) disproved the notion, it was felt that psychopathology expressing itself in adolescence could be attributed to developmental "turmoil" and ego regression which, allegedly, naturally occurred. Although adolescence is not without its age-appropriate miseries we now realize that the natural history of psychiatrically ill teenagers is to become psychiatrically ill adults.

© 1981 by The University of Chicago. 0-226-24054-1/81/0009-0007$01.00

The second widely held notion about adolescent depression is that it exists but as various other forms of behavioral delinquency such as conduct disturbances, delinquency, school phobia (Glaser 1968; Toolan 1962), anorexia nervosa, hypochondriasis, obesity (Malmquist 1972), school problems, and acting out (Bakwin 1972). Actually, masked depression probably represents two separate phenomena. In a scrupulously obtained history and mental status exam, a teenager will often assent to depressed mood and cognitive and vegetative symptoms that he might not have volunteered. Since he presents with other complaints and the depression becomes apparent only later, clinicians have felt the other problems "masked" the depression (Carlson and Cantwell 1980). It is interesting that certain kinds of problems are more often associated with a simultaneous or subsequent depression, problems such as school phobia, anorexia nervosa, some conduct disturbances, and stomachaches. Although the nature of the association is unclear in these cases, it is almost always possible to elicit the depression easily, hence the term "masked" is erroneous. There are some youngsters, however, who vehemently deny depression and anhedonia, and when examined a year or two later have had a depressive episode (Cantwell, Sturzenberger, Burroughs, Salkin, and Green 1977). Perhaps the term "masked depression" is more valid in these cases.

When one speaks of depression it is necessary to clarify whether one is talking about the mood itself, a combination of affective, cognitive, psychomotor, and vegetative manifestations, which may occur as a response to a variety of adversities and disappear when they do, or about depression as an illness. In depressive illness one has the depressive syndrome which is out of proportion to environmental stressors and is not relieved with environmental manipulation. Furthermore, there is ample evidence from the adult psychiatry literature that the entity of depressive illness has psychological, biochemical, pharmacologic, and genetic cohesion. The focus of this chapter will thus be on depressive illness in adolescents, distinguishing by definition these youngsters from those who are miserable and unhappy but do not meet DSM III (1980) criteria for depression.

It is possible to divide adolescent depression into primary and secondary types (Woodruff, Goodwin, and Guza 1974). By their definition, depressed people without preexisting psychiatric disorders were felt to have a primary affective illness: those with previous psychiatric disorders have a secondary (in terms of chronology not consequence) affective disorder.

412

Primary Affective Disorder

Until recently, bipolar affective disorder or manic-depressive illness was considered uncommon in teenagers, especially early adolescents. We now know that this rarity is accounted for largely by misdiagnosis (Carlson and Strober 1978). Of the ten young adolescents followed or consulted on by this author, only one whose manic episodes were rapidly recurrent was diagnosed correctly. Schizophrenia and adolescent adjustment reaction were the initial and often subsequent diagnoses.

An examination of the episodes of these subjects reveals that their symptomatology was similar to that of adults but in the context of adolescent turmoil were considered adjustment reactions in mild cases and schizophrenia in severe cases. Table 1 compares symptoms in six adolescents whose cases have been reviewed elsewhere (Carlson and Strober 1978) with those of adult manic-depressives (Winokur, Clayton, and Reich 1969).

One of the legitimate difficulties in diagnosing bipolar MDI in teenagers is that one is often seeing the first episode of a process which only in the future will become bipolar. Diagnosing with the retrospectoscope is infinitely easier than doing so cross-sectionally. There

TABLE 1
PERCENT OCCURRENCE OF MANIC-DEPRESSIVE SYMPTOMS
IN ADOLESCENT AND ADULT MANIC DEPRESSIVES

	Adolescents* (N=6)	Adults (N=27)
Dysphoric mood	100	100
Low self-esteem	66	91
Recent poor school performance	83	91†
Anhedonia	50	NR
Fatigue	NR	75
Insomnia	NR	100
Anorexia	50	97
Somatic complaints	NR	66
Suicidal ruminations	83	82
Agitation/irritability	50	75
Psychomotor retardation	83	75
Paranoid delusions	66	33
Auditory hallucinations	50	6
Confusion	66	13–24
First-rank symptoms	33	—

SOURCE.—Adapted from Carlson and Strober (1978).
NOTE.—NR = not recorded.
* Based on chart review.
† Poor concentration.

413

are no foolproof ways of making the diagnosis. Obviously, it is easier at times but difficult in other circumstances, and the more typical or adultlike the presentation the easier the task.

For example, a sixteen-year-old high school senior was having problems adjusting to her California surroundings, with the acute onset of troubles coming one year after the family's move from the East Coast. Given this girl's past history of serious medical illness, current family situation, and psychodynamics it was possible to formulate this case from almost any point. Her appearance was most striking. She looked almost like a zombie. Her attempts at smiling made her look sadder. Her chief complaint was that she could not concentrate and that school, the arena in which she previously excelled, was becoming a nightmare academically and socially. She said she had lost her confidence, lost her appetite, and lost her motivation. She was sleeping excessively, but was always tired, felt very slowed down, but was anxious inside. Although she had a number of interpersonal difficulties which were dealt with in therapy, her depression was the major problem. Interestingly, she did not describe herself as depressed though she assented gratefully when given the word. More significantly, her parents had not recognized her as being depressed (though they knew she was troubled). She is doing considerably better on amitryptiline (250 mg) and it is easier to work with and her family around other issues.

As this was M's first episode (with no prior history of depression or mood swings and a family history only suggestive for depression, and not manic-depression), one could not predict whether she would have a bipolar or unipolar course. The acute onset and the classical signs and symptoms made the depression diagnosis obvious.

Another fairly obvious case is exemplified by a college freshman who also had been a good student and who also was suffering severely from inability to concentrate and anhedonia. She, too, complained of fatigue and hypersomnia but had gained rather than lost weight. She noted both psychomotor retardation and internal anxiety. Unlike M, however, her symptoms had continued untreated for a year. She had a past history of rather striking cyclothymia, and there was positive family history for recurrent depressions, some terminated by ECT. This young lady is at risk for bipolar MDI. It is unclear whether she responded to a trial of imipramine or not as her parents terminated the medication prematurely. She had begun to improve and her improvement continued without medication. She lost the added weight, resumed her social activities, and reentered college the following semester.

414

In these two cases, and in the majority of teenagers given an affective disorder diagnosis noted in table 2 (Carlson and Strober 1978), we see the recent decline in school performance with impaired concentration and the loss of interest in previously pleasurable activities as very common presenting complaints in adolescent depression. The slowed thoughts and motor retardation are serious enough in the author's experience to drop a youngster's WISC scores twenty points and in several cases has been responsible for the erroneous diagnosis of mental retardation (Carlson 1979). These adolescent depressions otherwise fulfilled DSM III's operational criteria demonstrating that the core symptoms and signs of this disorder are similar in teenagers and adults (Baker, Dorzab, Winokur, and Cadoret 1971). Further similarities and differences are noted in table 2.

A more complicated diagnostic case is posed by L, a teenage girl with a childhood history remarkable only for the fact that she left her native South America at an early age and was without her father between ages eight months and four years. Her difficulties allegedly

TABLE 2
PERCENT OCCURRENCE OF DEPRESSIVE SYMPTOMS
IN ADOLESCENT AND ADULT
UNIPOLAR DEPRESSIVES

	Adolescent (N=28)	P	Adult (N=100)
Dysphoric mood	93	...	100
Loss of interests	71	...	77
Anhedonia	46	...	36
Hopelessness	43	...	56
Impaired concentration	82	...	84
Irritability	54	...	60
Problems making decisions	57	...	67
Slowed thoughts	46	...	67
Initial insomnia	61	...	77
Diurnal variation	25	...	46
Anorexia	68	...	80
Weight change	61	...	61
Suicidal thoughts	61	...	63
Auditory hallucinations	4	...	9
Depressive delusions	14	...	16
Feelings of worthlessness	64	<.02	38
Agitation	18	<.005	67
Excessive worry	39	<.005	69
Loss of energy	61	<.001	97
Psychomotor retardation	21	<.001	60
Terminal insomnia	39	<.02	65
Somatic complaints	50	<.02	25
Suicidal acts	32	<.05	15

SOURCE.—Adapted from Carlson and Strober (1978).

began on entrance to junior high school, when she claimed to be unhappy at school, reported that she "did not want to grow up," complained of being too fat, even though she was thin, and dieted down to seventy-four pounds at a time when she was five feet, three inches tall. She was ultimately hospitalized for about three weeks, treated only nutritionally, and reportedly gained weight. She was discharged and returned to finish junior high. She was given the diagnosis of anorexia nervosa.

In tenth grade, this previously compliant girl again complained of feeling ill at ease in school and responded this time by becoming truant. She was sleeping twelve to fourteen hours per day, began losing weight, was often tearful, and reported feelings of depression. She feared overeating would cover her heart with fat, and she exercised profusely. This process went on for a year. After quitting high school in the eleventh grade, she saw a psychiatrist who diagnosed her schizophrenic and treated her with 150 mg/day of thioridazine. There was no improvement.

Some months later her behavior dramatically switched; she slept only a few hours a night, was very energetic, grandiose, euphoric, intrusive, seductive, and occasionally bizarre. This behavior went on for about nine months, interrupted briefly by psychiatric hospitalization elsewhere, where readministration of thioridazine for her supposed schizophrenia did little.

She was ultimately hospitalized at age eighteen and given the diagnosis of bipolar MDI, a parsimonious and accurate way to explain one episode of anorexia nervosa, one of school phobia, and one of schizophrenia. A trial of lithium carbonate was helpful in returning her to reality although her relative lack of insight, her continued aversion to school, and an untenable family situation did not bode well for her.

According to her medical history, then, this girl has had two protracted episodes of depression. L's weight loss was obviously more purposeful than the result of simple appetite loss. Nonetheless, her other symptoms were more compatible with depression than anorexia nervosa. Her second episode was even more clearly depressive in nature and again we see school problems, both academic and social, as focal points for L's difficulty. It is sad that the early onset of her illness, the protracted nature of her episodes, and the fact that she received no appropriate treatment have led this young woman, with an above-average IQ, to be a high school dropout with a real distaste for school.

The natural history of bipolar and probably unipolar depressive illness in adolescents is similar to that for adults. That is, there are all degrees of severity and outcome, and the severity of a particular episode is not necessarily a clue to the prognosis (Carlson, Davenport, and Jamison 1977). Second, one can have any kind of personality, intelligence, and family situation and have an affective disorder. Although systematic research is lacking, the author's clinical experience is that youngsters with good premorbid adjustment and supportive families have better outcomes than the converse. A resolution of the affective disorder still leaves many of the coexistant problems, however, the less time an adolescent spends psychiatrically ill with depression or mania, the easier it is for him or her to try and solve these problems and to catch up developmentally with peers.

Secondary Affective Disorder

In a recent interview study of 102 psychiatrically referred children and adolescents, eight of fifty-one adolescents were diagnosed as having secondary affective disorder, that is, a nonaffective psychiatric disorder antedating the onset of their depressive symtomatology (Carlson and Cantwell 1979). Previous diagnoses included hyperactivity (two cases); drug use disorder (two cases); anorexia nervosa (two cases); severe learning disorder (one case); and grand mal epilepsy (1 case). Table 3 compares the depressive symptoms in adolescents with

TABLE 3
PERCENT OCCURRENCE OF DEPRESSIVE SYMPTOMS IN
ADOLESCENTS WITH PRIMARY AND
SECONDARY DEPRESSION

	Primary Depression (N=28)	P	Secondary Depression (N=8)
Dysphoric mood	93	<.05	63
Low self-esteem	64	...	75
Decreased school performance	82	...	75
Anhedonia	46	...	63
Fatigue	61	...	50
Sleep problem	61	...	75
Appetite problem	68	...	38
Somatic complaints	50	...	75
Suicide ideation	61	<.05	100
Hopelessness	43	<.05	88
Irritability	54	<.02	100

SOURCE.—Adapted from Carlson and Strober (1978).

primary and secondary affective disorder. Although symptom frequencies are similar, youngsters with secondary affective disorder are not surprisingly a more disturbed lot. They are more frequently aggressive, irritable, delinquent, hyperactive, and more frequently hopeless and suicidal. Many of these characteristics, often designated as depressive equivalents, probably reflect these teenagers' other psychiatric disorder. A comparison of frequency of the more common depressive equivalents is noted in table 4.

An additional difference in the primary and secondary disorder groups is in their family history of psychiatric illness. Five of the primary affective disorder patients had a family history of pure depression and only one had a history of depression and alcoholism. This contrasts with the secondary affective disorder subjects, five of whom had family histories of depression and alcoholism or sociopathy; none had histories of depression alone ($P < .01$). This greater saturation of familial illness may reflect the concurrence of psychopathologies in the secondary depression group. Except for the fact that half of our affective disorder patients fell into the secondary affective disorder classification, our findings are thus very similar to those reported by Andreason and Winokur (1979) for secondary affective disorder in adults.

These preliminary observations may bear directly on two issues in the literature on childhood and adolescent depression. The first concerns that of "masked depression." As Kovacs and Beck (1977) point out, many of the so-called masking symptoms such as fatigue, boredom, hypochondriasis, and irritability are actually well-documented

TABLE 4
PERCENT OCCURRENCE OF "DEPRESSIVE EQUIVALENTS" IN
ADOLESCENTS WITH PRIMARY AND
SECONDARY DEPRESSION

	Primary Depression ($N=28$)	P	Secondary Depression ($N=8$)
Truancy / school refusal	14	...	38
Disobedience / rule violation	18	...	38
Excessive drug use	21	...	25
Delinquent behavior	11	= .07	38
Hyperactivity	4	= .06	25
Aggressiveness	7	< .05	38
Excessive somatic complaints	21	< .005	75
One or more of the above	19	< .001	100

SOURCE.—Adapted from Carlson and Strober (1978).

symptoms of depression in adults. Additionally, in children with other psychiatric diagnoses, the primary diagnosis often distracts the clinician from concurrent depressive symptomatology.

These chronically disturbed youngsters may be less articulate about describing their distress than children for whom depression is an abrupt change from good functioning. However, careful, systematic questioning of parents and children frequently elicits an affective disorder where it might have otherwise been overlooked (Carlson and Cantwell 1979).

An opposite problem exists in potential overdiagnosing depressive disorder. Given the ubiquity of depression and low self-esteem, especially in disturbed children, it is important to try and distinguish environmentally responsive misery from true depressive illness. The distinction between hyperactivity and secondary affective disorder, for example, a hyperactive child with an understandable sense of discouragement and low self-esteem, is the most difficult and awaits further nosological clarification.

A final clinical vignette demonstrates the combination of attention-deficit disorder (ADD) and secondary affective disorder. H was a fourteen-year-old boy with a well-documented history of ADD and severe childhood asthma. As he entered adolescence he began to demonstrate minor antisocial behaviors. Long-term treatment with steroids had noticeably retarded his growth and while no longer taking steroids his growth had not compensated. With this background, H suffered the abrupt onset of insomnia, social withdrawal, phobic and somatic symptoms, and suicidal talk. When confronted directly about feeling depressed, he denied it, yet he admitted to hating himself, getting little pleasure from his usual activities, and that he felt tired and worried much of the time. His behavior was marked by noticeable restlessness, easy irritability, distractibility, and disinhibition. He presented, in other words, both his long-standing hyperactivity and short attention span and his more recent depressive disorder. His family history was replete with persons suffering from unipolar depressions, substance abuse, and sociopathy.

Although a systematic follow-up study has not been carried out on these adolescents to verify if, in fact, they have both diagnoses, the author's clinical observations note the following: The depression remits, either of its own accord or with antidepressant medication, and the original psychiatric problem remains unchanged. Second, these youngsters present more complicated treatment problems, are more often suicidal, and more often have chaotic family situations which result from and then perpetuate the inherent psychopathology.

Conclusions

Many questions remain in the search for the clinical boundaries, unique features of, and developmental contributions to adolescent affective disorder. It would appear, however, that a population of adolescents defined by adult criteria as being depressed, are not substantially different phenomenologically from their adult counterparts. Moreover, adolescent depression, so defined, is a significant psychopathological entity.

REFERENCES

Andreason, N. C., and Winokur, G. 1979. Secondary depression: familial, clinical and research perspectives. *American Journal of Psychiatry* 136:62–66.

Baker, M.; Dorzab, J.; Winokur, G.; and Cadoret, R. 1971. Depressive disease: classifications and clinical characteristics. *Comprehensive Psychiatry* 12:354–365.

Bakwin, H. 1972. Depression—a mood disorder in children and adolescents. *Maryland State Medical Journal* 21:55–61.

Cantwell, D. P.; Sturzenberger, S.; Burroughs, J.; Salkin, B.; and Green, J. K. 1977. Anorexia nervosa—an affective disorder? *Archives of General Psychiatry* 34:1087–1093.

Carlson, G. A. 1979. Affective psychosis in mental retardates. *Psychiatric Clinics of North America* 2:499–510.

Carlson, G. A., and Cantwell, D. P. 1979. Survey of depressive symptoms in a child and adolescent psychiatric population: interview data. *Journal of the American Academy of Child Psychiatry* 18:587–599.

Carlson, G. A., and Cantwell, D. P. 1980. Unmasking masked depression in children and adolescents. *American Journal of Psychiatry* 137:445–449.

Carlson, G. A.; Davenport, Y. B.; and Jamison, K. R. 1977. A comparison of outcome in adolescent and late onset bipolar manic-depressive illness. *American Journal of Psychiatry* 134:919–922.

Carlson, G. A., and Strober, M. 1978. Manic-depressive illness in early adolescence: a study of clinical and diagnostic characteristics in six cases. *Journal of the American Academy of Child Psychiatry* 17:138–153.

DSM III. 1980. *Diagnostic and Statistical Manual of Mental Disorders.* 3d ed. *Washington, D.C.: American Medical Association.*

Glaser, K. 1968. Masked depression in children and adolescents: American progress. *Child Psychiatry and Child Development* 1:345–355.

Hudgens, R. W. 1974. *Psychiatric Disorders in Adolescents.* Baltimore: Williams & Wilkins.

King, L., and Pittman, G. D. 1969. A six-year follow-up study of sixty-five adolescent patients: predictive value of presenting clinical picture. *British Journal of Psychiatry* 115:1437–1441.

Kovacs, M., and Beck, A. T. 1977. An empirical, clinical approach toward a definition of childhood depression. In J. G. Schulterbrandt, and A. Rasken, eds. *Depression in Childhood.* New York: Raven.

Malmquist, C. P. 1972. Depressive phenomena in children. In B. B. Wolman, ed. *Manual of Child Psychopathology.* New York: McGraw-Hill.

Masterson, J. F. 1967. *The Psychiatric Dilemma of Adolescence.* Boston: Little, Brown.

Offer, D. 1967. Normal adolescents. *Archives of General Psychiatry* 17:285–290.

Rutter, M.; Grahan, P.; Chadwick, O. F. D.; and Yule, W. 1976. Adolescent turmoil: fact or fiction. *Journal of Child Psychology and Psychiatry* 17:35–36.

Toolan, H. M. 1962. Depression in children and adolescents. *American Journal of Orthopsychiatry* 32:404–414.

U.S. Department of Health, Education, and Welfare. 1977a. Primary diagnosis of discharges from non-federal general hospital psychiatric inpatient units, U.S., 1975. *Mental Health Statistical Note,* no. 137.

U.S. Department of Health, Education, and Welfare. 1977b. Diagnostic distribution of admissions to inpatient services of state and county mental hospitals, U.S., 1975. *Mental Health Statistical Note,* no. 138.

Weiner, I. B., and Del Gaudio, A. C. 1976. Psychopathology in adolescence. *Archives of General Psychiatry* 33:187–193.

Winokur, G.; Clayton, P. J.; and Reich, T. 1969. *Manic Depressive Illness.* St. Louis: Mosby.

Woodruff, R. A., Jr.; Goodwin, D. W.; and Guza, S. B. 1974. *Psychiatric Diagnosis.* New York: Oxford University Press.

421

26   SEXUAL DIFFERENCES IN THE SUICIDAL
BEHAVIOR OF YOUNG PEOPLE

MAURICE J. ROSENTHAL

Statistics comparing suicidal behavior by sex usually show three important differences (Dublin and Bunzel 1933; Schneer and Kay 1961; Shneidman and Farberow 1961; Stengel 1974). First, more men than women commit suicide, three males for every female in the United States and most western European countries (Shneidman 1975). For white males ages fifteen to nineteen, suicide has become the second leading cause of death, eighty-eight per 100,000. Second, more women than men attempt suicide without completing it; again, about three to one. This is a surprising finding, reversing the sex ratio for completed suicides. Third, there is a difference in the methods used to perform suicidal acts. Males tend to use more violent and more lethal methods than females. To date, the reasons for such striking sexual differences regarding suicidal behavior among young people have not been adequately explained.

Those Who Attempt Suicide and
Those Who Complete It

This topic is relevant to our inquiry because the difference between the sexes shows up markedly when one compares statistically those who complete suicide and those who only attempt it. To begin with, there are far more people who attempt suicide than complete it. It is almost impossible to get a true estimate of the number of suicide attempts made since most incidents are reported as accidents. A great many suicide efforts are probably never reported, particularly when the risk of fatality or serious injury is low. In fact many authorities feel such cases should not be called "suicide attempts."

There is a wide discrepancy among published findings and estimates regarding the ratio of attempts to completed suicides. For example, Shneidman (1975) estimates eight to one, while Jacobziner (1965) estimates 100 to one. Some investigators claim that two different groups can be identified. As stated previously, among those who are suicide attempters there are more females than males. However, among adolescents the ratio may be much higher than three to one. Otto's study in Sweden for 1955 through 1959, involving 1,727 adolescents and children, found four times as many girls as boys attempting suicide. Relating his findings to the statistics for officially recorded suicides shows that boys made three to four suicide attempts per completed suicide, while among girls the ratio was twenty-five to thirty (Otto 1972; Waldenstrom, Larson, and Ljungstedt 1972). Most of the attempters indicated that they did not intend to die and accordingly did not use particularly lethal methods, or they arranged to be discovered before death could occur. Many consciously attempted to communicate with, influence, or impress a significant other by the act and thereby cause their relationship to be altered in a desired direction.

On the other hand, among those who completed suicide, most did not make any previous suicidal attempt; there were more males than females; most very clearly indicated a desire to die; and more used highly lethal methods to kill themselves.

However, the fact remains that far more completed suicides occur later from the group who began as suicide attempters than would be expected in the general population (Cohen, Motto, and Seiden 1966; Otto 1972; Petzel and Cline 1978; Pokorny 1966; Shneidman and Farberow 1961). Also, while not constituting a majority of the suicide attempters, a significant number used fairly lethal methods and did speak of a desire to die (Hendin 1976). Thus, it would be a serious clinical error to assume that cases of attempted suicide pose no risk of subsequent fatal acts. Clearly, to postulate the two groups as separate would be an oversimplification.

Some investigators and clinicians (Haim 1974; Hendin 1976; Meeks 1971; Pokorny 1966; Schneer and Kay 1961) believe that threats and attempts represent one end of a continuum that can lead to death by suicide. However, Shneidman (1975) and others interpret the above findings to mean that one could think of two sets of overlapping populations: (1) those who attempt suicide, few of whom go on to commit it;

and (2) those who commit suicide, many of whom had previously attempted it.

It should be noted that suicide attempts occur more frequently among the young than among the elderly. The peak age for attempts was thirty-two in males and twenty-seven in females. The modal age for completed suicide was older, forty-two for both sexes (Shneidman and Farberow 1961).

Jensen and Petty (1958) made a penetrating study of the interpersonal psychodynamics of attempted suicide, but without discerning any characteristic sexual differences among the attempters.

Previous Explanations of Sexual Differences

In most writings on the epidemiology of suicide, sexual differences are not mentioned. When they are, usually no attempt is made to account for the findings.

The incidence of suicide and the various ratios cited have been subject to considerable variation depending on the location of the study, the particular group studied, and the time of the study (Dublin and Bunzel 1933; Lin 1969; Petzel and Cline 1978; Waldenstrom et al. 1972). Shneidman (1975) states that in the 1970s there was a tendency for suicide rates among women to approach those for men. In western Europe and in America the rate of suicide was higher for women than for men until the 1930s (Dublin and Bunzel 1933; Mayer-Gross, Slater, and Roth 1969). Peck (1977) states that in recent years the suicide rate for young black women in Los Angeles county has become higher than that for black men in the same age group. These findings are exceptions to the nearly invariable finding that male suicide rates are higher than the female rates, which intimates cultural rather than biological factors.

But biological factors must be considered in a study of sexual differences in suicide behavior. One obvious factor to examine is that of pregnancy, particularly if it is illegitimate or otherwise unwanted. Most research minimizes the overall effect of pregnancy on statistics (Cohen et al. 1966; Kleinert 1979; Otto 1972; White 1974). Under certain sociocultural conditions, the fact of pregnancy may indeed provide a powerful incentive to suicide (e.g., Burke 1976), but this appears to be exceptional. Whitlock and Edwards (1968) found in a review of the literature that the proportion of pregnant women among suicide fatalities was 5 percent, the same as that for the general population of women of childbearing age. Kleinert (1979), who made an extensive review of the published findings, and some other investigators feel that in fact pregnancy confers some protection against suicide. This conclusion has been disputed (Gabrielson, Currie, Tyler, and Jekel 1970; Petzel and Cline 1978). Certainly such a statement ought not to be construed to mean that pregnant young women rarely attempt or complete suicide. Still others argue that it is not the pregnancy per se but the effect it has on the relationship with a significant male or with the parents that counts (Otto 1972; Teicher and Jacobs 1966; White 1974).

In any case, even among unmarried adolescent girls, the proportion of those who are pregnant does not seem nearly large enough to account by itself for the multifold higher number of suicide attempters among girls as compared with boys. In all studies of suicidal adolescents reported in the literature only a minority of females were said to be pregnant.

Gabrielson et al. (1970) found that the rate of suicide attempts among teenage girls who delivered babies was ten times higher than the rate expected for this age group. This finding must await replication and evaluation since most of the attempts were apparently made long after delivery, and this would mean that the role of pregnancy was indirect and certainly not a direct physiological precipitant of suicide. Possibly getting pregnant was in itself as much a symptom as was the suicide attempt the result of a psychological disturbance which preceded the pregnancy. As Toolan (1974) and others have suggested, many of the pregnancies may have been sought in the hope of alleviating unbearable dissatisfactions.

Lester (1972) felt that the evidence from several studies demonstrated that the premenstrual, bleeding, and ovulatory phases of the menstrual cycle were associated with an increased incidence of suicidal acts. But Lester concluded that direct confirmatory evidence for the proposed association of hormone level and suicide was at present not available.

Zilboorg (1937) attributed the greater number of completed suicides among males to their intolerance of traits suggestive to them of homosexuality. This speculation, however, would fail to explain the higher rates of suicide attempts among females. Nevertheless, Zilboorg's explanation does have much in common with the formulation which I will propose. I assume the intolerance to stem from another aspect of masculine standards, though Zilboorg from his perspective of the 1930s might not have agreed that there is any real difference between us.

Jacobziner (1965) asserted that the high incidence of suicide attempts among females was probably due to impulsiveness. However, other investigators doubt that suicide in adolescents is usually an impulsive act (Teicher and Jacobs 1966). Further, one could hardly maintain that females are more impulsive than males. Otto (1972) assumed that girls were more involved in suicidal behavior than boys because Western civilization did not offer them the same possibilities for outward-directed aggression. Their aggression, he reasons, turns more easily toward the self, increasing the suicidal tendency. On the grounds that boys were involved in suicidal behavior less frequently than girls, Otto also assumed that boys had to overcome a stronger "socially tinged resistance" to self-destructive acts than did girls. Finally, Otto found that boys had been more frequently sick-listed for mental causes than girls, and therefore he assumed that the males were more disturbed psychiatrically than were the females. This is debatable (Haim 1958; Mattsson, Seese, and Hawkins 1969). Furthermore, one should consider the possible role of compulsory military service in precipitating psychiatric disorders among Swedish males.

Lingens (1972) stated that the incidence of suicide among women was less than among men, in normal times, because the strong bonds tying mothers to their children deterred suicide. However, this reasoning would not apply to a majority of the young females and certainly not to those in the adolescent groups, most of whom were not mothers. Marks and Haller (1977) described a number of differences between adolescent boys and girls who had threatened or attempted (not completed) suicide. They did not, however, explain why many more girls than boys were represented in this group.

Hankoff (1979) suggests that adolescents are driven to explore deathlike experiences as rites of passage to adulthood. While Hankoff is correct in noticing that playing with death is a prominent part of contemporary adolescent pursuits in certain sports and in death-defying, risk-taking activities, similar dangers are involved in participation in warfare, revolution, and violent delinquency. It seems far-fetched to regard these latter as types of "play" and as preparation for adult life. He is right in saying that these activities are more usual for males than for females, but his conjecture that females are driven to attempt suicide as their main culturally approved avenue for exploring death seems unwarranted. Furthermore, as we have seen, many studies of attempted suicides in females have implicated difficulties in important relationships as the major precipitant of the act. To neglect this issue would be a serious clinical error.

If we reflect that many more females than males attempt suicide, and that suicide attempters are more apt than completers to feel closely involved in interpersonal relationships, even if these are strained or recently severed (Barter, Swaback, and Todd 1968; Davidson, Choquet, Etienne, and Taleghani 1972; Jacobziner 1965; Jensen and Petty 1958; Lukianowicz 1972; Otto 1972; Rubenstein, Moses, and Lidz 1958; Stengel 1974), we may assume that intense interpersonal involvement is truer of females than males as well. Indeed this was found by Peck (1977) and Weinberg (1970).

We then have both more frequent acts among females, largely because stresses from significant relationships are frequent precipitants of attempts, and fewer completed suicides because relationships per se provide some safeguard against the consummation of self-destructive urges (Durkheim 1951; Peck 1977; Tabachnick and Farberow 1961; Weinberg 1970).

The Explanations of Suter

Suter (1976) made a major contribution in explaining the differences by sex in the statistics cited at the beginning of this chapter. She stated that she saw suicide as the act of a person who saw no other viable option open. A suicide attempt in which the person did not fully intend to die occurred when a person was despairing about his/her own ability to cope, but still had the hope of being helped by others. In this sense, a suicide attempt was a particularly "feminine" act according to society's standards, since it combined a feeling of personal helplessness with the notion of being rescued by someone else. By these same social standards completed suicide was more "masculine," in that, if men felt helpless, they were not "supposed" to look for outside help. Correspondingly Suter noted there were many more women in therapy than men. She also cited writers on suicide such as Simone de Beauvoir, who hypothesized that women may use less violent methods of committing suicide than men because they are more concerned about what might happen to their bodies even after death and did not want to disfigure themselves. Less violent methods like drug overdoses (used by more females than males) also tend to be less lethal than methods like shooting oneself in that they provide more chance for discovery and rescue.

Suter's basic thesis is that the usual Western socialization process makes females more vulnerable to self-destructive behavior, particularly under stress. In this context, suicide may be understood as an extreme manifestation of a pervasively self-destructive pattern of be-havior. For instance, she asserts that females are brought up to believe that their self-worth depends on catching and holding a desirable man. But this overdependence on the other leads to rage—rage toward the self for being in the dependent position and rage toward others who have the power. However, this rage is generally repressed since it is "unfeminine" and would endanger whatever security women have if expressed. Anger is then apt to be turned against the self. Several other writers have also called attention to a likely consequence of the strong prohibitions against external expression of rage in women but without noticing this common source of rage. In any event, this is just one reason advanced for the greater vulnerability to depression and suicidal preoccupations of women.

Females, Suter continues, are likely to have great difficulties in de-veloping a sense of self-worth and providing inner sources of security. The socialization process can systematically develop in women the opposite of a sense of personal mastery. Moreover, many of the abili-ties that women do develop are sources of conflict rather than of strength, since these abilities may be considered unfeminine. Thus, they are deprived of an important means of staving off depression by their own efforts. Suter's paper goes into many similar considerations derived from recent studies of cultural pressures on females leading to increased difficulties in the handling of aggression and the regulation of self-esteem. Thus, it is the greater incidence of depression, difficulties in regulating self-esteem, and insecurity that lead more women than men to be preoccupied with suicide. In fact, the symptoms of depres-sion in mild form are considered feminine and laudable. A recent paper by Welmer, Marten, Wochnick, Davis, Fishman, and Clayton (1979) supports the high prevalence of depression among women. They note that the rate of depression among the general female population ranges from 3 to 25 percent. Robins, Gassner, Kayes, Wilkinson, and Murphy (1959) found that women were more likely than men to communicate their suicidal intentions to physicians. Similarly, Selzer, Paluczny, and Carroll (1978) found that women factory workers were more likely than their male counterparts to be depressed and to seek help because of it.

It is my impression that Suter has advanced powerful reasons for explaining the greater incidence of suicide attempts made by women as compared with men but has not adequately accounted for the greater incidence of completed suicide among males as compared with

428

females. In fact, according to Suter's main argument (that society adversely affects females), females ought to exceed males in completed suicides also. Why is this not so?

Hypothesis on Suicide Rates of Males

As a preliminary consideration, I suggest that when the thought of committing suicide becomes a serious intention for young persons of both sexes, it is simultaneously opposed by powerful wishes to go on living and by a dread of dying. The curtailing of the prospect, in years to come, of mind and body functioning at new high levels of excellence must surely add weight to the wish to live. Presumably the wish to remain alive ultimately ensures that there be more suicide attempts or gestures than completions for both sexes. I assume that it is principally the typical reaction by sex to the dread of dying which appears to differentiate the rates of completed suicides, so that more males than females go on to kill themselves. I believe that among males the awareness of this dread often gives rise to an inner judgment which decrees that now the fatal act ought to be carried out, because not to do so—to yield to the anxiety and continue to live—would not only perpetuate the seemingly intolerable conditions of life but would be deemed cowardly and unmasculine, adding this source of self-contempt to the torment already present. Among younger males this attitude is likely to be more forceful than in later years. Among females, on the other hand, this source of self-reproach does not appear to arise as a powerful influence. These differences in sexual attitudes appear to be profoundly affected by prevailing cultural positions, with the bravado and the phallic narcissistic defense among males in Western culture so familiar as to render documentation superfluous. What has not yet been demonstrated to my knowledge, however, is the key role this attitude may play in affecting the outcome among young males who contemplate suicide.

Fear and Shame in Males: Case Reports

It was during the following interview with an adolescent male that I first intuited some probable reasons for the differences between the sexes regarding completed-suicide behavior.

CASE 1

The patient was a sixteen-year-old male with a lifelong history of school difficulties who was on the verge of dropping out of school. He had been seeing me sporadically in joint sessions with his mother. On this occasion, he arrived shortly before his mother for the interview and began with remarking that there had been nothing new during the past week, that it had been an average week. However, he then told of a quarrel with his mother after which he withdrew to a friend's house. A short while later, when his mother arrived, she told more details about the incident. She was very angry when she learned that her son had been absent from school for several days and had lied to her about the matter. She noted, however, that one day he seemed to be very depressed. We turned to him. Suddenly his depression became apparent in the office. I urged him to report his thoughts and feelings. He felt dead, he said, like an egg. All alone. Everything seemed white. Now he felt it here too. It was scary. I asked what he felt like doing about it. He said unexpectedly: "Killing myself. But I don't have the guts to do it. I thought of my family and friends." Upon questioning, he revealed that he had thought of throwing himself off a high balcony in the high-rise building where he lived.

The fact that the session had begun with a statement minimizing any acute disturbance, but had led to a revelation of a serious suicidal consideration, does not seem all that unusual in such cases. What particularly struck me was the confession that he did not have the "guts" to do it. For the first time I appreciated some new implications of such a remark, banal as it was. His shame may well have been the main reason for initially concealing the matter. Perhaps this motive accounts for the reticence of many suicidal adolescent males as well. At any rate, not having the guts—that is, being a coward—appears to be a much more disturbing acknowledgment for males than for females.

CASE 2

At the age of fifteen a fearful, physically inhibited male was admitted to a psychiatric hospital because of a paralyzing anguish. He was immediately appalled by his situation. As a form of protest and to induce his parents to take him home at once he made an open suicidal gesture that was neither painful nor in any way dangerous. As he had hoped, his parents were notified promptly, and when they came to the hospital were readily persuaded to have him discharged in their custody. When I spoke with him afterward in the presence of his parents he acknowledged that he had been frantic to get out of the hospital. However, he was obviously so embarrassed by the feebleness of his ruse that he could hardly be induced to talk about it. It seemed he had no intention of dying; but in having relied on the threat of dying, he seemed deeply ashamed at the too obvious lack of risk of harm, let alone of death. That he used the occasion to triumph over various authorities might also have made the shame useful as a way of placating them. But my impression was that this played a minimal part in his mortification on this occasion. He was in fact very willful and openly defiant of authority figures without needing to resort to subterfuge in order to prevail.

CASE 3

This patient was a young man in his early twenties. His girl friend was visiting in his dormitory room just before he made his first suicide attempt. He told her he wanted to die but did not state explicitly that he intended to kill himself. After some discussion he ran out of the room. She started after him but did not follow him outdoors. He ran to an elevated station. Here he waited for a long time on the platform, saying that he hesitated because he did not want to be seen by other passengers. When the station became empty he got down on the tracks and placed his hand close to the third rail. "I wondered if I was man enough to do it." He remained there indecisively, and claims he did then touch the rail but that surprisingly nothing happened. Eventually he returned to the dorm and in a condition of extreme agitation told his girl friend what he had done. She brought him to the hospital. The examining psychiatrist felt there was a serious suicide risk and had the patient hospitalized. In the hospital he made several suicide attempts by strangulation using stolen materials.[1]

One may contrast these cases with the accounts of suicide attempts in young females where, to begin with, comments about lack of nerve are seldom made. When such statements are made, they are usually considerations which troubled the subjects far less than others, such as feelings of distress, dissatisfaction with self, and disappointment with some relationships (Jacobziner 1965; Jensen and Petty 1958; Lukianowicz 1972; Otto 1972; Rubenstein et al. 1958; Schneer and Kay 1961; Seiden 1969; Stengel 1974; Teicher and Jacobs 1966). Self-accusations of cowardice may occasionally be advanced as explanations for why dangerous suicide attempts were never made—even though the subjects had expressed a wish to die, threatened to kill themselves, or made some action of low lethality. But the self-accusations of cowardice are not then typically poignant, additional sources of distress. Of course, they may imply that they have deprived themselves of the benefits of suicide or jeopardized their credibility, and only in these ways may the trait assume great significance to the subjects.

CASE 4

A seventeen-year-old boy committed suicide a few hours after his fifth automobile accident. He left a note reading: "It is not because I have no courage, but it is because I know that I was born to come to a tragic end. This was my fifth auto accident, but I haven't been killed yet. No one could take my life but myself it seems, and I shall take it" (Ellis and Allen 1961). In distinction from the preceding cases this young man did kill himself. Nevertheless, the characteristic attitude was present. The protest about having the courage is actually clear inferential evidence that he was troubled by the inner reproach of cowardice and that he intended to remove this stain on his honor by taking his life. I submit that it is more characteristic of masculine than of feminine mentality for an individual in such circumstances in our culture to regard the necessity to kill himself as a duty.

Sociocultural Perspective

I have already remarked on the large variations present in suicide rates from place to place and from one time span to another and have indicated that such variations imply cultural rather than biological forces. Furthermore, we have seen that Suter (1976) has persuasively argued the powerful cultural role in the high suicide-attempt rate among Western women. These statistical tabulations and discussions, of course, do not totally negate biological factors, but they do limit their importance. I wish now to examine certain sociocultural attitudes and practices in the light of the hypothesis on completed suicides of young males.

The following excerpt appears in the psychological autopsy report of a sixteen-year-old white Protestant boy, Herman, who lived with his parents on a farm near a small town (Niswander, Casey, and Humphrey 1973). Herman had shot himself with a rifle. The excerpt illustrates the possible transmission from father to son of a "masculine mystique" approach to suicide. The father's evident eccentricity is responsible for the clarity with which he was able to express himself after the tragic event. Masculine pride or dignity "demands" suicide and an end to vacillation:

A clergyman reported the neighbor as saying Herman said his father told him, "If you are going to kill yourself, then go and do it." His father said nothing about a discussion of suicide having taken place that morning. He commented that there was one thing he had to see about Herman—his physical position at death—and he added, "If he learned nothing else from me, he did what I said, 'It's better to die on your feet than live on your knees.' "

The following newspaper item reported by Ellis and Allen (1961) shows the enormous social pressures which can be applied to a male who is contemplating suicide. To my knowledge, such pressure by threat of mortification is rarely if ever directed at a female in similar circumstances in Western culture.

For two hours yesterday a man perched precariously atop a twelve story building while crowds jeered "Jump, jump." Robert David Thomas, 22, was pulled off the roof by a policeman and a fireman. He told police he was despondent because he could not see his girl friend serving a 14 year jail sentence for forgery. A crowd of three thousand gathered in the street and some took bets on whether he would jump. "Make up your mind . . . Jump, man, jump . . . You're chicken . . . Why doesn't someone go and push him?" were among the taunts hurled at Thomas. At one time several hundred among the crowd chanted "Jump, jump, jump." Police said the mob apparently felt Thomas was only faking. As officers led Thomas away, a man tucked $7.00 in bills into his pocket. "Take this, son," he said, "and come back when you're a man."

It is relevant to the thesis of this chapter to examine certain features of counterphobic behavior toward danger. We have already taken note of risk taking in contemporary adolescent pursuits. Delk (1980), who compiled statistics of fatalities from high-risk sports, states that it is mostly males between the ages of fifteen and forty who are involved.

433

He notes that participation in these sports seems motivated by the pleasure gained when anxiety is ultimately reduced.

Ellis and Allen (1961) said of the well-known game of Russian roulette, where risking death does not even call for the chance to exercise a skill: "Although there are no figures to support the contention it is apparent from a large number of reports in the press over the years that so many young people kill themselves while playing this fantastic 'game' that it almost has a claim to a separate notation on standard lists of causes of death. In the 'game' a single bullet is placed in the cylinder of a revolver. The player spins the cylinder, points the gun at his head, and pulls the trigger. The odds of killing oneself are given as five to one. . . . 'The grisly game' also called 'Cossack poker' is almost the exclusive diversion of boys, though an occasional girl tries it."

Going even beyond the thesis here, Wolfgang (1959) proposed that a number of killings of Negro youths were victim precipitated and that such deaths were really forms of suicide. According to him, this form of self-destruction was due to an attitude that to die by suicide was cowardly and effeminate, whereas death by homicide was more masculine, hence, more acceptable!

In Japan suicide under certain circumstances is culturally encouraged for females as well as for males. This fact is responsible for Japan's relatively high overall suicide rate and for the finding that its suicide rate for women approaches that for men (Lin 1969). Conceivably, in such circumstances, the women are also subject to self-reproach for cowardice in the face of dread. Conversely, if a culture eases its prohibitions against males who turn to others for assistance with emotional problems, and if its intolerance of fear in males is reduced, the suicidal-behavior rates of males may become more like those of females.

The Psychodynamics of the Suicidal Act

A serious desire to kill oneself must arouse such intense fear that the fear itself must constitute a major deterrent to suicide. To my knowledge Spiegel and Neuringer (1963) and Trautman (1961) were the first clinicians to make this explicit and to insist on its importance. Spiegel and Neuringer argued that "an individual does not necessarily commit suicide when the urge to die becomes stronger than the urge to live, for everyone who has an overriding urge to die is able to take his own life. Most individuals find themselves overcome by dread as they approach suicidal action.'' To carry out a suicide, the dread (and guilt) must be reduced. This appears to require various psychological defenses. Denial, acting against the fear but not against the suicidal impulse itself, is especially important. The denial is facilitated by sleeplessness and the ingestion of alcohol, narcotics, sedatives, and hallucinogens (Dorpat 1968).

The following newspaper item was reported by Dublin and Bunzel (1933) as an example of how a suicidal person is determined to die only by the method of his own choosing. However, I wish to cite the same item as an indication of how a suicidally inclined person might still respond with powerful inhibition (presumably out of dread) against permitting his death if death becomes imminent. ''A man jumped off the Brooklyn Bridge but would not seize the rope that the policeman lowered in an effort to save him. When he refused to be saved the officer threatened to shoot him unless he complied. The man caught the rope and was pulled to safety.'' The same point is illustrated in a short story by Ambrose Bierce entitled ''Parker Adderson, Philosopher.'' In this story a captured military spy was able to discuss with his captors the knowledge that he would be hanged the following morning with philosophical detachment and equanimity. When, however, the officer in command gave orders to have him executed immediately, he abruptly lost his serenity and put up a violent struggle in the course of which he killed a young officer for whom he had developed paternal feelings.

Shneidman (1979) reports the case of a young girl who managed to survive a suicide attempt in which she got into her car, doused herself and the car's interior with gasoline, and then set fire to it. Her unexpected survival was due to the prompt action of strangers attracted by the blaze and required immediate and extensive treatment in a hospital. Her first thought when she began to burn (as told much later to Shneidman) indicated the undoing of a profound denial: ''I never expected,'' she said, ''that it would be painful.''

Trautman (1961) asked a number of suicide attempters (all Puerto Rican immigrants) to recall their thoughts before, during, and after the act. Before the act they had been involved in a state of severe and painful excitement, usually in a quarrel. This continued until their excitement reached a climax and they completely lost control over their feelings and actions: "The patients were out of contact with reality, their rational thinking impaired, their behavior like people in a trance." At the time when they took poison, "some patients said they had no thought of death; others said they did not care." The anticlimactic reaction set in as soon as the patient swallowed the poison or felt the first effects; at this point, the mind became alert again. Back to reality, the patients were suddenly aware of the deadly consequences of their act. Some, as soon as they tasted the liquid or felt a burning sensation in the throat or stomach, were thoroughly frightened and called for help. Several of those who took sleeping pills became terrified when they felt a wave of "weakness" coming over them. A few patients later died. "It is interesting to note the first sign of alert mental functioning is the return of the fear of death which was completely absent during the fit," Troutman reports. "The panic these patients displayed caused them to be rushed by ambulance to the hospital even though the danger may not have been serious."

It appears that it is rare for a person on the verge or in the middle of a suicidal act to be aware of death anxiety. This is true also of the contents of suicide notes (Spiegel and Neuringer 1963). Most of the evidence for this part of the thesis is derived from contemplators and attempters. Possibly depression and the prospect of putting an end to anguish have mitigating effects on the anxiety. However, Trautman's cases vividly illustrate that the absence of dread may be temporary.

As we have seen, there seems to be a characteristic sexual difference in the processing of this dread. In contemporary Western culture, males much more often than females react to the dread itself with shame and try to adopt a counterphobic attitude: "I will go on with it and prove I am not a coward or a sissy." Thus, the shame is used to counteract the fear of dying. If the shame motive does not prevail, the attempt may not be made.

To recapitulate, the sequence in suicide for the male is assumed to occur as follows: the wish to die becomes powerful → the decision to kill oneself is made, a plan for effecting the act is devised, the act is vividly imagined → dread is aroused → the plan is tabled → shame is aroused, reinforcing the urge to kill one's self → defenses against dread appear → the dread disappears or diminishes; the shame, too, disappears as the subject becomes firm in the decision to go ahead → the subject becomes preoccupied with the determination to act or becomes calm as he achieves confidence in his ability to carry out the plan (Keith-Spiegel and Spiegel 1967) → the act is carried out.

On the Manner of Suicide

The choice of a suicide method obviously depends on availability. Familiarity, physical vigor, and dexterity also play some part, and these factors are responsible to some extent for certain differences between the preferred methods of the two sexes. However, the principal statistical difference is that males choose more lethal methods than females. Thus, where females use overdoses of sedatives, males prefer firearms and hanging. At the Paris poison center the lethality of poisoning has been given as 5 percent (Soubrier 1972); at the Hôpital Fernand-Widal it is only 1 percent for adolescents (Frejaville 1974). Clearly, drug ingesters who get to hospitals usually survive. Tabachnick and Farberow (1961) present a ranking of the lethality of various suicide methods.

The point, however, may be that once the male has decided to act, he may force himself to do it in such a manner that he cannot fail, since failure could induce unbearable shame. However, we must bear in mind that males as well as females make more attempts than fatal acts. We assume that the dread of dying is the same for both sexes and serves as an equal deterrent to suicide. The male places more shame on surviving, however. It is interesting that jumping from high places, which is used by females more often than by males, is itself more likely to be fatal when performed by a male (Lester 1972). The same is true for poisoning. Hendin (1950) concludes that the intent has more effect on lethality than does method. A further conclusion can be drawn, that differences in choice of method per se cannot explain sexual differences in the rates of completed suicides.

As to the male choice of more violent methods of suicide, could it not then largely be accounted for by these methods (1) tending to be more lethal; (2) being more convincing as a demonstration of fearlessness; (3) expressing impatience with indecision; and (4) showing less regard for disfigurement of the face and body (Lester 1972; Suter 1976)?

Conclusions

The high female incidence of attempted suicide has been related to the cultural pressures of Western society, which foster in women the notions of personal helplessness and of turning to others for rescue. Related pressures lead to a greater frequency of depression among females and presumably a more frequent preoccupation with suicide

(Suter 1976). Another factor is the cultural disapproval of the expression of outward-directed aggression in females. On the other hand, such considerations do not explain the much higher rate of completed suicides for males than for females.

While all individuals of both sexes may be presumed to dread death, evidence is cited for believing that males to a greater extent than females react to the dread itself as a deplorable cowardly trait. Thus, a fear of death versus shame conflict is activated. The male is more apt than the female to consummate the act of suicide in order to avoid the self-accusation of cowardice, in addition to the other motivation for doing away with himself. Such attitudes are aspects of familiar masculine protest and are most conspicuous among younger males. It is presumed that this factor may greatly help explain the much higher incidence of completed suicide among young males compared with that in females.

This thesis could be checked by systematically asking key questions of survivors of serious suicide attempts with clear sensoria. As many writers have noted, even the information collected in this way could not automatically be regarded as accurate and thorough. Still, it may be the closest we can get to the emotional state of individuals on the verge of self-destruction.

In addition, the thesis of this chapter carries with it certain implications for the therapy of suicidal males. First, the point is well made by Spiegel and Neuringer (1963) that it would be therapeutic to persist in having the patient confront in detail the more dreadful personal ramifications of suicide to help curb the likelihood of further suicidal action. Second, males should be reassured that it is natural and mature to fear death—that having this particular fear does not imply cowardice but, on the contrary, believing that one should not fear and hesitate is unrealistic and immature because it demonstrates an unwillingness to accept one's imperfections. The patient's reluctance to discuss the matter may be largely based on a wish to avoid the exposure of feelings of humiliation over having failed to kill himself because of unmanly fear. Dealing with the patient's feelings may require considerable understanding without wavering from the bold and direct confrontation usually required in dealing with suicide issues. Third, one should vigorously counter the patients' self-reproach of cowardice when it has been accentuated by other individuals who challenged the patients' sincerity in threatening to kill themselves. This may necessitate undermining the authority status of the others; hopefully at a later time the matter may be discussed with them.

438

NOTES

I wish to thank Dr. Jay G. Hirsch and Dr. Norman R. Bernstein for their valuable suggestions in the preparation of this chapter.

1. Case of Dr. David Joel.

REFERENCES

Barter, J. T.; Swaback, D. O.; and Todd, V. 1968. Adolescent suicide attempts: a follow-up study of hospitalized patients. *Archives of General Psychiatry* 19:523–527.

Burke, A. W. 1976. Socio-cultural determinants of attempted suicide among West Indians in Birmingham: ethnic origin and immigrant status. *British Journal of Psychiatry* 129:261–266.

Cohen, E.; Motto, J. A.; and Seiden, R. H. 1966. An instrument for evaluating suicidal potential: a preliminary study. *American Journal of Psychiatry* 122:886–891.

Davidson, F.; Choquet, M.; Etienne, M.; and Taleghani, M. 1972. Contribution a l'etude du suicide des adolescents. *L'Hygiene mentale* 61:1–32.

Delk, J. L. 1980. High-risk sports as indirect self-destructive behavior. In N. L. Farberow, ed. *The Many Faces of Suicide*. New York: McGraw-Hill.

Dorpat, T. L. 1968. Loss of control over suicidal impulses. *Bulletin of Suicidology* July 1968: 26–30.

Dublin, L. I., and Bunzel, B. 1933. *To Be or Not to Be: A Study of Suicide*. New York: Harrison Smith & Robert Haas.

Durkheim, É. V. 1951. *Suicide*. Glencoe, Ill.: Free Press.

Ellis, E. R., and Allen, G. N. 1961. *Traitor Within*. Garden City, N.Y.: Doubleday.

Frejaville, J. P. 1974. Round table discussion: les tentatives de suicide de l'adolescent. *Revue de neuropsychiatrie infantile* 22:639.

Gabrielson, I. W.; Currie, J. B.; Tyler, N. C.; and Jekel, J. F. 1970. Suicide attempts in a population of pregnant teenagers. *American Journal of Public Health* 60:2289–2301.

Haim, A. 1974. *Adolescent Suicide*. London: Tavistock.

Hankoff, L. D. 1979. Situational categories. In L. D. Hankoff and B. Einsidler, eds. *Suicide, Theory and Clinical Aspects*. Littleton, Mass.: PSG.

Hendin, H. 1950. Attempted suicide: a psychiatric and statistical study. *Psychiatric Quarterly* 24:39–46.

439

Hendin, H. 1976. Growing up dead: student suicide. In E. S. Shneidman, ed. *Suicidology: Contemporary Developments*. New York: Grune & Stratton.

Jacobziner, H. 1965. Attempted suicide in adolescents. *Journal of the American Medical Association* 191:7–11.

Jensen, V. W., and Petty, T. A. 1958. The fantasy of being rescued in suicide. *Psychoanalytic Quarterly* 27:327–339.

Keith-Spiegel, P., and Spiegel, D. E. 1967. Affective states of patients immediately preceding suicide. *Journal of Psychiatric Research* 5:89–93.

Kleinert, G. J. 1979. Suicide in pregnancy. Paper presented at annual meeting of American Psychiatric Association in Chicago, May.

Lester, D. 1972. *Why People Kill Themselves: A Summary of Research Findings on Suicidal Behavior*. Springfield, Ill.: Thomas.

Lin, Tsung-Yi. 1969. Some epidemiological findings on suicide in youth. In S. Lebovici and G. Caplan, eds. *Adolescence: Psychosocial Perspectives*. New York: Basic.

Lingens, E. 1972. Suicide in extreme situations. In Waldenstrom, Larson, and Ljungstedt, eds.

Lukianowicz, N. 1972. Suicidal behavior: an attempt to modify the environment. *British Journal of Psychiatry* 121:387–390.

Marks, P. A., and Haller, D. L. 1977. Now I lay me down for keeps: a study of adolescent suicidal attempts. *Journal of Clinical Psychology* 33:390–400.

Mattsson, A.; Seese, L. R.; and Hawkins, J. W. 1969. Suicidal behavior as a child psychiatric emergency. *Archives of General Psychiatry* 20:100–109.

Mayer-Gross, W.; Slater, E.; and Roth, M. 1969. *Clinical Psychiatry*. 3d ed. Baltimore: Williams & Wilkins.

Meeks, J. E. 1971. *The Fragile Alliance*. Baltimore: Williams & Wilkins.

Niswander, G. D.; Casey, T. M.; and Humphrey, J. A. 1973. *A Panorama of Suicide*. Springfield, Ill.: Thomas.

Otto, U. 1972. Suicidal behavior in childhood and adolescence. In Waldenstrom, Larson, and Ljungstedt, eds.

Peck, M. L. 1977. Adolescent suicide. In C. L. Hatton, S. M. Valente, and A. Rink, eds. *Suicide: Assessment and Intervention*. New York: Appleton-Century-Crofts.

Petzel, S. V., and Cline, D. W. 1978. Adolescent suicide: epidemiological and biological aspects. *Adolescent Psychiatry* 6:239–266.

Pokorny, A. D. 1966. A follow-up study of 618 suicidal patients. *American Journal of Psychiatry* 122:1109–1116.

Robins, E.; Gassner, S.; Kayes, J.; Wilkinson, R. H., and Murphy, G. E. 1959. The communication of suicidal intent. *American Journal of Psychiatry* 115:724–733.

Rubenstein, R.; Moses, R.; and Lidz, T. 1958. On attempted suicide. *Archives of Neurology and Psychiatry* 79:103–112.

Schneer, H. I., and Kay, P. 1961. The suicidal adolescent. In S. Lorand and H. I. Schneer, eds. *Adolescence: Psychoanalytic Approach to Problems and Therapy*. New York: Harper & Row.

Seiden, R. H. 1969. *Suicide among Youth*. A review of the literature, 1900–1967. U.S. Public Health Service Publication no. 1971. Washington, D.C.: Government Printing Office.

Selzer, M. L.; Paluczny, M.; and Carroll, R. 1978. A comparison of depression and physical illness in men and women. *American Journal of Psychiatry* 135:1368–1370.

Shneidman, E. S. 1975. In A. N. Freedman, H. I. Kaplan, and B. Sadock, eds. *Comprehensive Textbook of Psychiatry*. 2d ed. Baltimore: Williams & Wilkins.

Shneidman, E. S. 1979. Suicide. Paper presented at annual meeting of American Psychiatric Association in Chicago, May.

Shneidman, E. S., and Farberow, N. L. 1961. Statistical comparison between attempted and committed suicides. In N. L. Farberow and E. S. Shneidman, eds. *The Cry for Help*. New York: McGraw-Hill.

Soubrier, J. P. 1972. Comment. In Waldenstrom, Larson, and Ljungstedt, eds.

Spiegel, D. E., and Neuringer, C. 1963. Role of dread in suicidal behavior. *Journal of Abnormal and Social Psychology* 66:507–511.

Stengel, E. 1974. *Suicide and Attempted Suicide*. New York: Aronson.

Suter, B. 1976. Suicide and women. In B. B. Wolman and H. H. Kraus, eds. *Between Survival and Suicide*. New York: Gardner.

Tabachnick, N. O., and Farberow, N. L. 1961. The assessment of self-destructive potentiality. In Shneidman and Farberow, eds.

Teicher, J. D., and Jacobs, J. 1966. Adolescents who attempt suicide: preliminary findings. *American Journal of Psychiatry* 122:1248–1257.

Toolan, J. M. 1974. Depression and suicide. In S. Arieti, ed. *American Handbook of Psychiatry*. Vol. 2. New York: Basic.

Trautman, E. C. 1961. The suicidal fit. *Archives of General Psychiatry* 5:76–83.

Waldenstrom, J.; Larson, T.; and Ljungstedt, N. 1972. *Suicide and Attempted Suicide*. Stockholm: Nordiska Bokhandelns Forlag.

Weinberg, S. 1970. Suicidal intent in adolescence. *Journal of Pediatrics* 77:579–586.

Welmer A.; Marten, S.; Wochnick, E.; Davis, M. A.; Fishman, R.; and Clayton, P. J. 1979. Psychiatric disorders among professional women. *Archives of General Psychiatry* 36:169–173.

White, H. C. 1974. Self poisoning in adolescents. *British Journal of Psychiatry* 124:24–35.

Whitlock, F. A., and Edwards, J. E. 1968. Pregnancy and attempted suicide. *Psychiatry* 9:1–12.

Wolfgang, M. E. 1959. Suicide by means of victim-precipitated homicide. *Journal of Clinical and Experimental Psychopathology* 20:335–349.

Zilboorg, G. 1937. Considerations on suicide with particular reference to that of the young. *American Journal of Orthopsychiatry* 7:15–31.

27 THE SYMPTOM OF DELICATE SELF-CUTTING IN ADOLESCENT FEMALES: A DEVELOPMENTAL VIEW

SHELLEY DOCTORS

The phrase "delicate cutting" was suggested by Pao (1969) to describe a form of suicidal gesture. It differentiates the type that makes superficial, delicate, carefully designed incisions (and who tend to repeat this act again and again) from those other suicidal patients who make single, deep, coarse incisions close to vital points. The larger group with which this particular group is often mingled are wrist cutters, in general. While it is known that many of the delicate cutters abuse alcohol, drugs, and pills and report overdosing at some time (Rosenthal, Rinzler, Walsh, and Klausner 1972), in evaluating the suicide potential of delicate cutting, Rinzler and Shapiro (1968) report that while the symptom is alarming, it is rarely life threatening. The wounds created by delicate self-cutting are shallow and superficial as opposed to deep and severe, they appear in number rather than singly, and, importantly, they reflect the maintenance of some degree of control rather than thoroughgoing abandon.

There is much to suggest that self-cutting is a phenomenon that has been known to the psychiatric community for over sixty-five years (Emerson 1914), and that it is likely universal, having been reported in Japan and Germany (Uemura 1975; Janus 1972) as well as the United States and Great Britain. The first report which delineated wrist cutting as a widespread phenomenon among psychiatrically hospitalized adolescents was made by Offer and Barglow in 1960. Repeated surveys at Mt. Sinai Hospital in New York City (Rinzler and Shapiro 1968) have established that between 5 and 20 percent of the patients admitted there exhibit the presenting problem of "wrist cutting." The behavior is not, of course, confined to those seen in hospitals, nor is it confined by site to the wrist. "Cutters" have been known to make incisions on face, chest, breasts, stomach, arms, and legs (Crabtree 1967; Emerson 1914; Kafka 1969; Pao 1969).

As there is high concordance among investigators regarding the phenomenology of the act itself, it is possible to offer a composite description. Therapists believe that the behavior occurs as a reaction to an actual or threatened separation (Pao 1969; Rosenthal et al. 1972), loss (Goldwyn, Cahill, and Grunebaum 1967; Grunebaum and Klerman 1967), rejection (Podvoll 1969), or disappointment (Novotny 1972), whether in reality or fantasy. What the patient is most aware of is the experience of feeling utterly alone and beginning to feel very tense (Pao 1969), or angry (Nelson and Grunebaum 1971). Following the period of tension, the patient decides to become isolated. There is striking uniformity to this finding—cutting is virtually always a solitary act. There is a shift to feeling "numb," "unreal," "empty" (Rosenthal et al. 1972), or "dead" (Asch 1971). One such patient said, "You feel a lot but then you don't feel anything." The patients, virtually uniformly, do not experience pain at the time of cutting (Graff and Mallin 1967; Grunebaum and Klerman 1967; Novotny 1972; Pao 1969; Rosenthal et al. 1972; Simpson 1975). The experience of pain is concomitant with the return of feelings of being alive and real again (Kafka 1969). Therefore, patients sometimes report cutting until they begin to feel pain or until they see the sight of blood (Asch 1971). While some patients may temporarily have feelings of disgust, regret, or guilt (Pao 1969), they give way to the typically reported experience of satisfaction, calm, and relief (Friedman, Glasser, Laufer, Laufer, and Wohl, 1972; Graff and Mallin 1967; Grunebaum and Klerman 1967).

As this symptom is reviewed, four areas of agreement emerge. First, the behavior is overwhelmingly a phenomenon of women (Graff and Mallin 1967; Phillips and Alkan 1961; Simpson 1975). Second, many investigators have pointed to the importance of disturbances in early object relations and the sense of self in these women (Graff and Mallin 1967; Grunebaum and Klerman 1967; Pao 1969; Rinzler and Shapiro 1968). In particular, early experiences of illness and injury are reported in the histories of such people (Kafka 1969; Rosenthal et al. 1972; Siomopoulos 1974; Simpson 1975). Third, the act seems related to conflicts around the experience of the genitals and genital sensations in an important way—it does not occur before the menarche (Siomopoulos 1974) but tends to occur around the time of menstruation (Crabtree

1967; Rosenthal et al. 1972). It seems to occur most often in women who are said to have problems with their feelings and attitudes toward their sexual selves (Gardner and Gardner 1975; Graff and Mallin 1967; Pao 1969; Rosenthal et al. 1972). Fourth, there seems to be considerable uniformity to the description of the act, including some shift during the course of the act which makes the act seem discontinous rather than continuous in time (Asch 1971; Grunebaum and Klerman 1967; Pao 1969; Rosenthal et al. 1972; Simpson 1975). This is usually referred to as depersonalization.

Toward Integrative Understanding

The study on which this chapter is based sought to provide some integration and focus for formulative understanding of these findings which emerge from the literature. Nine female hospitalized adolescents who repeatedly cut themselves superficially were studied using a broad array of clinical instruments. They were found to be similar to cases reported in that they had experienced difficulties early in life (relationship difficulties, but also experiences of illness or injury), had some disturbance in their feelings about menstruation and their relationship to their sexual selves, and were subject to the disturbances of consciousness typically referred to as depersonalization. In seeking to understand the relationship among these features, it was discovered that a common configuration of disturbances in early object relations, self-development, and in the female psychosexual (particularly genital) line of development was present in these young women.

It is my hypothesis that the symptom of self-cutting can be understood in the context of developmental disturbances which contribute to the clinical features seen in such patients: a heightening of feelings of frustration and simultaneously, a heightened intolerance for feelings of tension (experienced as physical tension); a lack of faith in others to provide help (and a markedly impaired capacity for self-soothing); a very limited capacity to verbalize affect and a deficiency in the capacity to represent experiences in higher symbolic modes; and a definite propensity to turn passively experienced diffuse distress into active, focal experiences designed to achieve a feeling of control over self and, thereby, a feeling of relief. While each of these elements can be seen to be one or another vicissitude of early object relations and self-development, the very same elements also characterized the vicissitudes of these patients' sexual development: the heightening of feelings of sexual tension and intolerance for such feelings; the lack of expectation of sexual relief and the absence of sexual self-soothing; the limited ability to use verbal and higher symbolic means to master feelings of sexual tensions; and the propensity to turn passively experienced diffuse sexual distress into active, focal experiences designed to achieve a feeling of control and relief.

The isomorphic relation between the features of object relations and self-development and the features of sexual development suggested common experiential origins. Both lines of development are intimately related to the experience of the body—object relations and a cohesive sense of self develop in the context of early experiences of bodily care and soothing. The task of progressively integrating the genital anatomy into the body image and assimilating genital tensions into a stable experience of self proceeds as well from bodily experience. This is a symptom which has its origins in bodily experience. Although the observer can provide higher-order abstractions, the essence of it remains tied to the physical level, never becoming sufficiently free of that aspect to be contained in the arena of symbolic thought. Ultimately, resolution is sought on the body. In this ordering of the clinical findings, the susceptibility to the cognitive and experiential dissociations which have been referred to as depersonalization is regarded as another result of the common configuration of developmental disturbances.

Object Relations Development

In the subjects studied, there would appear to have been some striking failures in empathy on the part of their mothers which would have made soothing far less than optimal and would have left them, as infants, feeling diffusely distressed. These failures to understand the wishes, intentions, and needs of the girls and, equally important, the mother's striking tendency to fail to respond constructively to those needs continued to define the mother-daughter relationship. Often, when these mothers poignantly showed their distress about their daughters, their expressions of concern were strikingly off the mark. Thus one girl's mother, when distraught and quite hysterical on the day her daughter was hospitalized (the daughter, too, was hysterical), frantically pressed the therapist for details of dental facilities at the hospital. Another mother, when concerned about her daughter's cutting, mounted a campaign to get the hospital to put her daughter on a diet. Quite the polar opposite from empathic relationship, these mothers seem strikingly alienated from their daughters' experience. The failure on the part of the mother to adequately sense the baby's needs, creates a need for the infant to react prematurely in order to provide for the missing mothering aspect. Such interferences in the process of gradual integration subject the infant, according to Winnicott (1962), to anxiety associated with disintegration, the fear of "going to pieces" or "falling forever." Certainly this remains the daughters' response to intense experiences of frustration, as many of them say, "I can't take it, I can't take it" at moments when they feel intensely frustrated. Furthermore, as we shall see, the unbearable feeling of being torn to pieces and a need to be "put together" lies at the very heart of the experience of self-cutting.

When these girls do express their feelings they tend to be regularly disconfirmed by their parents. None of the girls has any faith that expressions of their needs or wishes will be responded to positively. The simplest example was provided by one of the girls who recounted stories of going shopping with her mother in which she would select something saying, "I like that," to which her mother's typical response would be, "No, you don't; you like this," substituting something else. Thus the confident expectation of relief of tensions which ought to develop never takes place. When one or another of these girls begins to talk about something it is common for them to trail off saying, "Forget it, just forget it."

When earliest memories are elicited, these girls can tell stories which appear at first glance to be about mother and father. Yet, careful inquiry will establish that the remembered parental presence is not part of the actual memory. Such a finding suggests some interference with the achievement of stable objects and, thus, self-representations. The lack of internalization of a benign parental presence can be seen as related clinically to their discomfort with being alone and their inability to soothe themselves.

Winnicott (1971) has attributed the roots of the development of the capacity to use a symbol which both has meaning to the individual and to others to early experience with transitional phenomena. If, when the baby experiences tension and has some vague, diffuse idea that there is something to meet his need, the mother presents some kind of need satisfaction, the experience will give the infant the illusion that there is an external reality that corresponds to the infant's own capacity to create. Essentially, when the infant's gesture or wish is made real, the capacity to use a symbol is the result.

The inarticulateness of these girls, which colored all of the data collection, seems related to failures in the growth of trust and an associated capacity to perceive the symbol in its own right in a way that ordinarily enables the child to move beyond the illusion of omnipotence and beyond hopelessness about communication into real and effective communication. These girls have not given up the transitional objects. Not only do they cling to their stuffed animals and furry bathrobes, but the way in which they secrete glass and cutting implements conveyed a sense of fierce attachment to transitional objects imbued with the power to soothe them when all else failed. Clinically, they communicate the sense that one is expected to infer their feeling state from their grunts, shrugs, and generalizations. This lack of access to the use of symbols as abstract modes of expression limits their ability to ease their own feelings of frustration and is probably related to their propensity for motor expression of feelings of frustration, an example of which is delicate self-cutting.

According to Mahler, Pine, and Bergman (1975) the normal crisis of the rapprochement subphase of separation-individuation consists of conflicts that "hinge on the desire to be separate, grand, and omnipotent on the one hand and to have mother magically fulfill their wishes without having to recognize that help [is] actually coming from the outside, on the other." The normal manifestation of this conflict in the toddler is an alternation between "wooing" mother and "darting away" from mother. The heightening of these facets, dubbed "ambitendency" by the Mahler group, seems to describe well the pattern of recklessness seen in adolescence in the girls who engaged in delicate cutting. An early form of turning passive to active, the passive wish for mother is turned into behavior to elicit her attention and the passively experienced fear of engulfment is turned to an active running from engulfment. All of the girls studied showed this propensity for recklessness, incorporating this dynamic in their running away from home, running into traffic, and putting themselves in situations (such as hitchhiking) where they could be and often were harmed.

The girls studied had failed to develop emotional object constancy. The capacity to maintain a representation of an absent love object implies a firmly grounded unification of good and bad aspects of the object into a whole representation which then tempers hatred for the object when aggression is intense. Disturbances such as unreliability, unpredictability, and intrusiveness of the love object can interfere with this development such that the self-representation becomes identified with the "bad introject" and becomes confused with it. The experience of aggressive feelings under such conditions then inundates or sweeps away the representation of the good object. The disturbances in the development of both the cohesive object and the cohesive self-representation can be seen to characterize the identity development in the girls studied and to critically define their experience. Clinically, aggressive feelings in these girls quickly turn into intense hate which floods the object world, resulting in a feeling of hating everyone. Most importantly, however, the lack of sufficient differentiation between self and object representations and the parallel precarious state of both (the lack of unification of good and bad aspects of self and object representations) determine the clinically observed progression wherein hatred of everyone rapidly develops into painful feelings of being all alone. It is not only that the object world has been momentarily "wiped out," but that the individual experiences her own lack of a cohesive, temporally stable sense of self.

Experiences of Illness, Injury, and Physical Distress

These girls were found to have experienced a very large number and variety of kinds of experiences of physical distress, ranging from colic, high fevers, breath-holding spells, and motor seizures in infancy to falls requiring stitches, operations, and severe illness in childhood. Occurring early in the context of an already disturbed basis for body image formation (the disturbance in the mother-child relationship), such events may further contribute to such disturbances. Later experiences may serve specifically to organize the earlier experience of bodily tension originating in the mother-child relationship.

Hoffer (1950), in discussing the early organizers of body schematization, stated that in infancy, regardless of the cause of experiences of overwhelming bodily tension (i.e., constitutional or organic, failure of the self or the nonself), such events are experienced as if they were caused by the self and lead to an increase of active attempts to master the experience, including self-directed aggression. The paradigmatic example cited by Hoffer was of the infant who responded to pain attendant to severe colic by biting his own fist.

All of the girls reported experiences of being spanked, hit, or beaten during puberty. It is unclear whether these experiences are simply further instances of passively experienced bodily distress, increasing the propensity to turn passive to active, or whether, to some extent, these were already instances of abuse which the girls in some way provoked. Certainly there was an active component in the experiences which half of the girls had of beatings suffered at the hands of boy-friends.

The number of occurrences of rape in the lives of the girls studied was striking. Six of them had been raped, some two, three, and four different times. To say that these experiences contain elements of active provocation in no way is meant to imply that these girls were "asking for it," as is sometimes callously asserted. To be sure, many hitchhiked and repeatedly courted danger. However, reconstructing such experiences one could see that at several different junctures when the girl was frightened and overwhelmed by aggressive and sexual feelings, she would choose an action which would allow the experience to continue. In essence each time such a girl thought, "Oh, God, get me out of here," she reassured herself that she could handle it and stayed, in a move that seemed more fundamentally counterphobic than self-destructive, more based on turning passive to active than on a wish to suffer, be punished, or be hurt.

The synthesis suggested stems from the inference that earlier experiences of illness and injury heightened these girls' sensitivity to the experience of bodily tension, which for them, particularly, threatens bodily integrity and is intimately related to tensions originally experienced in the mother-child relationship. There is a progressive development of externalization and concretization of inner-tension states in which the psychological process of turning passive to active becomes increasingly important. The tendency to turn passive to active is over-determined, stemming both from the more distinctly physical disturbances and from the vicissitudes of the mother-child relationship. The element of hitchhiking relates the rape experiences to the "darting away" behavior (a forerunner of turning passive to active) now seen to take the form of extreme recklessness. Provocation of focal experiences of beatings and rapes serves (however misguidedly) to produce some feeling of control over aggressive and sexual impulses experienced as overwhelming tension states and thus can be seen to be functional analogues of delicate cutting.

The Sexual (Genital) Line of Development

The reconstruction of this developmental line is clearly more tentative and involves greater inferential leaps than the preceding one. In part this is due to the nature of the data. Interviews concerning the experience of the menarche, defloration, intercourse, sexual excitment, and masturbation (together with psychological testing) yield different results than the methods of child observation and psychoanalysis proper, from whose data the guiding theories of female sexual development have been constructed. Nonetheless, as striking disturbances in the postmenarchal years were clearly elicited, it was possible to attempt to integrate these findings with current theory and to hypothesize the major events in the genital line of development, knowing still that the earlier events are more speculative than later ones.

It is likely that by the second year, at the time of the naturally occurring efflorescence of genital interest and excitement, these girls have already experienced difficulties in the mother-child relationship (and possibly as well in regard to illness and injury) which have paved the way for disturbances in body schematization. It is posited that their discovery of the vaginal introitus is thus particularly distressing. Authors such as Horney (1933), Kestenberg (1956), and Fraiberg (1972) have written that this discovery leads little girls to believe that they have injured themselves, having "made a hole where no hole should be" (Horney 1933) and to typically consider the opening a "self-inflicted tear" (Kestenberg 1956). While none of the girls recalled such an event, all who would consider it resonated with the idea of "something being wrong," as one of them said "because you don't see any openings on your arms or your feet." Many (Greenacre 1958; Horney 1933; Kestenberg 1956; Kleeman 1977) have emphasized the little girl's real disadvantage in not having available to them the visual modality to check on the intactness of the genital apparatus and to incorporate the genital into the developing body schema.

Fears about destruction of a part of the body and concerns about bodily integrity occurring in girls who have experienced disturbances in the mother-child relationship and/or physical trauma (which can serve to magnify such fears) may serve to determine an extreme reaction to the discovery of the anatomical difference between the sexes, which can be experienced as a fearful confirmation of some damage having taken place (Galenson and Roiphe 1977; Mahler et al. 1975). These girls have a very poor understanding of their genital anatomy and their comments (such as those of one young woman who worried that her vaginal infection was related to her stomach ulcers) suggest diffuse concerns about damage.

The nature of vaginal sensations may be particularly difficult for these girls to integrate. For them, the diffuse genital feeling of being beset by simultaneous demands parallels their emotional difficulties with a mother who has failed to provide a model for the organization of stimuli. The little girl ordinarily has a greater propensity than the boy to externalize dissatisfactions and inner tensions onto mother because she is more beset by nagging inner genital tension (Kestenberg 1968). These girls may have had an even more difficult time. They certainly now demonstrate confusion in the face of sexual excitation, becoming hyperactive, spasmodic, and diffusely upset. They also seem to despair of achieving sexual relief. While most show the confusion of anger with sexual excitement, identified by Kestenberg (1973), it is common on closer contact to be privy to their despair. One of the girls reports that she cries when she becomes excited, feeling that there is nothing she nor anyone else can do to help her. She dreamed of going down some stairs and finding some unexpected things. The basement turned into an ocean populated with shipwrecked people who demanded that she get them supplies, which she experienced as overwhelming because she didn't know how to obtain them. When she tried, a sheriff told her that that was a dangerous place and she should stay away from there. While the dream may reflect concerns regarding genital anatomy ("finding unexpected things"), it is probably also related to her experience of genital sensations and their demanding, overwhelming nature.

Certainly all of the girls maintained a strict prohibition in their attitude toward masturbation. All were markedly phobic about the notion of touching themselves and all maintained that "only a boy should do that," or "you'd have to feel pretty ugly inside to do that," a comment which may suggest a link between concerns about the form of the genital and fears of self-damage.

The girls studied were quite unable to verbalize sexual feelings and sensations in the structured interview situation. While it may be that the nature of the sensations are to some degree refractory to verbal

452

description (Kestenberg 1968), one recalls that Galenson and Roiphe (1977) have also emphasized that severe reactions to discovery of the anatomical difference (therefore, possibly as well to the discovery of the introitus which is posited to likely precede this discovery) tended to constrict fantasy life.

As might be predicted from a reading of the literature (Benedek 1973; Haft 1973; Shainess 1961; Whisnant and Zegans 1975), for these girls the menarche most powerfully recalls memories of their relationship with their mothers. None of the girls experienced their mother as an active presence in helping them to learn about and integrate ideas concerning their developing bodies, and all had negative attitudes toward the menarche and menstruation. Further, as the menarche reawakens earlier conflicts regarding the vagina (Kestenberg 1961), the form of the conflict appeared to concern conflicts about control and perhaps as well about penetration. Their complaints concerned issues around soiling and their inability to anticipate a period and to control the flow.

All of the girls were sexually active; it was notable that all had begun having sexual intercourse within months of the menarche. However, while they would talk volubly about intercourse they rankled when the subject of defloration was raised. None reported bleeding in the first intercourse, but all said that they did in a subsequent experience. While one spoke of being embarrassed and frightened, the others said they "didn't remember," and one said she "didn't bother to look." One of the girls felt the very word was an outrage and finally dismissed it as ridiculous. Direct questions concerning penetration elicited counterphobic attitudes (e.g., laughter). Though they actively sought penetration, the experience of intercourse itself was found to be disappointing. Their concerns about penetration can be inferred from their refusal to employ contraceptive methods which involve putting something inside them, from their fears about injections, as well as from a broad range of psychological test data. It is suggested that the precocious seeking of experiences of sexual intercourse for these girls served not only to provide active focal genital experience (as opposed to diffuse genital excitation) but that such experiences turned the passive fear of penetration into an active control and seeking of penetration, providing thereby a relief of anxiety as well as genital tension. Early sexual experience is also posited to be a means of promoting body schematization and establishing firmer body boundries in girls who have earlier experienced genital sensations as threats to body integrity.

Clinical Vignettes

Both of the incidents which follow occurred to a fifteen-year-old girl who will be referred to as Carrie. She was at that time in the eighth month of her second psychiatric hospitalization which had been precipitated by her generally out of control behavior in regard to family, school, and societal rules which had progressed to the point of seriously endangering her. Several weeks before hospitalization she had been raped while hitchhiking 500 miles from her home. She is an attractive nonpsychotic girl of normal intelligence, who appears alternately perky and dejected. Though she talks volubly, she is often self-absorbed even while displaying labile and intense affect.

It was possible one day to observe the clinical development of an episode with Carrie which illustrates a form of object relations and self-development characteristic of the girls studied. She had been confined to her room following some infraction, was feeling increasingly frustrated, and continued to come out of her room to seek contact with her primary nurse, Jean. Jean tried many times to soothe Carrie and to return her to her room, but finally reprimanded Carrie and told her she had to stay in her room. The therapist, by chance, arrived at this point and was available to sit with Carrie in her room and be present while Carrie fumed. Carrie ranted on claiming that she "hated" Jean. She then, in mounting fury, listed more and more people she hated and the list rapidly grew to include virtually everyone, including the therapist. Carrie then reported, softly, with some perplexity and fear, feeling all alone. The therapist's empathic statements about Carrie's feeling of aloneness, emptiness, and panic served to consolidate a cohesive sense of self for Carrie. When her feeling of "falling apart" receded and more usual self-feeling returned, Carrie could again begin to think and feel about those around her in a more normal way.

It is my view that the foregoing illustrates the danger of intense aggressive feelings sweeping away the representation of the good object in patients for whom good and bad aspects of self and object representations have not become integrated. Further, and critical to the example which is to follow, the lack of sufficient differentiation between self and object representations subjects the individual not only to a momentary wiping out of the object world but threatens the individual with the experience of her own lack of a cohesive, temporally stable sense of self.

The following traces the development of an incident of self-cutting for Carrie. It occurred at a time when she was threatened with imminent separation from the hospital unit, as a result of having been a provocateur of behavior which endangered others. Her mood was sad, albeit expressed by angry affect. Yet her anger was threatening to her. Anger and blame were projected to the therapist and she thus decided that she could protect and preserve friendships (in which she was disappointed) by avoiding the "disapproving therapist:" Of course, this, too, constituted a loss and served to further structure her mounting sense of isolation. She began to report stomachaches. She felt agitated and diffusely upset. Reassurances given by important others that "things were going okay" were experienced by her as breaches of empathy. Misunderstandings emanated from her as well. She responded to friendly interest from the nursing staff with, "fuck you," later explaining that she meant that she needed help. She began to report headaches. Her parents were extremely anxious regarding the impending discharge, referring to the situation as "being on the brink of disaster," and said they were "feeling like they were falling to pieces."

A situation had developed in which the threat of separation, Carrie's anger, and her experience of the empathic gulf between her and others were combining to produce extreme feelings of tension which were experienced as bodily distress. She despaired of being able to obtain relief in her environment and was actively isolating herself.

The mood then momentarily changed to one of sexual excitement. The principal of the school called to complain about her "caterwauling"—a word which describes the discordant screeches of a cat in heat. On a pass home she was alleged to have had repeated experiences of intercourse. However, she was unable to achieve a feeling of relief either through focal somatic complaints or through focal sexual experiences.

When she returned to the unit she picked a fight and hit a patient whom she claimed had been threatening to her. She refused to talk to staff saying, "No one understands me." Externalization of blame and the weakening of self-object boundaries marked the beginning dissolution of the stable, reliable self and object representational world. She was placed in the quiet room where she says she cut herself slightly.

On the following day she fumed and raged, objecting vehemently to being kept on constant observation (C.O.) by the nursing staff. Approaching the therapist in a rage she threatened, "See what you've done to me? If you don't take me off C.O., I'll cut myself so bad, like you've never seen before."

She was demonstrating extremes of ambitendency—extreme approach and aggressive withdrawal from the object. The passive wish to be soothed was turned to angry, active attempts to elicit the care she wished for (paradoxically, to be left alone), and the passive fear of engulfment (should she allow closeness) was transformed into the active driving away of potentially comforting objects.

She appeared to have a storm brewing in her waiting to be released. Attempts to soothe her empathically were unsuccessful. She began to throw books around and overturn garbage cans. A social worker and nurse restrained her and insisted on her cleaning up the mess she made. They told her that they would control her until she could control herself, that they would not allow her to make a mess of the hall or to endanger herself or others. Immediately thereafter, when she again went to the quiet room she made numerous superficial cuts along both her arms, looking at her arms as she did this and saying to herself, "I'll show them, no one controls what happens to my body but me!" Fifteen minutes later, she was calm, lucid, and ready to review and discuss all of the events with her therapist.

In short, what Carrie then was able to communicate was that she had felt as if she were being torn to pieces, beset by a multiplicity of needs, and feeling abandoned at the same time. She wanted contact and rejected it, wished closeness and asked for separateness, wanted understanding and feared it. She felt she needed to be "put together" (and thought of wanting to be held tightly until she was calm) but experienced such rage that she could neither tolerate anyone coming close nor trust herself to let them try. Cutting, for her, dissipated the tension.

In retrospect one can observe the features contributing to her increase in feelings of frustration, experienced as bodily distress, her lack of faith in the surround to provide relief and the absence of her own self-soothing function, her lack of capacity to verbally and coherently express her distress (which became exacerbated as she progressively lost her sense of her cohesive, stable self), and the earlier abortive attempts to focus her diffuse bodily distress in experiences of somatic complaint and sexual activity.

The Function of Delicate Self-Cutting

Self-cutting served to express both the violation of boundaries she was experiencing and to concretely demarcate her disintegrating body boundaries. Sensations from the inside were concretized and localized at the wound (Schilder 1950). Carrie explained that when she cut herself, the tension came out. No doubt the visual element (she watched) was an ingredient in reconsolidating the body image. Self-cutting thus concretely represented the insult to self she experienced and her capacity to counteract it. To the extent that genital excitement had become a focus for her tension (and perhaps confused with her anger), the cutting could as well be conceptualized as a penetration which she controlled. She said, after all, that only she would control what happened to her body. This then was the function of delicate self-cutting for Carrie—in this concrete and dramatic act she consolidated her cohesive sense of self, managing both to soothe herself in the face of the terror of feeling that she was falling apart and to protect her relationships from the further ravages of her overwhelming anger.

Conclusions

The thesis presented is that the symptom of delicate self-cutting can be understood in the context of characteristic psychological features which can be seen as proceeding from developmental disturbances. An attempt was made to reconstruct the developmental disturbances thought to be related to the features which characterize self-cutting. It is not intended to assert that a developmental progression invariably predicts the behavior. Rather, given the behavior and some evidence of pathology in the spheres of object relations, self and sexual development, the foregoing is intended to expand a psychological understanding of the nature of the symptom and the functions it serves by considering earlier experiences which may have preceded it and the way in which character features which support the symptom may relate to those early experiences.

NOTE

The study on which this report is based was conducted at New York Hospital–Cornell Medical Center, Westchester Division, on the Adolescent Unit directed by Dr. Everett P. Dulit, who graciously supported and encouraged the research. The author wishes to thank Drs. Robert Stolorow, Jo Lang, and Martin Rock of Yeshiva University for their helpful comments on the original manuscript.

REFERENCES

Asch, S. 1971. Wrist scratching as a symptom of anhedonia: a predepressive state. *Psychoanalytic Quarterly* 40:603–617.

Bendek, T. 1973. Climacterium: a developmental phase. In *Psychoanalytic Investigations: Selected Papers*. New York: Quadrangle/New York Times Book Co.

Crabtree, L. 1967. A therapeutic encounter with a self-mutilating patient. *Psychiatry* 30:91–100.

Emerson, L. 1914. The case of Miss A: a preliminary report of a psychoanalytic study and treatment of a case self-mutilation. *Psychoanalytic Review* 1:41–54.

Friedman, M.; Glasser, M.; Laufer, E.; Laufer, M.; and Wohl, M. 1972. Attempted suicide and self-mutilation in adolescence: some observations from a psychoanalytic research project. *International Journal of Psycho-Analysis* 53:179–183.

Fraiberg, S. 1972. Some characteristics of genital arousal and discharge in latency girls. *Psychoanalytic Study of the Child* 27:439–475.

Galenson, E., and Roiphe, H. 1977. Some suggested revisions concerning early female development. In H. Blum, ed. *Female Psychology: Contemporary Psychoanalytic Views*. New York: International Universities Press.

Gardner, A., and Gardner, A. 1975. Self-mutilation, obsessionality, and narcissism. *British Journal of Psychiatry* 127:127–132.

Goldwyn, H.; Cahill, J.; and Grunebaum, H. 1967. Self-inflicted injury to the wrist. *Plastic and Reconstructive Surgery* 39:583–589.

Graff, H., and Mallin, E. 1967. The syndrome of the wrist cutter. *American Journal of Psychiatry* 124:36–42.

Greenacre, P. 1958. Early physical determinants in the development of the sense of identity. In *Emotional Growth*. New York: International Universities Press, 1971.

Grunebaum, H., and Klerman, G. 1967. Wrist slashing. *American Journal of Psychiatry* 124:527–534.

Haft, M. 1973. An exploratory study of early adolescent girls: body image, self-acceptance of "traditional female role," and response to menstruation. Doctoral dissertation, Columbia University.

Hoffer, W. 1950. Development of the body ego. *Psychoanalytic Study of the Child* 5:18–23.

Horney, K. 1933. The denial of the vagina: a contribution to the problem of genital anxieties specific to women. *International Journal of Psycho-Analysis* 14:57–70.

458

Janus, L. 1972. Personality structure and psychodynamics in dermatologic artifacts. (German—English abstract only.) *Zeitschrift fur Psychosomatische Medizin und Psychoanalyse* 18:21–28.

Kafka, J. 1969. The body as transitional object: a psychoanalytic study of a self-mutilating patient. *British Journal of Medical Psychology* 42:207–212.

Kestenberg, J. 1956. Vicissitudes of female sexuality. *Journal of the American Psychoanalytic Association* 4:453–476.

Kestenberg, J. 1961. Menarche. In J. Kestenberg, ed. *Children and Parents: Psychoanalytic Studies in Development*. New York: Aronson, 1975.

Kestenberg, J. 1968. Outside and inside, male and female. *Journal of the American Psychoanalytic Association* 16:457–520.

Kestenberg, J. 1973. Nagging, spreading excitement, arguing. *International Journal of Psychiatry and Psychotherapy* 2:265–297.

Kleeman, J. 1977. Freud's views on early female sexuality in the light of direct child observation. In H. Blum, ed. *Female Psychology: Contemporary Psychoanalytic Views*. New York: International Universities Press.

Mahler, M.; Pine, F.; and Bergman, A. 1975. *The Psychological Birth of the Human Infant*. New York: Basic.

Nelson, S., and Grunebaum, H. 1971. A follow-up study of wrist slashers. *American Journal of Psychiatry* 127:1345–1349.

Novotny, P. 1972. Self-cutting. *Bulletin of the Menninger Clinic* 36:505–514.

Offer, D., and Barglow, P. 1960. Adolescent and young adult self-mutilation in a general psychiatric hospital. *Archives of General Psychiatry* 3:194–204.

Pao, P. 1969. The syndrome of delicate self-cutting. *British Journal of Medical Psychology* 42:195–206.

Phillips, R., and Alkan, M. 1961. Some aspects of self-mutilation in the general population of a large psychiatric hospital. *Psychiatric Quarterly* 35:421–423.

Podvoll, E. 1969. Self-mutilation within a hospital setting: a study of identity and social compliance. *British Journal of Medical Psychology* 42:213–221.

Rinzler, C., and Shapiro, D. 1968. Wrist-cutting and suicide. *Journal of Mount Sinai Hospital* (New York) 25:485–488.

Rosenthal, R.; Rinzler, C.; Walsh, R.; and Klausner, E. 1972. Wrist cutting syndrome: the meaning of a gesture. *American Journal of Psychiatry* 128:1363–1368.

Schilder, P. 1950. *Image and Appearance of the Human Body*. New York: International Universities Press.

Shainess, N. 1961. A re-evaluation of some aspects of femininity through a study of menstruation: a preliminary report. *Comprehensive Psychiatry* 2:20–26.

Simpson, M. 1975. The phenomenology of self-mutilation in a general hospital setting. *Canadian Psychiatric Association Journal* 20:429–434.

Siomopoulos, V. 1974. Repeated self-cutting: an impulse neurosis *American Journal of Psychotherapy* 28:85–94.

Uemura, A. 1975. On a course of therapy for a self-destructive female student. (Japanese—English abstract only.) *Kyushu Neuro-Psychiatry* 21:37–42.

Whisnant, L. and Zegans, L. 1975. A study of attitudes toward menarche in white middle-class American adolescent girls. *American Journal of Psychiatry* 132:8, 809–814.

Winnicott, D. 1962. Ego integration in child development. In *The Maturational Processes and the Facilitating Environment*. New York: International Universities Press, 1965.

Winnicott, D. 1971. *Playing and Reality*. New York: International Universities Press.

28 THE LONER: AN EXPLORATION OF A SUICIDAL SUBTYPE IN ADOLESCENCE

MICHAEL L. PECK

More than 5,000 young Americans, age twenty-four and under, commit suicide each year. Suicide among this age group represents one-fifth of all suicides in the United States and is the third leading cause of death, preceded only by accidents and homicide (Holinger 1978).

Prior to 1965, suicide rates in the United States and in much of the world increased directly with age, with the lowest suicide rates among the young and the highest suicide rates in the older years (Seiden 1969). In the mid-1960s, however, the rate in young people began increasing. These increases, which have continued to the present, changed those relationships. Suicide rates generally increase rapidly in the teen years, reaching a peak sometime in the twenties, taper off and drop slightly in the thirties and forties, and then go up again, higher in the sixties and seventies (Peck and Litman 1974).

Many social changes occurred among youth in the 1960s and early 1970s that appeared to be dramatic departures from the past: increased activism in the antiwar movement; increased dropping out; and a dramatic rise in the use of drugs and, more recently, alcohol. The middle 1970s also saw a dramatic increase in crime committed by young people. It may be that some of these variables have contributed to the increase in suicide rates. We have observed (Peck 1980) that many suicidal youngsters abuse alcohol and drugs and become involved in criminal activities as a defensive system and a coping mechanism against their unhappiness and depression.

A substantial number of suicides occur in a group composed primarily of young white males who appear to be isolated in their life-style and relationships. It is from this group of suicidal youngsters that we have identified "the loner," who will be discussed in the following pages.

Description of the Loner

One of the earliest discussions of this category of youngster was by Jan-Tauch (1963). In a study of children who had committed suicide, he reported that these youngsters had no close friends with whom they might share problems or receive psychological support. He noted that the differences between those who attempted suicide and those who committed suicide centered on the former having had a close relationship that played a role in their rescue. Schrut (1964) points out that if the history of the youngster is one of progressive or continued isolation in early childhood, the prognosis for suicide is more serious than if the history includes the ability to have some relationships, at least, early in life. Peck and Schrut (1971), in studying a large sample of college student suicides, described the students who committed suicide as isolated, hopeless, and less likely to send out communication signals for help.

A behavioral description of the loner type would suggest that the behavior patterns manifested by this type of person begin to emerge in the early teens and seem to fit a fairly clear-cut symptom pattern. This adolescent frequently has a long history of spending much of his spare time alone. He is much more likely to be a male than a female, and white rather than nonwhite. These young boys tend to have very poor interpersonal relationships with peers and adults. They tend to feel isolated and lonely much of the time, with no one to confide in when they feel upset. When they do make friends, the relationship is often superficial. When friends are asked about this person, they often respond in vague terms, explaining they don't know him very well.

These boys appear to be very aware of feelings of sexual inadequacy and serious doubts about their ability to ever relate to women in the future. When these youngsters are seen psychiatrically, the most common diagnoses are borderline state, schizoid personality, and depressive character. Unlike other kinds of adolescent suicides, these youngsters are less likely to communicate or signal their impending suicidal attempt.

Most often, youngsters described as loners come from intact families with relatively normal parents. A closer analysis of these families suggests that the parents may have some difficulty with their self-image

462

as parents. These parents frequently interpret their child's complaints about problems and unhappiness as a statement about their own inadequacies as parents. They frequently respond defensively to their child, insisting that the child is not really unhappy or really has nothing to complain about. These parents require their children to be successful in order to compensate for their own feelings of inadequacy and insecurity. It is most important for them to view their children as an extension of their own fantasied successes, and therefore they are likely to screen out other kinds of communication, especially those implying failure. In these families, the children learn at an early age that what they think of themselves and what their parents think of them is different; and they come to distrust their own thoughts and feelings. A solution is often not to communicate unhappy thoughts and feelings to anyone.

As the adolescent boy approaches his middle and later teens, he becomes more and more aware of the discrepancy between parental expectations on the one hand and his own performance. He frequently feels as though the gap between what is expected of him and his performance is increasing. He grows increasingly more hopeless that he will ever be able to catch up. Often, when faced with increased stresses such as dating, graduating, getting a job, going to college, or going away from home, he becomes overwhelmed with the hopelessness of that situation. He is unable to share these feelings with anyone, and may enter into a full-blown suicidal crisis, feeling helpless, hopeless, and totally alienated.

Case Illustration of a Suicide

Larry, an eighteen-year-old white male lived at home with his mother, father, and two younger sisters. He was a senior in high school and had maintained a slightly better than average grade-point average for the tenth and eleventh grades, although there was a noticeable decline in the twelfth grade. Larry had shown little interest in extracurricular activities, although for a short period of time, in the tenth grade, he participated on the track team. He had few friends outside of school and none with whom he spent any serious social time. He had no relationships with girls other than for casual school related conversations. Larry never had had a date and was very much afraid of girls. He had been accepted by several colleges away from home, but was terrified by the thought of separation.

His parents believed that Larry had many friends, was very much involved in extracurricular activities in and out of school, went out on dates, and was looking forward to going away to college. His parents stated that he seemed like a happy young man and they had no idea why he would commit suicide. His acquaintances in school also had no idea why he would take his life, but admitted that they knew little or nothing about him, as did his teachers.

Clearly, Larry did not communicate to his parents, his sisters, his friends, or any significant others. His isolation reached such a point that he could not share his fears and inadequacies with anyone. He was terrified of growing older and hopeless that the way he felt about himself and about the world could ever change. His sense of hopelessness and his sense of helplessness that he could do nothing about his condition played a very important part in his shooting himself with his father's gun a month before his high school graduation. Few people who knew him felt that he evidenced any clues to his impending suicide, nor did they feel they knew him well enough to understand why he took his life. Only by talking to many people after his death and piecing together small parts of the puzzle did the whole picture emerge.

Treatment Problems of the Loner

Treatment of the loner may be long and difficult. Identifying this youngster is even more difficult. As stated, these youngsters do not communicate their suicidal intent in a direct fashion. Interrupting and preventing the suicide process in these youngsters is not particularly difficult once the youngster has been identified and brought into treatment. It is likely that one important reason that more of these youngsters do not commit suicide centers on the fact that they are by chance rescued by a friend or relative, usually an older person, who helps them to break through the pattern of not talking about their feelings, frustrations, disappointments, and failures. This rescuing person, in our experience, has been a relative, family doctor, clergyman, coach, teacher, or school counselor—someone who was able, somehow, to communicate to the youngster, "I know you are troubled, and I want to hear what you have to say."

Treatment of youngsters in this category is often in two phases. The initial phase is dealing with the immediate crisis which centers around the youngsters' long-standing fear of opening up and sharing any intimate thoughts and feelings with anyone. Once this is broken through, the terrors and inadequacies begin to spill out, and the suicide risk diminishes rapidly. Treatment has as its goal then to make a genuine change in life-style, including new social, psychological, and psychosexual adaptations. This requires long and intensive work. The focus is often on the buildup of trust, a working through of the inadequacies, with a stress on development of ongoing competence and mastery in a wide range of areas. Sometimes, an ego has been so assailed that intimacy and relationships can never be really attained. In these cases, the mastery and competence needs to center on other areas that are within the grasp of the youngster.

Case Illustration

Bill was referred to therapy after a suicide gesture in the home was aborted by his mother. He was nineteen years old, a sophomore in college. He still lived at home with his parents and a younger brother. Bill's entire history was one of social withdrawal and failure to develop relationships. He constantly depreciated himself for his lack of friends. His parents, too, made a great deal of his social inabilities and very little of the fact that he ranked in the top 2 percent in mathematics in his college entrance exams.

The therapy centered on his initial hopelessness that he would never be able to have a relationship. It had then moved from there, to the areas of mastery that he had already gained, that is, mathematics, with an effort to help him experience the importance of success in this area. Once this was accomplished, he was able to focus more readily on his social inadequacies and to lower his social expectations. He then dealt with his sexual fears. After two years of therapy he attended his first party. The success of this was in the sense that even though attending the party was not a successful experience, his expectations were such that he was not devastated. Bill did not become suicidal again, moved on to a successful career in mathematics, and seemed to come to terms with his own areas of weakness and his areas of strength.

Conclusions

Understanding and delineating certain characteristics of suicidal young people can be instrumental in the prevention and treatment of such problems. In this chapter, a category of youthful suicidal victims, the loner, has been delineated. The development and psychodynamics of these adolescents have been discussed, as have the prevailing presenting symptoms.

In discussing treatment, it becomes clear that recognizing and identifying these loners is a major consideration. The implication is that community education could become an important part of prevention and treatment. Long term treatment of these youngsters is usually essential because their lengthy experience of noncommunication and failure of ego development has led to great difficulties with identity formation and the ability to achieve intimacy. Hopefully, such a focus will ultimately have a favorable impact on decreasing the numbers of youngsters who attempt, or go on to commit suicide each year.

REFERENCES

Holinger, P.C. 1978. Adolescent suicide: an epidemiological study of recent trends. *American Journal of Psychiatry* 103:416–422.

Jan-Tauch, J. 1963. Studies of children: 1960–1963. *New Jersey Public School Studies*. Trenton: State of New Jersey, Dept. of Education.

Peck, M. 1980. Youth suicide: delineation of new classifications. *Roche Reports: Frontiers of Psychiatry* 10:2–3.

Peck, M., and Litman, R.E. 1974. Current trends in youthful suicide. In J. Bush, ed. *Suicide and Blacks*. Los Angeles: Fanon Research & Development.

Peck, M., and Schrut, A. 1971. Suicidal behavior among college students. *Health Services and Mental Health Administration Reports* 86:149–156.

Schrut, A. 1964. Suicidal adolescents and children. *Journal of the American Medical Association* 188:1103–1107.

Seiden, R. 1969. Suicide among youth: a review of the literature, 1900–1967. *Bulletin of Suicidology*. Washington D.C.: Government Printing Office.

29　THE INTERACTION OF DRUG ABUSE AND DEPRESSION IN AN ADOLESCENT GIRL

ROBERT A. CAPER

Depression is a normal part of adolescence, as it is of the phases of life preceding and following it. However, it is not unusual for depression to become so severe in adolescence that it erupts in some way which makes it impossible for those in the environment to ignore it. The fact that this eruption often takes the form of drug abuse or other delinquent behavior should not obscure our view of the underlying causes. In what follows, the description of a part of the psychoanalytic investigation of a case will illustrate some of the relationships between overt symptomatology, mostly of an acting-out type, and underlying depression. It will also describe some implications of these relationships for the treatment of similar cases.

Case History

When first seen, the patient, whom I shall call Alice, was fourteen years old, the eldest of three children of an attorney and his wife. Her parents sought professional help for her because they had become increasingly concerned about her use of drugs, truancy, promiscuity, defiance of parental authority, and general unmanageability, all of which seemed to be getting worse despite their best efforts to control her. She would stay away from home for long periods of time without permission, occasionally overnight, causing her parents to worry about her physical safety, especially in view of her provocative behavior at home and with her friends. Matters came to a head when the public school authorities informed her parents that she would not be promoted to the next grade because of academic deficiencies. This shocked them and forced them to realize how far things had deteriorated since two years previous her grades had been excellent and she had displayed outstanding mathematical ability.

When Alice was nine years old, her parents began to be involved, along with many of their friends, in the recreational use of marijuana and cocaine. They made no attempt to conceal this from their children and on occasion would invite Alice and her friends to join them. At the time of the consultation, the parents were having serious marital difficulties and neither of them felt able to manage Alice's behavior.

When seen in consultation, Alice was a poorly groomed, moderately obese girl who glanced suspiciously about the room and was clearly very frightened. She maintained that there was nothing wrong with her. She went on to tell a rather touching story about the family dog (she had a great interest in dog breeding), a poorly behaved animal and a nuisance to the family. All the dog needed, she went on, was some understanding and a good course of training, since it was really still a baby despite its chronological age.

Alice's early development was described by her parents as that of a model child who did not appear to have any emotional problems. She was quick to learn, but having done something once she would firmly insist that she could do it ever after without help, despite all evidence to the contrary. Both parents seem to have been rather preoccupied when she was little. She was cared for much of the time by an aunt with whom she seems to have had a good relationship. In school, she had a winning way with her peers and usually had an entourage of friends. She was somewhat tomboyish, however, and would frequently provoke fights.

In view of her parents' concern about her safety (which turns out to have been justified as several of the friends who were involved with Alice in the drug scene are now dead) and their inability to cope with her, it was decided to hospitalize her and to treat her along psychoanalytic lines. Following her eventual discharge from the hospital, she arranged to live with some friends of the family in order to continue her treatment, her parents having moved out of town in the meantime.

Course of Treatment

The first six months of treatment were characterized by her prolific, ingenious, and occasionally violent attempts to disrupt the organizational structure of the hospital and of her treatment. These took the form of arriving at sessions late, leaving early, shouting her analyst down, attempted escapes from the hospital, and forcing hospital staff into restraining her rather than utilizing their ability and willingness to understand her. Alternatively, she would become docile and well mannered, a "model child," while secretly violating some major hospital rule, usually after recruiting other patients in the effort.

This behavior was an early indication of a part of her personality which took great pleasure in deceiving and secretly triumphing over authority. In fact, she was a captive of this aspect of her personality, which was also responsible for her insistence as a child that she could do everything she needed for herself, and which came to be referred to in treatment as the "do-it-myself" part.

The power this aspect of her personality had over her was revealed in a session during her sixth month of treatment. An interpretation was made connecting her secret triumph over her parents with her subsequent fear of them. She became quite confused in contrast to the usual clarity of her thinking, despite the fact that the interpretation itself was quite simple and straightforward. It was suggested that she felt the interpretation was correct (and there was plenty of evidence for it), which made her aware of her dependence on the analyst as a source of correct information. This led the "do-it-myself" part of her personality to mangle her ability to think and be aware of what was correct. She reacted to this further interpretation with anger and contempt. The following day, however, after her therapist announced that he would be taking a one-week vacation later in the month, she became acutely depressed and lamented that all she ever loved was always getting lost, denying, however, that it had anything to do with the break in treatment.

The understanding of how strongly this "do-it-myself," omnipotent aspect of her personality affected her, even to the point of depriving her of her ability to think, led her to a series of insights about how humiliated she felt if she was forced to wait for what she wanted. She felt she was a "sissy" if she did not get stoned when on pass from the hospital, but she gradually became better able to withstand the taunts and assaults, which originated more within herself than from her peers.

Her parents and hospital staff noted a new stability, seriousness of purpose, and trustworthiness about her. At this point in her treatment, she expressed "heartache" at the slowness of her progress and had two associations to this: suffering frustration at the hands of her mother and kicking a soccer ball and hurting her ankle, which slowed her progress when she tried to walk. This was interpreted as a communication about a part of her that kicks her mother and her therapist inside her in response to frustration, causing a bad relationship with them. These actions slow her attempts to grow and cause heartache for having hurt someone she cares about. Her immediate response was to become offended, as though she had been assaulted.

A few months later she described a "crazy guy" whose car she had bumped in a parking lot, causing no visible damage. He accused her of "gashing" his car, chased her, and actually dented hers. The analyst connected this to her reaction to the interpretation concerning her heartache, saying that it must have made her feel guilty, and that she experienced that as a very damaging assault (actually it was the omnipotent part of her that felt that way), which was why she had stormed out of the session. She responded by saying, in a sad and thoughtful way, that she did not see how doctors could stand to see people who are dying. This was taken as an expression of appreciation for the difficulties which her parents and therapist had to tolerate in order to help her, including having to face the realization that she may never recover.

This phase was followed by a renewed series of complaints and accusations about her treatment. Her by now undeniable improvement, obvious to everyone, was attributed, when it was acknowledged at all, to a constantly changing list of factors in her life. On this list her treatment appeared near the bottom, if it appeared at all. This led into a prolonged period of grievances about narcissistic wounds—nobody understood how she felt, people only saw the bad in her, etc. As long as these were looked at as responses to unempathic parents and analyst, the sessions were smoother and agreeable. If any suggestion was made that her expectations might be somewhat unreasonable she became angry. In her behavior outside the sessions, however, she was much more reasonable and had better relationships with friends and parents following stormy sessions. Her acting out was now confined to periods of separation from treatment and to periods following quiet sessions.

The full extent of her enslavement to the omnipotent part of her personality was revealed in a dream which occurred rather late in her treatment, following a piece of acting out which gave her real reason for seeing how much her behavior was costing her. She dreamed she had been kidnapped by a cult where she was bullwhipped. She escaped and took her father back to show him, but the cult members had disguised themselves as a sort of agricultural commune. He could not recognize the danger and dropped her off at an ice-cream store. The counterman turned out to be a cult member who threatened her for trying to expose the cult. The cult was connected to the drug culture and also to that part of her that used drugs. Both disguised themselves as free spirits while secretly engaging in extremely destructive and sadistic practices. By this time the life-threatening aspects of her acting out had abated as a result of her growing insight and had begun to be replaced by frightening dreams such as the one mentioned.

Discussion

In the process of formulating a model which would clarify an understanding of this case, it has been useful to think of the patient's personality as divided into two parts. These are not multiple or split personalities, but rather two parts of a single personality coexisting, in conflict, and interacting with each other in complex ways. The division is most clearly indicated in the patient's cult dream, where one aspect of her personality—an omnipotent and sadistic aspect—is represented by the cult. The other—a healthier part—is represented by the girl who tries to get help from her father in dealing with the cult. This latter aspect is capable of healthy dependency and was essential to her recovery. In formulating this model, the author has used his experience with this and other patients, as well as Klein's (1940, 1946) differentiation of the paranoid-schizoid and depressive positions, the work of Rosenfeld (1960) on drug addiction, and of Meltzer (1970) on adolescent perverse sexuality and delinquency. This model has shed some light on the problem of the causes of depression in adolescents, its relation to drug abuse, and contains some significant implications for the management and treatment of these patients.

In one aspect, the girl's drug abuse, running away, and promiscuity were defenses against a profound underlying sense of depression and worthlessness. The drugs functioned as an anesthetic or a euphoriant. The promiscuity brought at least the illusion of closeness. The running away reassured her of her competence in coping with the world on her own.

At the same time, however, the omnipotent, "do-it-myself," or "cult" aspect of her personality was providing quite a different motivation for her behavior. By holding her parents' child hostage and exposing it to great danger she could force her parents to experience the guilt, frustration, and depression that she would otherwise have to

471

experience herself. In addition, like the cult in the dream, she would, when confronted, make her dangerous behavior appear harmless or even beneficial. Thus, serious drug abuse was labeled "experimentation"; running away from home or "getting out on my own"; exposure to serious physical danger, "learning to take care of myself,"; and sexual promiscuity, "developing a sexual identity." This deception enabled her to triumph over her parents and to feel that they, and not she, were helpless, stupid, credulous infants. This part of her personality subjected the healthy part of herself to the same treatment, intimidating it and calling it "sissy" and "baby" if it did not go along. This was quite a different kind of defense against her feelings of helplessness, both in its mode of operation and in its effects on her development.

One consequence of the latter type of defense was a profound unconscious sense of guilt and depression caused by the damage the "cult" part of her was doing to her object relationships, which she dealt with partly by projection. Her friends, especially her boyfriends, tended to treat her in a rather cruel way, and she was unable to defend herself because of her need to be a victim. This was also a factor in her periodic exposure of herself to extreme physical danger.

Her parents' difficulties, including their abuse of drugs, affected her in a complex way. The healthy aspect of herself recognized that something was wrong with her parents. She became depressed both because she was deprived of her "good" parents and because she knew how little she could do to help them. The omnipotent part of her personality, because of its tendencies to deal with her infantile weaknesses and inadequacies by making her parents appear inadequate, made her fantasize that she had therefore caused their difficulties. This was a source of a painful and deep sense of guilt. These fantasies, which seemed to be supported by some reality, exacerbated her depression and sense of badness which then had to be dealt with by renewed delinquent behavior—a vicious cycle.

One implication of these findings is the importance of recognizing and dealing with both aspects of the depressed, drug-abusing adolescent's personality. The depressed infant must be recognized, acknowledged, and treated appropriately. At the same time, we must bear in mind the possibility that the patient's behavior may represent, not just a defense against depression, but also a constellation of conscious and unconscious fantasies that, by attacking the internal parents, can be an important source of depression.

The importance of correctly differentiating these aspects of the patient's personality and of dealing with each appropriately becomes clear if one considers the consequences of neglecting either. If the depressed infant is not recognized in treatment, the patient will not feel that it is acceptable and will eventually feel hopeless about its ever being understood and dealt with. On the other hand, if the unconscious, sadistic, triumphant aspect of the personality is not sufficiently recognized and dealt with, then it will be strengthened by the belief that it has succeeded in blinding the therapist and its secret claims that triumph and deception are superior to healthy dependency will increase. Of these two types of therapeutic oversight, the latter appears to be more common: we have greater difficulty detecting our patients' desire to have us fail than their desire for us to succeed. But if the therapist does not have a balanced view of these coexisting unconscious currents in the transference and in the patient's overall emotional life, then treatment of this type of patient will be a very partial success at best.

The problem which confronted the analyst in this case was thus twofold: how to recognize the roles various aspects of the patient's personality played in her emotional life and how to deal with each. Some light is shed on this problem by the portion of the treatment described above in which the patient complained of never being understood and of people only seeing the bad in her. A pseudoempathic response (agreeing that her suffering was due to failure on the part of her objects) led to a smooth session which was, however, usually followed by an increase in unreasonableness and paranoia in the transference and in her relationships outside of treatment. These sessions were also characterized by a lack of any sense of real emotional contact with the patient. Once this became clear, it was possible to interpret the situation to the patient in a different way: that her characterization of her objects was perhaps intended to make them look bad in order to prove her moral superiority over them. This type of interpretation generally led to a stormy but far more genuine response, followed by an improvement in her relations with her external objects and an increase in positive transference. A sequence of events such as this is quite good evidence that one is at least approximating a correct clinical differentiation. The cult dream gives an indication of why this pseudoempathy fails. If the analyst-father does not recognize the true nature of the cult, the patient is exposed to great anxiety and danger. Recognition of what they are (she is) up to consciously or unconsciously, while eliciting a temporary wounded reaction, also produced great relief on a deeper level, with subsequent clinical improvement.

Another indicator that the differentiation mentioned above is being made correctly, shown rather clearly in this case, is the progressive appearance of the capacity for concern for one's objects which Klein (1940) has called depressive anxiety. This developed in the patient over the course of several months' work and can be seen clearly in the material centering around the soccer ball, her difficulty walking, and the "crazy guy" who dented her car. Her response to the analyst's interpretation about the damage that her paranoia does to herself and her objects (which, in marked contrast to her usual way of considering her feelings, was quite thoughtful) contained a poignant element of concern for her objects, both internal and external, and guilt over the pain she had caused them.

The appearance of a capacity for genuine concern is, in the author's experience, firm evidence of progress in the treatment and an indication that one is on the right tack. The failure of such evidence to appear after an extended period of treatment is a bad prognostic sign and should spur the therapist to examine whether he is not perhaps missing something important. In this connection, an interesting feature of this case, which could be fully appreciated only in retrospect, was the patient's initial concern, touchingly expressed, about the family dog, which was connected to her interest in dog breeding. This seems to have been founded on an identification with a pair of good, creative parents who were concerned about their child. This identification played a role in her eventual recovery, which was based in part on her capacity to experience concern about the pain she had caused her parents and the danger she had placed their child in.

The second problem faced by the therapist in addition to differentiating these two aspects of the patient (among others) is how to deal with them. In a sense, this problem cannot be clearly separated from the problem of identifying them, since the more clearly they can be identified the easier it is to know how to treat them. However, a major technical problem still exists even after one can see to some extent that one is dealing with, say, an unconscious sadistic aspect of the patient which enjoys causing suffering in her objects, including the therapist. The problem is primarily an emotional one, and was also well illustrated in this case: the therapist, at certain points, would find himself increasingly anxious about the patient's safety. The patient, at such time, saw to it that the anxiety persisted by making veiled references to some dangerous, secret activity. At other times, the therapist was made to feel guilty over the "needless" restrictions that the treatment was placing on the patient's life and the suffering that resulted from them.

Numerous other examples of difficult counter-transference feelings could be mentioned, but these two must serve as representative. In the first instance, it turned out that the therapist was being made to bear the anxiety that the patient would otherwise have to experience over the danger in which she placed her internal and external objects, for which she felt responsible and about which she felt unable to do anything. In the second, the therapist was having put into him the guilt that the patient could not experience over the way she sadistically controlled and restricted her objects.

The temptation facing the therapist in the first case is to impose more and more restrictions on the patient in an attempt to save her from herself and to relieve himself of the anxiety he is bound to feel lest some harm should befall a patient for whom he is responsible. However, if this is done, the patient is then able to spurn the treatment with the justification, reinforced by the extraordinary measures that the therapist might sometimes feel compelled to take, that it is after all just an attempt on the part of the adult world to control her. There ensues a power struggle, one of the most frequent causes of treatment failure with adolescents. Its frequency reflects in part the frequency of this type of transference-countertransference dilemma. In the second case, where the therapist was made to feel guilty about even the necessary restrictions placed on the patient by the treatment, the temptation was in the opposite direction: to shorten or even abandon the treatment on the grounds that it was too much of an imposition on such a young patient. This might have been rationalized, at certain points, on the ground that she had made considerable improvement already, which may have been quite true, however irrelevant to the question of a stable recovery.

The therapist must thus be prepared to experience forcefully both the guilt which the patients should be experiencing over their unconscious sadism and the unconscious anxiety and powerlessness which they feel when their sadistic attacks are felt to endanger their objects, both internally and externally. In short, he must be able to bear all those feelings which the patients find unbearable, until they are able to bear them themselves, that is, until they have made considerable progress, by becoming more fully aware of their inner world and the forces in it. Failure of the therapist to do so runs the risk of a series of modifications of the treatment which may reflect more an acting out of the countertransference than considered clinical judgment. In the experience of the author, which supports that of Rosenfeld (1960), if the analyst attempts to fill a role for the patient other than that of providing understanding by interpreting the patient's unconscious, the treatment will suffer, probably by being deprived of the chance to reach the depth and intensity necessary to enable the patient to achieve genuine integration.

Conclusions

When the therapist was able to use his counter-transference as a basis for understanding what the patient was doing to him, why she was doing it, and could interpret this to the patient, modification of the analytic approach was found to be unnecessary. Understanding arrived at in this way represents genuine empathy. If a consistent analytic approach can be maintained, a kind of working through occurs even with quite disturbed patients which we have ordinarily associated only with less disturbed patients. This has important implications both for the extent of improvement that we can hope to bring about in such patients and for the durability of such improvement.

NOTE

The author would like to thank Susanna Isaacs Elmhirst and Charlotte Riley for their helpful discussion.

REFERENCES

Klein, M. 1940. Mourning and its relation to manic-depressive states. *International Journal of Psycho-Analysis* 21:125–153.
Klein, M. 1946. Notes on some schizoid mechanisms. *International Journal of Psycho-Analysis* 27:99–109.
Meltzer, D. 1970. *Sexual States of Mind*. Perthshire: Clunie.
Rosenfeld, H. 1960. On drug addiction. *International Journal of Psycho-Analysis* 41:465–475.

30 FEELINGS OF POWERLESSNESS AND THE ROLE OF VIOLENT ACTIONS IN ADOLESCENTS

IRVING H. BERKOVITZ

Adolescence, more than any other developmental stage, involves swings of mood from feelings of powerlessness to feelings of powerfulness. In between, there are moments of feeling reasonably competent. When events and conditions interfere with development toward autonomy and competence, feelings of helplessness, often with hopelessness, may abound. Therapy when successful can help to rediscover paths of action which can restore feelings of power and control.

Related to these feelings are the emancipatory imperatives of adolescence. Emancipation from parental and familial ties, and the consolidation of identity are prime tasks. This involves furthering the separation-individuation begun in childhood and advancing the development of a stable self. A large element in emancipation at this period is the lessening of the power of parental introjects and the formation of a new individualized superego. These imperatives continue into later adolescence, having first appeared after puberty in early adolescence. If the actions begun earlier have not resulted in competent autonomy by the late teens, the feelings of failure and of "time running out" can be extreme. In late adolescence, especially, a chronic state of powerlessness, helplessness, and hopelessness can lead to actions; violent or controlled, intentional or accidental, random or a mixture of these.

In some adolescents achieving adequate autonomy requires overt rejection of parents, including at times the option for excessive hostility. Reciprocal, gradual withdrawal by parents is helpful. Earlier childhood development, allowing effective expression of anger to a dependable and responsive adult group, will influence the degree of rage and emancipatory intensity generated in adolescence. The fear that movement to emancipation will lead to death for self or parents is often an unconscious (or conscious) obstacle to development of autonomous identity.

The three males presented here were entrapped during late adolescence in moods of powerless depression and mutually reinforced bonds of hostile attachment to parents. Among other familial factors, there was fear of and difficulty in expressing anger to fathers. The three fathers involved could not receive, allow, or facilitate the anger of their sons. Other family members, especially mothers and older brothers, had important roles as well. The experiences to be described suggest that the inability to be fully aware of and achieve adequate expression of this repressed rage aggravated the feelings of powerlessness and interfered with development of autonomous identity.

Such situations of depression, frustrated growth, hopelessness, and repressed anger may set the stage for the unpredictable eruption of strong, occasionally violent, uncontrolled impulses. Impulses of homicide and suicide may alternate, and fate may determine which will emerge. Drug use will often be called on to blunt the impulses, slow the rate of change, and reduce drives. At times, drug use will lessen control of impulses.

If impulsive violent actions do occur, these may contain an attempt to assert power, make a decision, exercise control, and/or deny helplessness. Often the action may be intentionally or unintentionally destructive to significant others directly, indirectly, and/or symbolically. Such actions, whether suicide attempts, or at times homicide attempts, may also set into motion corrective changes in the unsatisfactory life equilibria. These changes may lead then to relief of stagnation and impasse, often restoring a sense of power.

The three adolescents to be described here experienced many of these feelings. In that context each performed individually relevant violent actions. Two of them had several years of treatment with different therapists, individually and in family modes, in office and hospital settings, but effective life changes did not occur until the occurrence of violent action and subsequent events. For one, the action was shooting both parents, inflicting nonfatal injuries. For the second, the action was involuntary manslaughter while driving under the influence of alcohol. For the third, a fall from a fourth floor window served to break an emotional impasse, especially in his sense of self in relation to father.

These acts seemed to function almost as traumatic events around which external as well as internal changes become organized, especially the formation of a new, more responsible, less narcissistically oriented superego and a new relationship to family and society. Certainly many young men, with or without psychotherapy, achieve character change without such events. On the other hand, many go through such actions without subsequent positive developments. Probably the special individual and familial circumstances of these three young men, including the previous psychotherapy, helped stimulate subsequent growth.

Some hypothesis is in order to attempt an explanation of the mechanisms underlying these psychological changes. The first two actions are among the most heinous and forbidden in our society, especially when committed by the young. In addition, these men had strong beliefs against interpersonal violence. This belief system, instilled by their intellectually oriented families, could be also seen as a defense against expression of murderous rage in their families. Inadvertently breaking this taboo therefore could be seen to have set into motion the need to reintegrate this rejected part of themselves. This in turn could lead to a reappraisal of their previous restraints on effective self-assertion and their continual use of masochistic, self-punitive defenses.

The Case of Greg

Greg's family moved from the east coast to California when he was eight. He described himself as "a most precocious delinquent who could get away with things. I had the family brains and talent but the least motivation." An older brother was less assertive, but was infantilized and favored by the parents. He described his father as "the softest person I know. He was not a person you could argue with . . . he never took sides. He's always been a very gentle person. Sometimes it was beautiful, but sometimes it was uptight and confusing. Like once when he was really pissed, all he did was ask me to read the definition for respect from the dictionary. I mean, that might have started my career as a writer, but it didn't tell me why I had to respect him. He was a totally nonviolent parent, but I think more from fear than any religious convictions."

About his mother he said, "Whatever she made up in strength, she lost in doting. I've never met anyone as convinced of my genius as she is."

He said their attitude made him feel "completely lost. Like I could drop dead and they wouldn't know it until I started to stink. My being fucked up just didn't fit into their life's dream. It would have blown their minds if they really understood what was going on in my head. They had to minimize it; they were true experts in public relations.''

Greg was frequently in conflict with the school authorities. He also made explosives in his home chemistry lab and exploded them in the neighborhood. Peers scapegoated him and his parents feared him. Some indication of Greg's tentative self-definition and tenuous object relations are indicated by quotes from an autobiography written at age sixteen for a high school class. While typical of many adolescents' writings, it seems more extreme.

> As an introductory thought before attempting this brief autobiography, may I caution the reader that if he refers to the coldest wind, the wildest mountains, etc., he will probably find that my autobiography is best written without words at all, and that the most successful understanding of my transcending subjectivity is obtained through the reader's inner perception of my subjective symbols. It is because of the transcendent state of my definition that I can find love at the present time only with nature.

About his parents he wrote,

> I do like my parents, and undoubtedly enjoy the sense of security I gain from their existence. . . . The various conflicts I have with my parents arise from such trivial things as my need for a haircut or shave, and the need of coming home before sunrise. Such problems are quite disturbing, for I resent terribly the fleeting attempts to pollute me with the superficial values of society. I will do what I damn well please, but I will never intentionally harm another or blindly let one go without a true attempt at befriending him and showing some understanding.

Greg left home to go to college at eighteen. There he felt alienated and was scapegoated as different. Several students even forcibly shaved his beard. Several months later he developed severe abdominal pain diagnosed as ileocolitis, a chronic disease of the intestine causing pain, anemia, weight loss, occasional bleeding, and arthritis. He did not return to school and required many medical procedures, frequent brief hospitalizations, and numerous medications including codeine.

480

He was referred for psychiatric care when he became depressed and angry on the medical ward. Admission to the psychiatric ward was necessary several times for depression and to reduce drug use. Office psychotherapy was difficult due to intestinal exacerbations and absences from the city. He was seeking new adjustments and relief from symptoms. He had literary goals and wrote much poetry as well as several short stories. As his emotional and physical condition worsened, entry to a hospital for long-term care was considered. Supportive psychotherapy sessions continued in the meantime. He continued living at home, using tranquilizers and pain medication. There were periods of anger but also closeness with his concerned but helpless parents. He busied himself writing poetry.

After five months of this aimless routine, the following event occurred. One evening he stopped at the scene of an auto accident to offer assistance. Police noted his unsteady speech and gait and arrested him, suspecting narcotic abuse. He was kept in jail overnight and released next day after lawyers' and parents' efforts. The event seemed to exacerbate a paranoid ideation and anger with police and society. He talked of "shooting all the police," words not unlike others he had used over the previous years. He did possess firearms, which had been locked away by his family.

Five days later while at the city attorney's office with his father, a fire in his room at home destroyed some books and highly valued photographic negatives. His room as a refuge was now less available, especially with workmen coming in to repair the damage. He had previously been spending much time in his room under the influence of tranquilizers.

He now complained of increased stomach pains due to withdrawal of codeine. He was tearful concerning the loss of his negatives and was angry at his parents' increased concern about his driving ability. They wanted him again to go to a local hospital, which increased his resentment. Eleven days after the arrest, he shot his father in the arm. When mother came to investigate, he shot her in the chest. Both recovered. Police used tear gas to subdue him and remove him from his home. He was incarcerated in the state hospital, in their therapeutic prison, for two years. There he worked on an autobiography describing his experiences. In his book, he stated that he had swallowed pills the evening before the shooting in an attempt to commit suicide, and had the loaded gun ready in case the pills failed. When he awoke the next day he was disappointed to find himself still alive. He wrote:

481

Well, at first, in a literal sense, I was trying to commit suicide.
That was my primary goal; it never occurred to me to shoot them or
anything. I mean, they were so nice to me . . . the rest was pure
release. My father started hassling me about not working . . . he
figured if I went out and got a job, everything would be all right. . . .
At that point in life my profession was pretty well established and it
was too bloody late to go out and become top boxboy. His timing
really pissed me off, telling me to work while I was committing
suicide. As I took the gun out I told him something like that. . . .
Soon I'll be dead and you won't have to worry about me not
working. . . . But before the gun reached my head I flashed on all the
suffering I'd already gone through, and I completely unhinged the
blame; they became the ones who deserved to get hurt. In that
second, I must have felt all the things about them that are beginning to unravel now.

Fourteen years later, at age thirty-six, he wrote:

There was no premeditation involved when I nonfatally shot my
parents. After five years of a severe gastrointestinal illness which
had made me totally dependent upon parents and doctors, I was
merely attempting suicide with my many medications; the back-up
system was loaded next to my bed—one of several gift guns from
my parents. When the pills didn't work, and the following morning
I turned that gift from my temple to my parents, I was acting on an
impulse which appears to have logically followed an upbringing as
primary scapegoat in a family that refused to face reality.

In these same later writings, he detailed some of the events subsequent
to the shooting.

I was found not guilty by reason of insanity and committed to [the]
State Hospital, where I'd still be if my brother hadn't convinced
the folks to hire the lawyer who filed the writ that got me out in
1967. . . . That cooperation marked the beginning of a new family
closeness which has slowly grown over the past twelve years.

While I was writing *Exile's End* and having it regularly rejected,
Dad was working on a musical that was chronically rejected before
being accepted, only to bomb. For the first time, we shared a
public sense of failure; no doubt we were both working hard . . .

482

Dad gradually exerted more effort as a father, having more faith in his opinions, and more opinions than ever, and in general we've felt more in common, perhaps even a sense of being rival scapegoats.

I've also grown closer to Mom's mixture of mysticism and pragmatism. . . . By the time I was on welfare in Denver, I even believed in God. I've shown my appreciation by being discreet enough to not ask for so much as a car, satisfied with a roof over my head, and for the past few years, a bad marriage.

They are unswerving friends, sometimes my only phone call in months, always with something good to say no matter how bad things seem. They read everything I write carefully enough to know it's good; even their lies are honest, and just when it all seems impossible, they convince me to try another day.

Perhaps the most decisive influence in recent years has been my parents' forgiveness and support; they may have never faced the basic issues of our tragedy, but they've surely suspected our shared responsibility sufficiently to forgive me, and this forgiveness has become both a control and a model for all my actions and insights ever since. Society and parents alike don't ordinarily acknowledge any responsibility for the misdeeds of misfits, but my parents did. . . . After all, with parents like this, how could I ever really lose?

His brother also was now having difficulties in his academic career and personal affairs. Ironically, when Greg committed the near suicide-homicide, his father and brother had both been at successful points in their careers. After his release, Greg discovered family therapy literature, especially Ackerman (1958), and proceeded to examine his family dynamics in a very valid and useful way. It was a thorough analysis which had not been possible in his earlier therapy. He concluded that he had been the "scapegoat" of the family neurosis. In sharing these writings with family members, it was like a literary family therapy, as well as helping him to work out some of his guilt. His writing also had a confessional quality. He became active in prison-reform activities and studies of violent behavior.

In 1979, after ten years of noncommunication, Greg contacted the author, noting from a professional journal a shared interest in the study of violence. He shared some of his recent writings which are quoted above. He was proud of being employed as an ombudsman in a mental hospital, and wrote in a letter:

I started my new ombudsman job last month, and already it's taking interesting directions. I've been initially assigned to the Forensic and Admissions units, though for obvious reasons have been concentrating on Forensic so far. It's an inherently stimulating and unusual position to find myself in—perhaps the first ex-forensic patient to ever be working on a forensic ward, with the full knowledge of the hospital administration to boot. Of course, us ex's tend to be rather idealistic, so it's also important to maintain an adequate balance of social reality while furthering my bias towards the patients.

There are many speculations one could raise about the period leading to Greg's violent action. One is that it was a period of therapeutic and life hiatus where his only recent attempt at activity—offering help at the scene of an accident—was rebuffed and punished. He felt useless and, after the fire in his room, displaced. The decision to suicide was a drastic decision to take control and resolve the impasse. When that failed he countered his father's appropriate anger with the surfacing of a latent anger never before expressed. This broke the impasse in a way that was ultimately constructive and changed his life.

The Case of Mike

At his parents' annual Christmas party, Mike, age twenty-two, had consumed a great deal of alcohol. Driving back to his residence he struck another car on the freeway. This car went off the road and the woman driver was killed. Mike had struck his head. The next day the awareness of his action broke through. He became depressed and suicidal. He was admitted to a private psychiatric hospital.

Approximately six weeks previous, Mike's best friend Gus had killed himself with a shotgun. Mike was not able to show feelings at the time of the death, but felt responsible, guilty, and burdened since he had been with Gus two hours previously. They had used drugs together in younger years and Mike had identified with Gus, seeing them both as equally desperate. A few days prior to the auto accident Mike learned that another friend had committed suicide. This rekindled grief about Gus. Mike had a long-standing history of drug abuse beginning at age fifteen, including virtually all drugs. He felt pride and identity as the "biggest drugger" on his street and used amphetamine, heroin, and barbiturates.

He had attempted suicide twice: once at age sixteen, when he slashed his wrists while his parents were in Europe; and at age eighteen he took an overdose of pills and required intensive care for several days to save his life. This latter attempt occurred the evening preceding a scheduled first entry into psychiatric hospitalization. Hospital had been recommended to reduce drug dependence, a persistent feeling of failure, and fear of close emotional relations. In this first hospitalization, the testing psychologist noted the following:

Mike discussed this suicide attempt and his chronic drug usage and reported almost proudly that some people thought him to be incurable. He is also filled with self-blame, describing himself as unable to cope with society, unable to achieve successfully—"everything I have touched has turned to shit." He described himself as apathetic and lethargic, a thinker but not a doer. He described his parents in glowing terms, as remarkable for their tolerance, but he reports repeated incidents of conflict with authorities at all levels outside the home. His disturbance surfaced early, beginning with agoraphobia or dyslexia in elementary school. His relationships with peers was not good, and he was teased by his classmates for being a "fatty" weighing more than 200 pounds in junior high school, although he is now a trim and sturdy young man. One of the problem areas for the patient, is that of finding a level of operation comparable to the achievement of his brilliantly successful father. The patient wants to be a winner or else withdraw from the race. Up to now he has withdrawn from competition but has fought his battles indirectly, scrapping with authorities and power figures outside the family setting.

After discharge he maintained his gains very briefly. Two other hospitalizations were necessary over the next year. He did make some changes, but further relapse led to his entering a drug rehabilitation therapeutic community out of the city, twenty-one months after his suicide attempt.

In the behaviorally oriented therapeutic community setting he ac-

cepted many new group and work responsibilities. The ability to express anger and affection in group confrontations seemed more effectively mobilized than in the previous psychiatric experiences. The
center's ethos rejected psychiatry, and he had no psychotherapy during this period. He was able to give up drug use. He became respected
and a helper to others. After twenty-one months in the therapeutic
community, he graduated, returned to the city, found a job, and shared
an apartment with a peer who had also been part of the center. The
auto fatality occurred five months later in December.

Many aspects of Mike's highway manslaughter action were random
misfortune. He could have crashed without injury or killed only himself. However, there were several dynamically relevant features. Mike
had not been doing well emotionally since his departure from the
structure of the therapeutic community. He missed the group support,
and the relationship with his roommate was deteriorating.

Mike had been close to Gus since return to the city, but he had also
become aware of Gus's homosexual trends. Gus's suicide left Mike
with guilt and loss of the relationship. Mike could not return to former
psychiatric assistance. Effective liaison with and support from the
therapeutic community staff was poor. Additionally Mike's dog died
shortly before the accident.

The consequences of the accident were far reaching. For one of the
first times in his life, Mike had to be fully accountable for a hurtful
action to another person. When hospitalized three years earlier, he had
seen the hospital staff as people to be manipulated. Now he saw them
as people whom he needed to keep him out of jail. He couldn't maintain
the self-contained omnipotent defenses he had previously in his life.
Fortunately the several supports in his life united. The therapeutic
community personnel accepted his return to psychiatric care and kept
contact during the hospitalization. The need to undergo legal de-
positions, stand trial, and receive sentence provided a repeated blunt
confrontation with a less yielding authority. Also his father and mother
became closer to him in helping him. This bridged some of the previous
gap, especially between Mike and his father. Father and mother had
changed over the years, with the aid of their therapy.

Mike had changed as well. The same psychologist who tested him
three years earlier now reported:

> The most striking feature about the present test results is the
> softer, more benign cast to the entire protocol, contrasted with

previous testing. Whereas before, his associative material dealt with hostile, regressive, primitive, and destructive feelings the content now centers about more controlled and adult concerns. His focus is contemplative regarding the future, uncertain about his own adequacy, and still tempted to engage in regressive play, but there are consistent themes of wanting to perform at a high level and to avoid further failure. He is still sensitive to early hurts when he was teased and felt isolated, but rather than wish retaliation, he now expresses fantasies of wanting to help others who have been troubled or hurt like himself.

His attitude toward his father is characterized by greater tolerance, respect, and recognition of the differences between them. He sees himself as more capable of emotionality and intimacy and his father as more experienced, more patient, and wise. He views his older brother as somewhat like his father in terms of drive and lack of warmth. Attitudes toward mother are not clearly defined. She may be a very indulgent person, and if so, at least one of his test themes suggests that he is closer to being able to give up the indulgence that she has provided. Overall, he gives a picture of much better personality integration, greater control, and better use of affect than when tested in 1971. He shows greater stability, maturity, and greater capacity for self-direction. His basic orientation remains dependent and nurturant-seeking and uncertain of his own capacities as a productive, effective male, but he is much better able to accept responsibility and has fantasies of responsible adult achievement and contributions to society. He does not currently appear seriously depressed, nor does he show evidence of organic brain syndrome. Signs of a serious underlying personality disorder which were noted on earlier testing are now less obvious.

While the driver's being a woman was completely coincidental, one could draw some dynamic relevance. In some ways, for Mike it represented a resolution of his anger toward women. Mike had felt at the mercy of women, and often those women he had been close with would leave him feeling impotent. He did feel sincerely sorry for the woman victim and her family and could identify with children being deprived of a mother. At times he feared retaliation from the victim's family.

Mike was found guilty and sentenced to thirty weeks of weekend jail time. This began after some months in the hospital. He learned much from the people he met in the jail. In the meantime he continued a closeness with Gus's girl friend, and they married after he left the hospital. Mike has held a semiskilled job for the five years since the accident, earning promotions and recognition. For four years he refused to buy a car and used public transportation. He has remained drug and alcohol free and has continued psychotherapy once per week. Rage at the early scapegoating by peers has emerged as a continuing strong affect.

The Case of Dave

By contrast, Dave did not have the same ability of expressing open anger at extra-familial authority figures. His anger was more passive. He too feared, hated, and loved his demanding, distant, successful father. Dave's situation included several differences from those of Greg and Mike. Dave's parents had divorced when he was seven. His mother was more punitive and demanding, arousing greater justified (though still guilty) hatred in Dave. Dave had a stronger identification as a student. He did well at school and college, motivated by family scholarly and religious values. These values had been passed on from a successful and demanding grandfather, as well as father and older brother. His older brother, while also successful, had been a polydrug user, unlike Mike's and Greg's older brothers, but had been helped in therapy to control the drug abuse. Dave was depressed and used marijuana. Also Dave was the youngest of the three subjects by about six years. Thus he came into adolescence when adolescent societal drug mores had changed to some extent.

Dave did not have a physical illness as did Greg. He did have poor peer relations, but had not developed a negative identity as scapegoat or "biggest drugger on the block." Depression, marijuana, and social withdrawal had helped to avoid open anger but did arouse concern in his family. His verbal skills did allow him to make greater use of psychotherapy, aided also by brother's example. Gradually he came closer to confronting his intense hostile feelings, first to mother and then to father. But he still feared direct confrontation. He finally did confront his mother, who was in a distant city, first by letter and then by phone, but with great fear of irreparable alienation. He was relieved at mother's ultimate acceptance. Open confrontation of father was still feared. Yet of the three men, this was the most appropriate and effective emancipatory anger any had expressed.

At this time his daily use of marijuana had been reduced after discussion in therapy. This probably brought closer awareness and less dampening of the anger. However, direct dialogue with his father was still difficult. It was in this context that the following action occurred. Dave was sitting at the window of his fourth-floor dormitory room studying for a final exam and feeling discouraged. The book he held fell from his hand to a ledge under the window. He stepped out on the ledge to retrieve it, slipped, and fell. Later he stated he could have knocked the book off the ledge to a roof three floors below. While falling, he took several lifesaving measures. He pushed himself away from the building, thus avoiding the metal awnings over the windows, which would have inflicted serious cuts. He recalled what he knew of how paratroopers land on their feet and managed in fact to land on his feet, incurring only a broken metatarsal. He was released from the hospital on crutches in three days, to the marvel of the medical staff.

Several factors seemed to have added unconscious self-destructive currents to this event. Over the previous six months he had come to the difficult point of realizing the need to verbalize old angers to his mother. His father was now threatening to reduce his funds for school, as well as to prevent him from spending the summer abroad with his mother, sister, and older brother. Dave had too much difficulty facing his father to disagree with this decision or to negotiate a compromise. One of his problems had been difficulty in speaking up in class or to instructors. This he related to the difficulty in talking to his father. His older brother was more aggressive to the father and often spoke for Dave, while dominating him as well. Dave was reducing the tranquilizing use of marijuana. His therapist was away for the weekend. An optional extra session might have been used otherwise, since he was depressed.

As a result of the fall, Dave was evicted from his dormitory room by the school authorities. While still hospitalized, Dave was called by the school representative and given this news. Dave was incensed at this announcement and found himself protesting the action with more assertion and confidence in his own behalf than ever before. In a similar, almost reflex manner, he found himself provoked into confronting his father on the phone when the latter incorrectly accused him of using marijuana which had contributed to the fall. While in the past Dave had used marijuana excessively, he had decreased this use the two weeks before the fall.

When interviewed ten days after the fall Dave recalled: "First of all I think the most important thing to me that happened was just the fact of having my life threatened. I was putting myself down, cutting myself down. To me the ultimate put down and ultimate cut down is death. And I realized right then that the unpleasant connotations and stuff that went along with it were so great and so horrifying to me that it almost made my whole attitude take a total turn around. All of a sudden I realized if you keep putting yourself down and keep doing this, this is your inevitable end, this is what you will come to."

When asked if stepping out on that ledge was like being willing to give up his life, he agreed. He talked of his father: "I felt like he once again had control of me and I felt helpless and like there was nothing I could do. And my life seemed at that time like a relatively cheap price for me to pay, because my life didn't seem to be worth that much at the time anyway."

It would seem that having faced death and having the power to survive, made it unnecessary to fear human authority—college or paternal. Dave did not return to therapy after the fall, other than for the session when he made the quoted comments. He felt no further need.

Discussion

These three men show gradations of powerlessness and reactions to it. Greg was the most powerless. He was weakened by dynamics in his family, as well as his unpredictable, unremitting, untreatable gastrointestinal illness. The arrest by the police, the fire in his room, and the failure of the suicide attempt all added to the frustration. Pulling the trigger, shooting his father and mother, was his first clearly assertive action to change his predicament and to pull himself out of the morass.[1] Possibly he startled himself with his power. Fortunately the family's anger against this action was expressed by the legal system. The family could thus resolve the ambivalence and group around Greg to support and succor. This family had shunned any previous open expression of anger. With his action Greg had deviated from a family taboo which exceeded society's taboo. Surfacing this anger allowed more realistic relating in the family.

By the time of his accident, Mike has recovered some from the feelings of powerlessness which had existed at the time of his suicide attempt. The therapy, the hospitalizations, and the therapeutic community experience had all contributed to some repair of feelings of power, fostering ability to help others and to control his use of drugs. However, he had not yet attained the power to resist alcohol, the family nemesis. He had overpowered his own generation's substance abuse, but the ability to confront and reject the family social lubricant had not been a prime goal in the drug-focused therapeutic community. Unfortunately this last residual of his chronic oral addictive need for relief of tension required a fatality and legal consequences before Mike could gain effective power. The differential gain in ego strength is reflected by Tabachnik, Gussen, Litman, Peck, Tiber, and Wold (1973, p.199). They relate that the suicidal person feels he has completely "lost his self-esteem" while auto accident subjects have not given up and "seem to be involved in life." They feel less like "losers."

It is probable that both Greg and Mike could be considered borderline personalities (Masterson 1972). According to Masterson, persons in this diagnostic category very likely had difficulty with separation-individuation in childhood, at ages eighteen to thirty-six months, but, unfortunately, knowledge of Greg's and Mike's early childhood is only fragmentary.

Dave on the other hand was the least powerless of the three. He had just confronted his mother with anger. He had survived and felt effective. He still feared the greater threat of facing the powerful father. However, contrasted to Greg and Mike, Dave had achieved his educational goals, and he had not been humiliated by scapegoating from peers. He did feel low power socially and in facing his teachers. His falling from the window was not a deliberate suicide attempt, though unconscious intentions could be inferred. The power to save his own life during the fall seemed to give him the momentum to defy the college administrator and then his father, thus freeing himself from the power of frightening male introjects.

Anthony (1975) has described several examples of "self therapy":

> With the development of crisis, the individual becomes conscious of the incompatibilities and disharmonies between inner and outer worlds. Finally, a synthesis takes place between the apparently disparate parts, and this may then be externalized in the form of some life occupation symbolizing reconstitution.
>
> In interpersonal terms, the self-psychotherapeutic process may include a better acceptance of others, better acceptance by others, and consequently greater acceptance of oneself. Roles are clarified, remodeled, and adapted to a new interpersonal situations.

It was fortunate that similar changes were able to occur for the three young men described here.

Conclusions

These three men had shown a power to survive and persevere in the face of difficult life situations. Their energies, however, up to the moment of the crucial turning point had been expressed in self-defeating directions. Therapy had brought to each a new awareness, but not the ability to translate this awareness into action changes. It would seem that these examples attest to the power of an accidental action and the sequellae in helping young people to reach deeply repressed murderous anger, in order to change previously harmful life patterns. In many therapies, interventions of various types often can reach this anger and repair the feelings of powerlessness, without the need for such catastrophic life events. Whether other types of therapeutic interventions could have been possible with these three men can only be speculated. In many therapies, intellectual awareness can occur without effective behavioral changes. In some cases, one may learn that events later in life did facilitate and integrate fuller action usage of the awareness.

The lives of the three men described represent examples of change effected by a combination of planned and unplanned events. They are similar in some ways to the examples of self therapy cited by Anthony (1975) but with the addition of psychotherapeutic self-awareness which facilitated beneficial characterologic reactions to the catastrophic events.

NOTE

1. Allan Rosenblatt, M.D. (San Diego), helped in the formulation of this dynamic.

REFERENCES

Ackerman, N.W. 1958. *The Psychodynamics of Family Life*. New York: Basic.

Anthony, J.B. 1975. Self-therapy in adolescence. *Adolescent Psychiatry* 3:6–24.

Masterson, J.F. 1972. *Treatment of the Borderline Adolescent*. New York: Wiley-Interscience.

Tabachnick, N.; Gussen, J.; Litman, R.E.; Peck, M.L.; Tiber, N.; and Wold, C.I. 1973. *Destruction by Automobile, Accident or Suicide*. Springfield, Ill.: Thomas.

THOMAS MINTZ

Nietzsche (1886) wrote, "Suicide has saved many lives." He meant by this that for certain people in distress the recognition that their pain and anguish was not interminable—that they could control their own destiny—allowed them to fight through or at least endure their pain, and to wait for a better day.

Thoughts about suicide are universal in childhood and adolescence. As with masturbation, an individual who cannot remember such adolescent thoughts has probably repressed them. In addition, we must recognize that the abuse of drugs, alcohol, and marijuana and the practice of reckless driving and habitual accidents are suicidal equivalents.

It is apparent that life, death, and time begin to come together during adolescence. Many suicidal problems evolve from the adolescent's realization that life is finite and one can kill. These concepts can be approached clinically from three points of view: frank suicidal cases, covert suicidal cases, and the therapist's countertransference reactions to suicidal issues.

Frank Suicidal Cases

If suicide is the main presenting problem, when there has been an attempt at or threat of suicide, the symptom becomes the predominant concern. Parents and caretakers become worried and call in a therapist. These frank cases, in some respects, are easier to deal with because the presenting problem is clear. The immediate task is to elicit enough history from the patient or parents to ascertain the cause of the present situation. A thorough history is necessary to discover what early developmental faults, failures, or disruptions may have predisposed the patient to illness during the stress of adolescence. There are several crucial areas to be explored: Does the history indicate a lack of good internal objects or introjects? Is the patient suffering from a deficiency disease or a toxic disease? Has the ego become depleted owing to a normal or an accelerated adolescent process of withdrawal of investment from internalized objects? Have certain external events depleted the sense of self? Has there been rejection by a friend or peer group or absence or illness of either or both parents? Has the particular age of the adolescent caused a reawakening of old, unresolved separation anxiety showing itself for short or extended periods prior to graduation? Has age forced on the adolescent a new life crisis such as that which accompanies menses or a sexual experience?

Once the therapist determines what has brought things to a head—this can usually be accomplished in one or two hours—he can proceed in the following crisis-treatment direction: Interpret the situation to the patient and/or the parents in an attempt to give them some intellectual awareness of the problem's origins and point the way for a new solution. Understanding or clarification inspires hope in both the patient and therapist. In the very common situation where there is a loss which has precipitated the crisis, the therapist can attempt to correct the loss by filling some need or place in the patient's psyche, or advising the parents to change their behavior in some fashion. The therapist may recommend hospitalization if the situation is too acute.

Covert Suicidal Cases

The issue of suicide may present itself in equivalent forms at first, becoming explicit only after certain defenses have been worked through. There is the danger in this covert suicidal situation that the seriousness of the problem may not be apparent until after the therapist is involved with the patient. In contrast to the frankly suicidal cases which we can take up with a full awareness of the immediate concern, these covert cases may reveal the suicidal problem only after a period of treatment. This breakthrough usually occurs because the patient now trusts us enough to tell us what was or is really bothering him; we have freed up certain blocks and the true feelings are now surfacing; we have removed, or the patient has been able to give up, certain behavior patterns (e.g., drug taking), which we can now recognize to be suicidal equivalents; and life events continue to intensify the patient's conflicts before the therapeutic relationship has taken hold.

Countertransference Issues

Countertransference issues are of paramount importance to the therapist treating a suicidal youngster. The therapist's well-being is crucial if he is to have the stamina to see the patient through the crisis. A therapist working at an in-depth psychological level with such adolescents must not take on more than one or two at a given time because of the enormous demands. The therapist must have worked through a number of personal issues around death and dying in order to be effective in dealing with suicidal patients. The following considerations should be weighed:

1. The fear that the patient might kill himself may inhibit a therapist from exploring the frank suicidal problem, thereby increasing the patient's feeling of isolation and explosiveness. Sometimes it can cause one to underestimate the danger of suicide because we are afraid of the conclusions. Fear can lead to denial of the real dangers involved. As an expression of that fear, we might become worried that the patient will die, that we will be blamed by parents, relatives, and colleagues as well as our own conscience.

2. We have tried to help the patient with our thoughts, our feelings, and our empathic suffering—why is he doing this to us? Why is he placing this burden on us? Why does he not get better? Such illness can mount an attack on our personal and professional pride. Sometimes, though not always, patients can sense (unconsciously or consciously) our state and can deliberately attack us with their suicidal thoughts. They need more, want more, and believe we are not doing enough. They attack us and our sense of well-being with all the fury they themselves experience from their hostile superegos. Searles (1965) wrote, "In general, if the patient's illness is causing more suffering to the therapist than to the patient, something is wrong." Sometimes, in the inexperienced therapist, anger shows itself in hostile comments or provocative actions: "Well, why don't you kill yourself?" These statements can add fuel to the patient's self-destructiveness. In fragile situations, such comments may be all that the patient needs to kill himself.

3. We may be blind to the inertia in the patient, to the fear of change he or she has, to the anguish that he or she is attempting to avoid through death, or to the patient's need through suicide to control his or her own life and destiny. One patient, early in treatment, was continually confronted by suicidal thoughts whenever she became afraid of dying. Death at her own hand was preferable to handing herself over to fate (which to her was represented by her malevolent parents). "Pas-

495

sive to active," at any price, is an old psychological truism and may be denied by the therapist as he struggles to establish a relationship.

4. Our feeling of the loss of control, of impotence, of loss of our own sense of omnipotence—this is the greatest single problem. Our own expectation to heal all wounds may create an impossible bind. If we can't be successful, we may feel helpless and the situation becomes hopeless.

Conclusions

In general, in uncovering the roots of the patient's problem, the hard work, effort, and purposefulness can inspire hopefulness, optimism, and control. Letting the parents know clearly and sensitively in the early consultations that there is a significant suicidal risk is of great importance in shifting the balance of forces. As to fear, Fenichel (1945) said, "He who cuts must not fear blood." We have to go ahead with therapeutic intervention despite the fears.

As to anger, our recognition that the patient's hostile superego is looking for an ally will help our restraint. We have to remember that the patient's anger is part of his illness, something over which he has little or no control. Examining our own internal attitudes will help clear up any countertransference induced blind spots. Consultation with a colleague or supervisor will at least share the burden even if no new solution is found.

The frequency of contact—by session or phone calls—with a suicidal patient is extremely critical. The more contact there is, the more time to work towards establishing a relationship, lending ego strength, and filling up the adolescent inner void. Thus, the therapist is able to provide another calming introject to mitigate against the pleading voices inside.

Each of us has to accept our limited power. We cannot control or fix everything, even though we might hope that we can.

REFERENCES

Fenichel, O. 1945. *The Psychoanalytic Theory of Neurosis*. New York: Norton.
Nietzsche, F. 1886. *Beyond Good and Evil*. New York: Boni & Liveright.
Searles, H. 1965. *Collected Papers on Schizophrenia and Related Subjects*. New York: International Universities Press.

PART V

PSYCHOTHERAPEUTIC ISSUES IN ADOLESCENT PSYCHIATRY

EDITORS' INTRODUCTION

A major task for the psychotherapist is to establish a working therapeutic alliance with difficult patients. The alliance may need to be reestablished many times due to repeated breakdowns before successful therapy can ensue. The successful therapist will be able to see the patient's primitive defenses, to have an awareness of his own countertransference reactions, and to conceptualize treatment process from an overall developmental perspective.

E. James Anthony describes difficulties in the treatment of the paranoid adolescent and the modifications necessary in psychoanalytic process owing to the necessity to deal with preverbal material. He reviews problems in the opening phases of treatment. The paranoid patient's more typical reactions include a predominant use of projection, narcissism, latent homosexuality, absence of guilt and remorse, a fear of being watched, and a disposition to magical thinking. A triad of character traits—ego-suspiciousness, sensitivity to contact, and defensive aggressiveness—present themselves almost immediately in treatment and need to be dealt with to avoid flight from therapy. Further techniques for treating a paranoid adolescent analytically are discussed and include resistance issues, difficulties with containment, sensitivity to pressure, the strategies of interpretation, and countertransference problems.

Susan Fisher discusses creativity as a proper experience of the developing human being at every level and a goal of all parents for their children and all therapists for their patients. She sees the sources of play and creativity as unconscious fantasy. Inner experiencing can substitute for relatedness to real objects in the world and be a means of avoidance; active fantasies can be adaptive and help ease a traumatic experience. She sees the therapist's function as engendering a sense of spontaneous, integrated wholeness. Early infantile creativity remains in the imaginative use of fantasy throughout development, and it is this usage that is once again revealed in successful psychotherapy. Fisher decries considering creativity only a talent to be exploited. She believes all people are potentially creative and that it is this creativity that should be unleashed.

Allen J. Cahill considers the expression and mastery of aggression as important in the treatment of children and adolescents. He differentiates between the aggressive sources of anger and destructive hostility and describes the aim of anger as mastery; the aim of hostility as destruction. Anger is used to overcome differences and deficits during the development of intimacy; uncontrolled hostility leads to the accumulation of hurts that eventually destroy an alliance. In treatment both the patient and the therapist have to deal actively with their aggression; anger is needed to deal with resistance while hostility must be recognized so that its destructive potential can be neutralized and positive ego defenses can further develop.

Theodore B. Cohen presents examples from the psychoanalyses of adolescents who manifested slow neurological and psychological maturation, mild ego distortions, and the self-pathology of developmental arrest. He interrelates self and drive theory and identifies low self-esteem, rage reactions, failure to develop self-object differentiation, bisexual conflicts, and omnipotent and grandiose defenses which interfere with both reality testing and good object relations.

David Halperin, Grace Lauro, Frank Miscione, James Rebhan, Jan Schnabolk, and Burt Shachter discuss countertransference issues in a long-term residential facility for severely damaged late adolescents. They found that the psychotherapeutic expectations of the program placed the therapist in a coercive role. The therapist in turn had to strike a balance between rigid expectations concerning the work ethic and the tolerance of a more flexible therapeutic model. Reconciling and integrating these attitudes was reflected in the work of the entire interdisciplinary staff, who must be aware of the potential for different role delineations that may foster countertransference splitting. Case illustrations of splitting, projective identification, and intense displacements on the part of staff are presented, and principles of the individual management of countertransference are discussed.

32 TREATMENT OF
THE PARANOID ADOLESCENT

E. JAMES ANTHONY

Whenever I am confronted with a paranoid adolescent in the analytic situation—a relatively infrequent circumstance presumably because of mutual avoidance mechanisms at work—I become uncomfortably aware of the deficiencies in my theoretical and technical resources. The experiential aspects of treatment predominate over work-engendering insight and frustrate any efforts to deal with these patients on the basis of a classical approach. On the conscious level, there is a deliberate and persistent effort on their part, or so it seems, to thwart the setting up of an analytic situation, and I sometimes find myself reacting non-therapeutically to the apparently willful sabotage that goes beyond neurotic resistances, although I am not unprepared to encounter predictable irregularities in response to the usual treatment procedures and processes.

Like adult analysts, child and adolescent analysts have generally been brought up on a fairly strict training schedule and tend to adhere to this model in their work with adult patients. Subsequently, in learning to treat the immature psyche they find that certain modifications become a legitimate necessity and are accepted as such by institutional authorities. This, however, means that the primary treatment model is often at variance with the secondary ones that evolve later and may generate philosophical conflicts within the analysts in relation to their cherished analytic ideals; at the same time, the experience with additional parameters furnishes them with a capacity to adjust themselves to unusual requirements in therapy.

In the special instance of the paranoid adolescent, my primary training urges me to trace the disturbance back along its line of devel-

© 1981 by The University of Chicago. 0-226-24054-1/81/0009-0005$01.00

opment as far as theory and technique will allow. I find myself curious to find out how the paranoid propensity will manifest itself in the process of treatment and in the transmutations of the transference, and whether it is susceptible to dissolution by the analytic method. Would the aim of analysis need to be modified in any way? Would the pursuit of insight and a widening consciousness demand curtailing? Would the major work of interpretation concern itself more extensively with primarily rather than secondarily repressed material that can only be relived and not remembered within the transference? And, finally, to what extent would the exigencies of the external world be brought into meaningful juxtaposition with the chaotic and confused emotional states that exist within these patients?

Thus, when I am brought face to face with the paranoid adolescent, I am motivated by a degree of curiosity stemming from many sources, and my first lesson in practice was to learn that this in and by itself constitutes a profound threat to the patient, particularly during the opening phases of treatment. An obtrusive inquisitiveness can rapidly disrupt and destroy the analysis of the basically mistrustful and suspicious patient, especially if one also bears in mind that adolescence is itself a time when the adult is no longer a persona grata with ready access to the secret life of the child. As with parent figures, the analyst can expect to be ruthlessly investigated and scrutinized through the same distorting lenses of disillusionment and deidealization. Furthermore, adolescents, aware of their own inner turmoil, are fearful that the clinician will confirm their own worst fears and deem them "crazy."

Nonetheless, there are also plusses. Although with these patients we may often have cause to regret their defective sense of reality when they set out deliberately to hurt us, as the analysis becomes an inquisition and the analyst a hated persecutor, there are times when we are startled by the profound insights directed inwardly into the psyche or outwardly (as an outsight) into the difficulties experienced by the analyst and into his countertransference. We may even sometimes wish that our neurotic patients had some of the same insights into the equation of treatment with attack and mutilations (Glover 1955).

Psychoanalytic Research into the Psychopathology of Paranoia

Freud (1893–1899; 1911; 1917; 1933) maintained a lifelong interest in the psychopathology of paranoia, constantly discovering new facets to it. Initially (1895), he referred to it as a neurosis of defense, with projection as its main mechanism. A year later (1896) he made the daring suggestion, based on careful and detailed family studies, that sexual abuse before the age of fifteen to eighteen months (that is, while the psychic apparatus was still largely unformed) led to psychosis. Exposure to "scenes" of seduction later on were more likely to result in neurosis. Four years onward (1899), brought a cryptic comment that paranoia involved a return to an early autoerotic stage. In 1906, he presented a case of female paranoia before the Vienna Psychoanalytical Society, and in 1908 and 1909, in letters to Jung and Ferenczi, he began to formulate his main generalization, linking paranoia with repressed passive homosexuality, which was confirmed by the publication of the Schreber memoirs and his analysis of the unconscious processes at work in the illness (1911). In 1931 he went a step further in his examination of paranoia in females and reported some important theoretical additions to the genesis of paranoid disorders, including new preoedipal data, that proved a stimulus to later workers in the field and that can be summarized as follows:

1. The preoedipal attachment and dependence on the mother was the "germ" that led to later paranoia.

2. This "germ" stemmed from the regular dread of being killed and eaten by the mother.

3. This dread of being devoured was itself derived from hostility toward the mother caused by her restrictiveness (which was more rigorous toward the daughter than toward the son).

4. The psychic immaturity at this early age favored the mechanisms underlying paranoia, such as projection.

5. The paranoid fear of being poisoned was connected with the trauma of weaning following the birth of the new baby and a rage of accusations against the mother in consequence. These controlling, condemning, and criticizing elements then became permanently incorporated into the psychic life of the child, dominating his characterological responses.

The preoedipal interplay of hostility between mother and daughter was further complicated by the sexual activity of the little girl toward the mother in the oral, sadistic, and phallic sequence; and, sometimes, these were transferred to the later father object "where they [did] not belong" (1933) and where they seriously interfered with the understanding of the Oedipus complex. The oral-aggressive and sadistic wishes, appearing as a fear of being killed by the mother, justified the death wishes toward her, if these became conscious. In return, the

503

mother had ample conscious and unconscious reasons for feeling and acting in a hostile way toward her little daughter, and not infrequently acted these out. In a more actual and traumatic sense, the intense fear engendered by her could also have to do with the enemas in great vogue at the time that were often resisted and reacted to with fear, anxiety, and rage. The intense passive stimulation of the anal zone inevitably came to serve as a developmental fixation point to which regressions later returned.

I found Freud's reconstruction of the preoedipal phase of the future paranoid individual very helpful. This is not to deny the importance of oedipal fantasies in the illumination of the total picture. "Those who have any doubts about the central significance of the Oedipus complex in the psychoses and particularly in the paranoias should observe (for they will have difficulty in analyzing) the reactions of erotomanic paranoias . . . in which the homosexual core . . . is covered by a layer of positive Oedipus phantasy thinly disguised" (Glover 1955).

The Primal Scene and the Formation of the Paranoid Superego

Kanzer (1952) also concurred with this view that the phallic stage of the Oedipus complex constituted the nucleus of the psychoses, but added the further component of the "primal scene" to the clinical picture of paranoia. According to him, it is this experience that embodies all the perplexities troubling the developing mind of the child, namely, sex differences, pregnancy, hitherto vague incestuous wishes and urges, and uneasily sensed distrust and hatred of the parents. The experience not only clarifies but traumatizes. It brings into nearer awareness the powerful and exclusive collusion, but at the same time it generates a sense of irreparable alienation, fears of retaliation for desiring to intrude erotically and aggressively, castration anxieties from the observation of genital differences in operation, and a disruption of infantile ties. A flight into regression ensues in an attempt to deny the reality of the "scene." (As often reiterated, the experience may not be an actual but an unconsciously constructed one with possible constitutional roots.)

However, the sadistic and aggressive fantasies associated with paranoid developments tend to prevent the formation of a normal, well-internalized superego. The voyeuristic impulse connected with the "discovery" and representing the ego witness to the act, together with the memory of the bad sexual parents are projected outward to embody the "persecutors" and thus complete the make-up of the paranoid superego. The "persecutor," who is the incarnation of the warded-off drives, constantly tries to reenter and fragment the improvised system. The ensuing conflict is reflected in the profusion of anal fantasies.

The clinically recognized failure of the paranoid patient to experience guilt stems from a combination of different defense mechanisms that include the *projection* of forbidden impulses, the *identification* with the desexualized parental images, the *regression* to infantile omnipotence, and the *masochistic submission* to the "persecutor," all of which has an unconscious punishing and atoning effect, but at the expense of reality testing. It is "out there." Inevitably, the analyst in the analytic "trial" for the unknown crime becomes the "persecutor," threatening both the paranoid system, so carefully but unconsciously constructed and defended, and also, at the same time, bent on punishing the patient. From the beginning he is feared and hated and has strong allies within the patient in the form of the observing and criticizing ego. The patient becomes fearful of being watched, of being found out, and may exhibit agonized compulsions to confess.

We have now accumulated a composite picture of the paranoid patient's more typical reactions: the predominant use of projection, the narcissism, latent homosexuality, the absence of guilt and remorse, fear of being watched, and a disposition to magical thinking. The triad of character traits, manifested by his ego-suspiciousness, sensitivity to contact, and defensive aggressiveness (Glover 1955) present themselves almost immediately in treatment and need to be dealt with quickly before the patient takes flight. The dream material provides a good but paradoxical monitor to the intrapsychic status (Freud 1900) and frequently shows a curious intermittency: when the patient is in a stage of remission, his dreams are flagrantly violent and sadistic; when frank paranoia intervenes the dream material becomes altogether more subtle and symbolized.

Infantile Paranoia

We have now to deal with where and when the paranoid propensity begins, which is also the point where controversy starts. Abraham, in his papers on the anal character (1921) and the development of the libido (1924), emphasized a sequence of starting points for the mental disorders. Paranoia had its origin at the anal level and consequently anal erotism was prominent in the psychogenesis of paranoia, with feces being unconsciously identified with the penis of the "persecutor," who is therefore not a part of the patient's body that he carries within himself but also "someone" he cannot get rid of. Later theorists, like Glover (1955), have also subscribed to the theory of psychotic fixation points at different developmental levels and with different defensive operations.

Such a theory might explain, through the mediation of a deep regression, the reappearance of subsequent psychopathology in the child, adolescent, or adult; but it would also imply the existence of a cluster of paranoid elements in the infant that could only be regarded as something more than a paranoid "point." The preoedipal infant would need to be in some form of quasi-paranoid status at the time. An alternative view might be that a gross oral/anal psychopathology was actually present in a particular infant during this period and that the reactivation of this gross material in later life underwent adultamorphic transmogrification, that is, psychosis.

As previously mentioned, Freud (1931) took the view that regressions to preoedipal fixation points were more frequent in females and associated with fears of being poisoned and eaten; he quoted a case of Brunswick's who never developed beyond the preoedipal stage. The clinical picture in the adult was one of paranoia (1933).

Let us now examine some recent paradigms of infantile paranoia that might help us understand the nature of subsequent paranoid developments.

KLEIN

Picking up from Abraham and Freud, Klein (1948) described a sequence of psychotic developmental "positions" that she had uncovered by child analysis and that not only amplified and added to the earlier work but gave a much more complete, internally consistent, comprehensive, and metapsychologically sound progression of normal preoedipal development with its inclusion of a "normative" infantile psychosis that antidated Freud's nuclear infantile neurosis and was based on his concept of a "death instinct." A picture was offered of the baby in the paranoid-schizoid position in whom the central anxiety was concerned with the destruction of the self- and ideal-object by "persecution" (fragments of bad objects and ego disintegrated by the "death instinct'' and then projected). Against this, schizoid mechanisms were brought into play, leading to an increasing split between good and bad objects, to excessive idealization, and to omnipotent denial. Infantile experiences of hunger, pain, and frustration were all felt as persecutions. A nonresolution of Klein's psychotic positions, it is claimed, may lead to excessive anxiety and excessive use of defenses (although it is not clear why this should be the case), and an interplay between the paranoid-schizoid and the depressive positions may in turn interfere with this essential resolution. When the phase of persecution anxiety is inordinately long, fantasied suspicions become fixated and manifest themselves later in paranoid states, phobic anxieties, and hypochondriacal fears. Furthermore, the persecution anxiety restricts the development of a whole-object relationship in order to avoid the additional burden of depressive anxiety and the associated guilt and remorse.

WINNICOTT

Accepting some of the basic tenets put forward by Klein, Winnicott (1952) has added elaborations of his own. Characteristically, he has likened the infant in his infantile predicament to the uncertainties of the nursery figure, Humpty-Dumpty, who has just achieved integration into wholeness, having emerged from the "environment-individual set-up." He is no longer devotedly held and is therefore "in a precarious position," and "liable to irreversible disintegration." At this point in developmental time, he is "a potential paranoiac." What normally saves him from the "persecutors" (and every infant is in essence a "survivor" if he negotiates this hazard) is his mother's compendium of loving care (holding, understanding, empathizing, and sensitively adapting). Should the environment fail him at this juncture, he starts his life with a paranoid potential. Winnicott emphasizes that this is a matter of infantile experience, not genetics.

He does, however, add a paranatal factor to this development. The birth experience itself places the baby in a helpless situation, at the mercy of external forces, and so provides a "model of persecution" that further determines the pattern of future persecutions and future interferences with "basic being." He terms this "congenital paranoia." All this constitutes the "natural history" of infantile development and we, as parents, need to accept it and "allow the infant this madness" before reality takes over. What we can do is to support him in this initial developmental struggle and guard against environmental failure. Psychosis arises out of "delays and distortions, regressions and muddles" at the early stages of the "set-up."

During later childhood, "latent paranoia" can be discerned in a type of play characterized by intense preoccupation, lack of beginning and end, lack of any patterning, a high degree of magical control, and apparent inexhaustibility.

Winnicott thus gives us here a series of steps along the developmental line of paranoia: "congenital paranoia" set into motion by birth, followed by the part-whole dangerous period of "potential paranoia," succeeded by indications of "latent paranoia" in "paranoid play," and giving place, in adolescence, to paranoid ideation, paranoid attitudes, paranoid acting out ("senseless destructiveness"), and systematic delusional thinking.

ERIKSON

Erikson's (1950) description of infancy has highlighted issues of basic trust and autonomy in the absence of which mistrustfulness, shame, and doubt develop. His portrayal of paranoid development, however, is somewhat skimpy and certainly less dramatic when compared with the descriptions furnished by Freud, Abraham, Klein, and Winnicott. The psychosocial crises cast a pale shadow in comparison with the terrifying persecutions postulated by the others and are less clinically significant. Furthermore, there is no account of the "persecutor." The epigenetic snowball, rolling down the developmental hill toward adolescence, and accumulating only negative outcomes, would gather up a nucleus of mistrust, lack of confidence, helplessness, pessimism, shame and doubt, low self-esteem, inhibition of initiative, poor peer relations, feelings of inferiority, and finally, confusions of identity, a sense of isolation, and an inability to withstand closeness. This "negative identity" is the outcome of rearing procedures with an overuse of shame as a controlling device and may aggravate the "life-long paranoid trends such as are present in everybody." Clinical paranoia is regarded as an extreme accentuation of the obsessive and suspicious doubt about what is done behind one's back, or by the shattering sense of shame engendered by the loss of self or body control under everyone's eyes. Erikson would therefore agree with Winnicott that there is a paranoid potential "present in everybody," and this fits with everyday experience.

JACOBSON

But does one need to postulate the existence of infantile paranoia? Jacobson (1971) has attempted to forge clinical links between shame, guilt, depression, paranoia, inferiority, and problems of identity. These form a syndrome in which "guilt conflicts may be absent or recede in favor of paranoid fears of exposure while feelings of shame and inferiority, self-consciousness and fears of feeling a loss of identity frequently appear as a characteristic triad of symptoms" in the adolescent. In no way, however, does she subscribe to the Kleinian formula connecting paranoid-depressive outcomes to paranoid and depressive "positions" in the infant. It is difficult to understand how she manages to bypass the commonly accepted proposition by Jones (1922) of recapitulation in adolescence of the infantile stages of development in the individual. "The precise way in which he will pass through the necessary stages of development in adolescence is to a very great extent determined by the form of his infantile development—the autoerotic, the anal-sadistic, the narcissism, the homosexual and the heterosexual." Why then have Jacobson and other classical analysts of this period not seen the necessity for postulating an infantile precursor of paranoia? Benedek (1956) and Mahler (1966) have injected depression into the preoedipal phase, but not paranoia, and for them depression is not an integral part of normal ontogeny but an expression of environmental failure.

SCHATZMAN AND SULLIVAN

And what of environmental failure during the infantile stage? Following on the discovery of the details of Schreber's infancy and childhood, the importance of a persecutory child-rearing practice in the genesis of paranoia has been raised (Schatzman 1973). Was Schreber "born into a conspiracy against him . . . into a microsocial despotism?" Did he feel persecuted because he *was* persecuted, and were his realistic feelings of persecution later denied and transformed into paranoid delusions? Was his father not actually an archpersecutor responsible for a "household totalitarianism" who used his infernal machines on his own children, driving one of them into paranoid schizophrenia and the other into suicide? If Freud had been aware of this would he have incorporated it into a theory of paranoia based on the notion of the "complementary series?" Sullivan (1953) was also of the opinion that in any form of child rearing in which there was a systematic rejection of the child, the sense of safety and security was inadequate and required bolstering by paranoid projections. Thus the individual developed a need to blame others, to feel himself persecuted, and to draw into his "self-system" anyone or anything that appeared to threaten his psychological survival. When shame was linked to this paranoid circuit, the patient became hyperalerted to minimal slights and reproaches. At some point in this type of life history, a "malevolent transformation" took place and paranoia ensured.

Techniques for Approaching a Paranoid Adolescent Analytically

In general, adolescents are resistant to the analytic process, and those adolescents, suffering from a shame-paranoid syndrome, become extremely difficult to contain within the analytic situation. At the onset, their sense of persecution and their sense of shame are so intense that the situation of exposure becomes far too threatening for them to tolerate before the therapeutic alliance can help to withstand them.

What can be done about this therapeutically? According to Freud (1917) the most that one can do is "to cast an inquisitive glance over the top of the wall and spy out what is going on on the other side of it. Our technical methods must accordingly be replaced by others; and we do not know yet whether we shall succeed in finding a substitute." Here Freud was clearly speaking of what is now referred to as a "parameter"—an adaptation of classical procedures to nonclassical patients.

His suggestions may not be good advice for the paranoid adolescent; the "inquisitive glance" and the "spying out" would reflect a state of mind in the therapist that the hypersensitive patient would pick up only too quickly and take to his heels—"treatment interrupted by the patient's flight," as Freud (1893–1899) once put it.

The amount of pressure that a paranoid patient will tolerate is surprisingly little, and when he seems to be most accepting of what the analyst is giving out is a time to be especially wary. The "malevolent transformation" can take place within seconds. I am reminded here of Winnicott's (1971) work with Sarah, a sixteen-year-old who had intelligence and a sense of humor but was basically "very serious."

He started her on the squiggle game and during it she began to make comments. "I believe I came to see you when I was two, because I didn't like my brother being born; but I can't remember." He asked her, "do you mind playing this game?" and she said: "No, of course not." But she had difficulty with it and eventually said, "It's all cramped up, it's not free and spreading." He saw this as the main communication and said: "It's you, isn't it?" To which she replied "Yes. You see I am a bit shy." To which he said: "Naturally, you don't know me and you don't know why you've come or what we are going to do." She answered: "I am all the time trying to make an impression because I am not sure enough of myself. I have been like it for ages. I can't remember being anything else." To this he said: "It's sad, isn't it?" as a way of showing that he had heard what she had said and that he had feelings about what she was telling him.

She became eager to reveal herself further to him. "It's stupid, pig-headed. I am all the time trying to make people like me, respect me, not make a fool of me. It's selfish. . . . I sit around all the time wondering what impression I am making." He said to her: "But you are not like that here, now." And she said: "No, because it doesn't matter. Presumably you are here to find out what's the matter, so you make it possible for me not to have to do all this."

He then began to press her about her dreams, about her sexual identity, about her father, and about her mother. She told him a re-current dream in which she is being chased by a man and is running—running through mud, through treacle; then another dream about a witch in the cupboard. This was followed by silence.

When she began again, she talked about lying to her mother, about being unhappy, and about growing up too quickly. And she told him about a peculiar sensation: "I feel as if I am sitting or standing on top of the spire of a church. There is nothing anywhere around to keep me from falling and I am helpless." Winnicott reminded her that her mother had held her until she became pregnant and had then ceased to hold her. She listened, but her thoughts appeared elsewhere. Then, quite suddenly, she said "it's bigger than that. That whatever is chasing me, it's not a man chasing a girl, it's *something* chasing *me*. It's a matter of people *behind* me."

At this point Sarah became manifestly ill in a paranoid way. She began to talk about being laughed at from behind, about feeling worthless, scared physically, and expecting to be stabbed, shot, or strangled; especially stabbed. "Like having something pinned on your back and you didn't know about it." And then she asked: "Are we getting anywhere?'' When she spoke of the fact that she was sometimes very depressed, Winnicott said to her: ''The depression means something, something unconscious'' (he could use this word with this girl). He told her that it took the place of feeling hate for someone who had been reliable but who had changed. And this seemed to help.

She began to talk about disliking people who hurt her and went into a vituperation against a woman at school. For the first time he learned why she had been referred to him. She had thrown a knife when the woman, a teacher, told her that she must be out of her mind. The girl became very excited as she described how she was ordered to take off her ''ridiculous hat,'' and had screamed and screamed and screamed! (Winnicott then remembered that he had first seen her as a little girl, hardly two years old. Her mother was pregnant, and Sarah had changed from a normal child to an ill one.) Sarah said that the woman teacher was as insecure as everyone else and gradually began to reveal her ambivalence to this person. (At this point, he felt it advisable to stop making notes.) He then pointed out that she was always repeating something that had happened in the past. Her mother and father had loved each other, but her mother had then become pregnant and changed. Being so young she could not deal with this except by developing the conviction that whatever was good would inevitably change and would cause her to hate it and to want to destroy it. A good person changed into a bad person; a reliable one into an unreliable one. He then told her that her job would be to live through relationships that did go bad, that did make her angry and disillusioned, and to realize that somehow everyone survived. When she asked how she could stop bursting into tears, Winnicott became aware that she had come through an experience that he had shared with her. Her final remark to him was, ''I think I must have exhausted you.''

In thinking about the case, he thought that if he had known that she was going into psychoanalytic treatment, he would have said much less and behaved more like a human mirror. One would not question this afterthought had Sarah been in a state of neurotic conflict, but as the case (to be described later) will demonstrate, one needs more than mirroring to tide someone through a paranoid crisis. One has to reciprocate, however exhausting it is for therapist and patient.

With paranoid cases, Glover (1955) recommends that at the beginning the therapist should deal with a reduction of initiation stresses before going into the analysis of the defenses interfering with the transference contact. Only then can one begin to deal with the sadomasochistic elements distorting the oedipal pattern. Suspiciousness has to be ventilated from the first session, although transference aspects can be introduced indirectly by allowing the patient to bring out reactions to treatment. The therapist can start to explore with caution and care the paranoid predisposition, working mainly on the level of anal sadism. In this manner, the patient gets the feeling that the analyst is talking his, the patient's, language. It is a procedure that helps to reduce resistances before they harden "to an impenetrable negative reaction." Glover also mentions that the unconscious frustration of the paranoid individual is on a homosexual level, hemmed in by pregenital defenses. He cautions strongly against the interpretation of near-delusional material during the early phases, treating it instead with "non-committal receptivity."

The place of guilt in the analysis of the paranoias can be measured by the tense traumatic anxieties of a persecutory nature that is often masked by equally intense hostility in response to any form of contact. The error lay in regarding this aggression as primarily sadistic and not as a defense against the anxiety.

When one comes to the "third phase," one can begin, belatedly, to retrace the course of the Oedipus situation and deal with the sadistic type of superego that has been introjected. The relationship to the mother will then be found to be heavily charged with ambivalence and only by attempting to reduce the projections associated with this can a more positive reaction toward objects be established. Work here, however, is frequently interrupted by periodic regressions during which the defense of suspiciousness returns with apparently full force, and during any one of these regressive episodes the patient can abandon treatment. Analysis of such cases is always "touch and go."

The countertransferences that are roused can be at times almost intolerable for the analyst to bear and he needs to pay constant attention to his own reactions when confronted by the malignant negative transference. As Glover put it: "The analysis of a paranoiac is undoubtedly the most severe test of the analyst's capacity to sustain the impact of a steady current of hostility. Only those who can withstand such hostility should undertake the analysis of a persecutory anxiety" (1955).

The Case of Helen

Helen was fifteen when she was presented to me as a candidate for analysis. She was described as being extremely nervous and self-conscious; had the constant fear that everyone was looking at her; was unable to eat in front of other people; feared getting into a crowd and imagined that everyone was out to harm her. She also had a number of nervous tic-like mannerisms and at times felt that her legs were too weak to support her. Her peer relations were uniformly bad; she not only mixed poorly, but appeared actively to dislike young people of her own age and experienced great difficulty in talking with them. Her mistrustfulness was persistent and pervasive; she suspected everyone, especially those who tried to be nice to her, since she regarded this as a sinister manipulation. She saw her father as weak and inconsequential and her mother as a self-absorbed woman who had little time for her children and occupied herself writing novels. The family had been afflicted with mental disorder through several generations, and Helen's maternal aunt had gone through a similar "catatonic" phase when she was an adolescent. Her parents had separated when she was age seven.

THE INITIAL INTERVIEW

What was striking about Helen was not so much her suspiciousness, which was manifest, but her excruciating sense of shame. She said to me: "I've been ashamed since I was born. Everything was wrong with me from the beginning, and my appearance did not make things any better." She sat in a stiff, uncooperative posture and warned me not to stare at her or else she would leave immediately. She said that she was afraid of losing control because she might kill someone. She did not think that she would get along with me. "I don't like you; I don't like doctors and, in fact, I don't like men. They make me feel stupid, as if I was a nothing." Her earliest memory was running into a spider's web, at the center of which was an enormous spider. She associated the memory with her mother, but could not tell why. Ever since, she had had a great fear of spiders. She said that she found the treatment situation very unpleasant. She had a strong fear of being looked at and being "found out." She had an equally strong desire to look at me and make me cringe. She insisted on staying at a safe distance from me. Since childhood she had never allowed anyone to touch her. She could not bear the thought of anyone "slobbering" over her. She also talked of her fear of committing suicide, of going crazy, and of getting caught in a crowd.

THE FIRST PHASE

During the early sessions, she was tense and apprehensive. She felt

514

sure that I was trying to get at her brains, and she hated my smugness and air of superiority. She said that I made her feel more inferior than she felt outside, even more inferior than she felt with her mother. She could hardly bring herself to speak because of what might come out. There were prolonged silences during the sessions, sometimes brought to an end with the remark, "I hate coming to see you." Yet she continued to bring her dreams, which were generally horrifying, mostly of people being drowned. There were no associations except to drowning: "You kept swallowing water until you could swallow no more and then you swelled up and died." I did nothing at all with the dreams, maintaining a "noncommittal receptivity." She appeared to wallow in the topic of death, dying, drowning, being buried alive, and of killing someone. She thought that they would not hang her because she was a juvenile but only put her in prison for about fifteen years. She began to talk about her blushing and about how badly she felt about it. She said that she was hot all the time that she was in the office with me and that this was because I made her feel ashamed. "You think yourself wonderful just because you are a doctor. I think you are very conceited: just about as conceited as my father."

She brought two more frightening dreams with identifiable people: one involved the image of her mother's drowned body floating in the water; the other of a dog biting her and of a man coming up and starting to stick pins into her. I said that she was still experiencing me as a hurtful figure, taking over, as it were, from her father. Generally she would make no response to such transference clarifications but would continue to stare fixedly at me.

I wondered about the adolescent girl described by Abraham (1913a, 1913b) who likened her glance to the Gorgon's head: people exposed to it could die on the spot. It made people afraid of her and necessitated her withdrawal from society. Helen was also completely isolated. She had no contact with the outside world apart from the journey that she made from home to my office and back—a journey that terrified her, yet she too felt that everyone feared her because of the destructive ideas that occupied her mind. This was a variant of the "omnipotence of thoughts" that she had in abundance, and that included the omnipotence of dreams. According to Abraham, the extravagant sadistic fantasies involved in the Medusa theme appeared to occur only in women with whom the eye was identified with the destructive penis. It later became clear that Helen's delusional penis was her "secret weapon." The matricide that appeared manifestly in her dreams was denied in consciousness but undoubtedly added to her tormenting anxiety. My own association to the dream image of the mother's body floating in the water was to possible "primal scene" experiences. Needless to say, I kept this to myself at this stage.

Her moods alternated suddenly without warning: she either flopped forward, blushing, in a posture of shame, or sat stiffly, looking extremely suspicious. Her openly expressed hate for me began to grow rapidly. She accused me of keeping notes about her and demanded to see them. She threw a book at me and laughed in grimacing fashion (she seemed incapable of normal laughter) when I stopped to pick it up and replace it. She said she wanted me on my knees, scared and ashamed. She would like to get rid of me, just as she would her mother and father.

At this point, she asked me to get out of the room because my very presence offended her. I spoke to her quietly and encouragingly *and then did as she requested,* telling her that I would come back in a few minutes to see whether she felt a little better. She seemed astonished at my compliance and, on looking back, I would regard this as the first mutative point in the treatment.

THE SECOND PHASE

She had always come every day on time, but now she took to coming earlier and waiting for her appointment. She also began to talk more freely. When I had to leave for a week, she asked whether she might write to me, but then added, mistrustfully, that "they" would probably open her letters and read what she said and would then put her away in a mental hospital. The drowning and murder themes and the dreams of being tortured became less frequent, and her almost built-in suspiciousness and hostility were gradually replaced by periods of sadness and the beginnings of self-reproachfulness. I was no longer faced daily with impenetrable negative reactions and bristling defensiveness. She said she wished that she had never been born because life had been such an unhappy time for her. I suggested to her that she probably had many painful feelings buried deep inside her, as indicated by her dreams, and that these came to the surface whenever she got upset with me. She should know, however, that I would be there when she needed me.

Her reaction to this overture was almost predictable. The next session was full of silent hate. After a while, she was able to reveal another dream in which she was drowning in a large bath and no one seemed to be around. I suggested that the dream might be a response to what had happened the summer before, during which I had left her at a critical time, and that she was probably expressing doubts about my trust-worthiness. Once again I repeated that it was my aim to make her feel safer both with me and outside the treatment situation. Considering the extent of her shame and insecurity, I said that I appreciated just how much personal courage it took for her to be able to leave her home and come by herself to her session. Under the pressure of her traumatic anxieties, I clearly overdid my comforting move toward her. Rather than being reassured, she flared up and said that she could in no way believe what I was saying to her and that I was just playing at being a doctor. I could afford to gloat since I was not the one who was suffer-ing. I admitted that I was certainly not suffering like her but that, like everyone else in the world, I too had experienced moments of shame, humiliation, and embarrassment and knew how painful it could be. It was because of this that I could share her feelings and perhaps help her to understand why they happened. She said grudgingly, "I suppose so." Again, retrospectively, I came to see this as the second mutative point.

For the next two sessions, she sat silently, but without shame and without suspicion. She appeared to be working something out within herself. When I asked her how she felt about coming in the face of so much shame, she burst out angrily that she had always come for her sessions and that it was I who kept questioning her wish to come. Perhaps I did not want her to come. Perhaps I could not take her. I remarked sympathetically that she must have experienced the same sense of rejection at home when she was little and expected to be rejected once again. (As always, I was struck by her sensitive "out-sight" and alertness to every move and feeling.)

THE PHASE OF DISCLOSURE

She now seemed to be feeling very much "at home" in the session. She sat more comfortably in her chair and was able to talk without "affective storms" disrupting her communications. She said that she wanted to tell me about "deeper" things that she had never told to anybody else. She was aware that she caused a great deal of her own suffering in her everyday life by the provocative and crazy way in which she behaved. My ears pricked up at this, thinking or hoping that some degree of internalization was beginning to replace the inexorable stream of projections. She then compared her visits to me with a period of tutoring that she had received from her father, who was a teacher who did only tutorial teaching because he had an aversion to groups. She had also gone to see him every day at the home to which he had retreated after he had separated from his wife and family during her latency years, and every day, she said, had been a torture of shame, ignominy, and humiliation. The sessions had always ended in a big upheaval because neither of them could stand the tension. He would refer to her as mentally defective. "And you," she said to me, "think that I am mentally insane."

Her resistance to treatment reached a new level. She said that there were things about herself that she could never reveal to anybody. She would sooner die. There was no one in the world that she could trust sufficiently to tell. I interposed as gently as I could: "Even someone who might want to help you with them?" She bristled with rage. "I am fed up with people trying to help me. The more they try the more I hate them. The more you want to help me, the more dumb and crazy and useless you make me feel." She said that if she told me her secrets, she was afraid that she might have to kill me since there would be someone walking about in the world who knew all about her shameful life. I remarked that when one was fifteen, many things about one's body seemed to be shameful. For example, things to do with sex often made one feel embarrassed. She said quickly, and in some confusion: "No, not that!" and was then silent. After a while, she said: "I am not afraid of crowds anymore. I go to work and I feel all right. Yet you keep nagging me and digging into me when I come here. Even if you do cure me, how do I know that I shall like what I become?" I asked her what kept her coming now that she felt so much better. She admitted that she no longer was afraid to come but now even wanted to come sometimes, "because you never know what's going to happen next. I wanted to get better and I wanted to come and see you. There's like a big hole in the ground between us and if I told you some things I would just go into it and get covered up and never come out again." I was buoyed by her new insightfulness that there was something the matter inside her, that she wanted to be cured of it, but she was afraid of what this might entail.

Although I was inactive for the next few sessions, she kept up a barrage of accusations, as if every step forward needed to be followed by a step backward. There was no need to interpret since she made the transference connections herself. "I hate you nagging me. You want to make me feel ashamed like my mother. You are just like my mother, always nagging until I feel that I could kill her. You are both exactly alike." She was then lost in thought for a few minutes, before she added: "But then you also put me down like my father and make me feel dumb. Mother makes me feel dirty and my father makes me feel dumb and you make me feel both." I simply echoed these last thoughts: "You have now made me into a combination of your mother and father, and you expect me to shame you as they once did even though you never told them things that you were really ashamed about." She once again reiterated that she would almost certainly hate me if she told me her secrets, and I replied that if it helped her to feel better, I would not mind being hated. She said at once: "I hate you for not minding being hated. I want you to feel hurt. I want you to be upset like I am upset. I want you to be ashamed like I am ashamed." She was again silent and then added: "But you never seem to feel ashamed at anything I say to you and I want to be like that. I don't want to hate everybody. I want to have friends. I want to feel happy." I noted the idealization of myself as the good object, and again experienced a feeling of hopefulness.

PHASE OF A PREDOMINANTLY POSITIVE TRANSFERENCE

She was now, in the middle of her second year, talking much more freely, spontaneously, and unself-consciously. She even laughed at times, and the outbursts of violent rage had almost ceased. She was now working in the evenings to obtain money to help with her treatment because she felt that she could mix with people without intense embarrassment and fear. Toward the end of this year, she said that she was more contented now than she had ever been in her life, adding with satisfaction: "I know I have surprised you. I am doing much better than you ever expected me to do. You thought I was going to be a hospital case." She was now sitting closer and on one occasion asked me whether I would like to share an apple that she had brought with her. I said that I would like to share certain things which she still did not feel quite ready to share with me, but the apple was a good beginning and I would be glad to have half of it. She was able to smile at this and added humorously: "All in good time. You mustn't try to run before you can walk." She sounded like a schoolteacher and I, in turn, had to smile. This was a side to her that I had never seen. Later, this seemed another critical mutative point in the treatment.

At the beginning of her third year, the question of a vacation break arose. I asked whether she would like to have the name of someone she might call in case she needed to do so. She threw up her hands in horror. "What do you mean? I am not going to see any other doctor. I just got over being ashamed with you and you want me to go through all *that* again." I said soothingly that it was only a suggestion. "It had better be!" she said, and then added with a teasing smile, "Better the devil you know . . . !" There was laughter on both sides.

The paranoid and shame reactions now conspicuously absent, the situation was still far from stable. For example, she missed several days and blamed me for confusing her about her appointments when I had only made a small change in the time of her sessions. She could still become very angry. "Nothing is ever right when I come to see you. Everything seems to go wrong. You still blame me for everything. You always did."

I could sense that something was coming up that was taxing the good therapeutic partnership that had now been established. After one or two very silent sessions, she said that she wanted to tell me something and then never to see me again. When there was no response from me about this, she turned her chair around and talked quietly and rapidly to the wall. She said that sometimes she felt very nervous and would take a razor and cut her arms and legs until the blood came. It always seemed to be when she was having very angry feelings toward her mother. She sometimes thought of doing it to her mother and, once or twice, she had thought of doing it to me. She wanted to see my blood flow. She wondered why men did not bleed every month like women. It made her feel like a pig. She thought that everyone in the street would know that blood was running down from her body and that they would despise her. She could not bear me to know that she was bleeding under her clothes. I would just throw up. She knew that her brother did not bleed and that she would like to cut him with a razor. I listened to her quietly and then remarked that I understood about her shameful feelings now and was glad that she was able to talk to me about them. Sometimes such feelings covered over other feelings that could also be very upsetting: not only that I might despise her as she despised herself or felt that others despised her but that I might leave her. She said that sometimes she had felt that if she could kill somebody, she would never have to feel inferior again in her life. "My brain has always been slow because of what that woman (meaning her mother) did to me. She must have hurt me when I was coming out of her. That is what one book said. When I feel inferior I feel that no one wants me and that I'd better be dead or else they'd better be dead. I can tell what people think of me because I can see it in their eyes."

Feeling much more confident about the strength of the relationship, I suggested that some of her aggressive feelings toward me were a cover up for warmer and more sexual feelings she did not want to admit. Her answer to this was, "I am afraid of loving and hating people. I just want people to be neutral and I just want to be neutral."

A little later, she informed me that her mother wanted to come and speak with me but she had vetoed this vehemently. "If she comes, I go. It's either her or me. I am not going to share you with her. She has always taken everything away from me because she only loves herself. She never even wanted me to have lessons from my father." I noted the positive elements of the Oedipus complex that were beginning to emerge but made no comments. She went on to say that when she was about ten years old, she became extremely religious and thought of God as a very kind person who would forgive everything. She soon realized that this was quite untrue and that he could be very cruel and punishing like her parents. In fact, he made her feel so ashamed that she could no longer go to confession. She knew that if she had died then, she would have gone to hell and that the devils would all be laughing and jeering at her for the bad things that she had done. She had a strong feeling, too, that her mother never wanted her to be born, that she was ashamed of her because she was such a peculiar baby. She wondered how it was that I could like her when she was so peculiar now. She wished again that she could be like me and like everybody, even when they were mean and hated everybody. She wanted her mother to die, but she could not think of living without her. She some-times thought that I might die and then she knew that she herself would have to die because she could not live without me. There was no one else who cared about her because she was peculiar. She recalled how much torture it was for her to come to see me in the early days and how wounded she always felt after the sessions. She remembered leaving and walking down the street feeling that everyone was staring at her and could see that her face was red and hot.

There was a silence in which she seemed to be weighing something in her mind. She then said that she wanted to tell me something, and then hesitated. I waited, holding my breath for fear of offsetting her train of communication. She said that when she was about three years old, she remembered playing a game with another little boy about a year older.

She had forgotten all about it until just now. He did "very dirty things" to her and she could hardly bear to think about it. Then, when she was about thirteen, she played the same sort of game with another girl who was only seven. She had met her again a few months ago and when the girl said to her: "Do you remember the games we used to play?" Helen had been terrified and told her that she must never mention this to anybody else or else she would kill herself. I said that it was now our secret and that we could talk about it between ourselves only and try to understand why it had made her feel so very ashamed. She said that the little boy had tried to rub his "thing" into her and that sometimes she now tried to do the same thing with her finger. At this point, she once again turned her chair around and faced the wall. I pointed out how difficult it must have been for her to tell me and that it was a mark of our good friendship that I realized now how much she trusted me. She said that she was sure that somewhere inside me I hated her now that I knew the dreadful things that she did. Most of the thoughts that she had about me now when she was at home were bad thoughts. She wanted to cut me and watch my blood flow, and she wanted me to cut her and make her bleed. She wanted us to be the same. She told me that she had had a dream recently in which a man had been cut in half and his bottom half had disappeared. I wondered whether she wanted my bottom half so that she herself would not need to bleed anymore. However, my bottom half was not right for a girl and her bottom half was just right for a girl and something that she could be proud of. I reminded her that she was one of the people in the world who could produce beautiful babies from inside their bodies whereas my bottom half could never do that. She listened silently.

A little later, she began to talk about playing with dolls when she was little and giving it up because it bored her. She now thought that she would like to adopt a baby and wondered whether I could arrange this for her. We could look after it together. No one else need know about it. It would be our secret. She could live in a cottage in the country, and I could come down and see her there and play with "our" baby. It surprised me to hear this manifest oedipal transference material coming from such a preoedipal girl.

She again talked about how much better she felt and how after her sessions she even ran down the street feeling very light as if all the badness had gone out of her. She could not have said this a year ago and would have killed herself rather than let me know about it. This morning, she had actually thought that she would visit her father again.

She had been avoiding him for many months feeling that she could not bear to be with him in the same room. Now she wanted to see him and to see how he really looked. She then said that she had forgotten to tell me a dream recently that had made her feel very sad. While I had been away on vacation, she had had quite a number of nightmares in which she was running away from something horrible and was looking everywhere for me. This had happened again the other night. She added naively: "I often dream about anything that I want very much and that I can't get." I pointed out that this was the first time that she had admitted dreaming about me, looking for me in her dreams, and telling me that it was because she had wanted me so much that she dreamed about me. She blushed at this but kept silent. I talked about the many secrets that she had revealed to me and that we now shared together without feeling bad and ashamed about them. When she left the session, she was smiling broadly and in a very loving sort of way.

The next day she remarked that she had seen another patient leave the office and admitted to feeling very jealous even though she realized that I did see other people. She had also been rethinking her thoughts about her parents. She was now aware that both her father and mother had their problems and that she even found herself feeling sorry for them. It was a funny sort of feeling, as if she was coming out from inside herself and looking at people for the first time. I said to her, half humorously, that if she continued like this, she would soon start feeling sorry for me. She considered this very seriously and said that she could never imagine feeling sorry for me. I was such an all-right sort of person; nothing ever seemed to worry me or make me feel ashamed, even when she was being most horrible to me, hating me, and wanting to kill me. I said that we had become close friends and understood each other much better and were not thinking wrong things about each other and certainly not imagining things about each other. She looked at me and smiled spontaneously, making a sudden contrast in my mind to the first picture I had had of her as a frozen, rigid, tense, and very disturbed girl, wracked with paranoid anxieties. In her present relaxed state, she was looking pretty and was certainly dressing herself much more attractively. When the sessions were over now and it was time for her to leave, she showed increasing reluctance to go and would maneuver in several ways to stay. She said that she could now ask me how I felt about her because she knew that it would be true and she knew it would not hurt her. The confidence and trust in me was a constantly growing factor, and what was perhaps most striking was the emergence of her feminine psyche. In the course of her treatment she had ranged between severe paranoid reactions, intense shamefulness, feelings of inferiority, murderous rages, depressions, remorsefulness, and a consciousness of herself as a person.

In the final phase, we were no longer dealing with "an externalized form of unconscious conscience" but with what seemed to be genuine guilt reactions. She recalled again the early memory of visiting the new home when she was about four years old, when she had walked into a spider web with a large spider attached to it. She recalled screaming with horror trying to get the web out of her face. She had always been afraid of spiders and felt that it was due to this incident. I again recalled the work of Abraham (1922) that had sustained me through this analysis. It was he who first investigated the spider symbol as the phallic organ of the mother. As he pointed out, the spider represented the dangerous mother and the patient's unconscious fantasies were concerned with the danger of being killed by her. The spider killed its victim by sucking its blood. This brought us to the theme of her menstrual shock, her self-incisions, her wish to draw my blood, and for me to draw blood from her.

CONCLUSIONS

The case exemplifies the type of syndrome described by Jacobson (1971) in which guilt, shame, inferiority, paranoia, and depressive reactions distort the process of identity formation. In such very disturbed patients, one is confronted with gross immaturity of the psychic systems and their extreme proneness to regression leading not only to the experience of object loss but also to a "loss of the self." In Helen's case, the mother was a narcissistic character disorder and completely self-absorbed, while the father was a schizoid, ungiving, and unloving teacher who could not handle a normal classroom but could only deal with the situation of private tutoring.

In Winnicott's diagnostic session, Sarah (who seemed better adjusted than Helen) was able with the help of Winnicott to bring together the change in the teacher and the change in her mother at the time when her sibling had been born. Helen also had a displacing sibling, a younger sister, and it is quite possible that the change in Helen occurred at this time, although I was unable to uncover this. Winnicott had the advantage of having seen Sarah during the infantile stage. Therefore he was able to say to her: "I do want you to know that I can see one thing you can't see, and this is that your anger is with a good and not with a bad woman. The good woman changes to bad . . . your job will be to live through some relationships that do go a bit bad, when you do become a bit angry and a bit disillusioned, and somehow everyone survives." I too felt that Helen and I had both survived a very trying, exhausting, and disheartening relationship. I had the advantage over Winnicott in that he only had one session (and he did wonders with it), whereas I had almost four years.

Since shame and paranoia feed into each other, dealing with the shame becomes as important as dealing with the suspicion.

In his first draft on paranoia (1896), Freud suggests that shame must be "relocated" from the outside to the inside implying that what he wanted was for the patient to make use of introjective rather than projective mechanisms and to develop depression rather than paranoia, perhaps feeling that the former was less difficult to treat. As a consequence of this therapeutic maneuver, the patient dropped out of treatment complaining that it upset her too much, drawing from Freud the expostulation of "defense!" Since he was using a rather rapid and dramatic technique of "concentration hypnosis" (a transitional combination of hypnosis and free association, soon to be abandoned), one might be inclined to think today that the patient knew her own level of tolerance better than the therapist. I think that if Sarah had continued with Winnicott on the same level of her diagnostic session, she too would have most probably dropped out. Winnicott knew this and acted accordingly.

As Freud would have stated it, I was able in this case "to cast an inquisitive glance over the top of the wall to spy out what was going on on the other side of it." I would agree with him that "our technical methods must accordingly be replaced by others; that we do not know yet whether we shall succeed in finding a substitute." Finding a substitute is the task of the analyst who deals with children, adolescents, and the so-called "narcissistic neurotics."

REFERENCES

Abraham, K. 1913a. The observation of sexual intercourse. In *Selected Papers on Psycho-Analysis*. London: Hogarth, 1948.
Abraham, K. 1913b. Transformation of scoptophilia. In *Selected Papers on Psycho-Analysis*. London: Hogarth, 1948.

Abraham, K. 1921. Contributions to the theory of the anal character. In *Selected Papers on Psycho-Analysis*. London: Hogarth, 1948.

Abraham, K. 1922. The spider as a dream symbol. In *Selected Papers on Psycho-Analysis*. London: Hogarth, 1948.

Abraham, K. 1924. A short study of the development of the libido, viewed in the light of mental disorders. In *Selected Papers on Psycho-Analysis*. London: Hogarth, 1948.

Benedek, T. B. 1956. Toward the biology of the depressive constellation. *Journal of American Psychoanalytic Association* 4:389–427.

Erikson, E. H. 1950. *Childhood and Society*. New York: Norton.

Freud, S. 1893–1899. Early psycho-analytic publications. *Standard Edition* 3:3–325. London: Hogarth, 1962.

Freud, S. 1900. The interpretation of dreams. *Standard Edition* 4:88–92. London: Hogarth, 1953.

Freud, S. 1911. Psycho-analytic notes on an autobiographical account of a case of paranoia. *Standard Edition* 12:9–82. London: Hogarth, 1958.

Freud, S. 1917. Introductory lectures on psycho-analysis (Part III). *Standard Edition* 16:243–463. London: Hogarth, 1963.

Freud, S. 1931. Female sexuality. *Standard Edition* 21:223–246. London: Hogarth, 1963.

Freud, S. 1933. New introductory lectures on psycho-analysis. *Standard Edition* 22:7–182. London: Hogarth, 1964.

Glover, E. 1955. *The Technique of Psycho-Analysis*. London: Bailliere, Tindall & Cox.

Jacobson, E. 1971. *Depression*. New York: International Universities Press.

Jones, E. 1922. Some problems of adolescence. In *Papers on Psycho-Analysis*. London: Bailliere, Tindall & Cox, 1948.

Kanzer, M. 1952. Manic-depressive psychosis with paranoid trends. *International Journal of Psycho-Analysis* 33(1):34–42.

Klein, M. 1948. *Contributions to Psycho-Analysis 1921–1945*. London: Hogarth.

Mahler, M. 1966. Notes on the development of basic moods: the depressive affect in psychoanalysis. In R. Loewenstein, ed. *Psychoanalysis: A General Psychology*. New York: International Universities Press.

Schatzman, M. 1973. Paranoia or persecution: the case of Schreber. *History of Childhood* 1:62–88.

Sullivan, H. S. 1953. *Interpersonal Theory of Psychiatry*. New York: Norton.

Winnicott, D. 1952. Psychosis and child care. In *Collected Papers*. London: Tavistock, 1958.

Winnicott, D. 1971. *Playing and Reality*. London: Tavistock,

33 SOME OBSERVATIONS ON PSYCHOTHERAPY AND CREATIVITY

SUSAN FISHER

My friend, dreams are things hard to interpret, hopeless to puzzle out, and people find that not all of them end in anything. There are two gates through which the insubstantial dreams issue. One pair of gates is made of horn, and one of ivory.

Those of the dreams which issue through the gate of sawn ivory, these are deceptive dreams, their message is never accomplished. But those that come into the open through the gates of the polished horn accomplish the truth for any mortal who sees them.

HOMER

This analysis of fantasy, perhaps the oldest in all of Western thought, proposed that dreams that came through the gate of horn were to be trusted and attended to; dreams that came through the gate of ivory were to be foresworn. Horn, we may note, was the stuff of everyday life, of reality, of wakefulness. Hence dreams coming through that gate would connect with the real world and be fulfilled in it. The brilliant, exotic, and special light of the more precious ivory was self-reflective and did not lead to useful connections with experience; hence those dreams were illusory and life rejecting.

When Penelope awakens after dreaming that her husband Odysseus has come home, after twenty years of being away, she is suspicious that her dream is a vain wish, in which case she would be better off looking for a new husband. But she also knows that if her husband is alive the dream or fantasy of his return could nurture her and give her strength to continue the long wait.

528

The problem for Penelope is a perennial one. Everyone knows that some fantasies are invigorating, enlivening, and motivational; we also know that some fantasies or dreams represent avoidance, escape, and, if acted upon, would be disastrous. The problem for Penelope, and for the developing child, is to be able to distinguish which is which. Penelope awakens and asks, Which gate did the dream come through? And she knew. But Penelope is perhaps the most mature woman in all of literature, and her ability to use the dream and to assess its origin—the gate of horn—is both a manifestation of her creativity and a reflection of her maturity. Both creativity and maturity in Penelope have to do with the relationship between inner experience and outer reality. The dream, after all, is a creation of great complexity for Penelope. Of course, it is her greatest wish that Odysseus come home. Is it a mere wish? Is it born of signals that are coming from her responses to the subtle, subliminal clues that Odysseus is near? Is it an attempt to sustain her from within by vivid expression of her hopes, as she weaves and unweaves, by day and by night, holding off the suitors in another act of creativity?

In the strongest sense, to create means to make something from nothing; to make something absolutely new. Creativity is the power to do this, and significant creativity occurs in some potential space, linking inner and outer reality. Creativity occurs in the psychological activity in which inner life—its images, fantasies, dreams, perceptions, and populations—and the outer world—its new information, experiences, impingements, and surprises—mutually inform and mold each other. It is fairly clear that if either one of these regions, inner life or outer world, dominates there is a loss of creativity. Mere compliance with the external world is an uncreative act. Retreat from the world to fantasy-hallucination and more purely interior experience is an uncreative act. The creativity, the making of something new is not, for the human being, limited to what is given from the outside. It need not be something never before achieved. It is simply the original, what comes from oneself, the creation or the re-creation, the "finding or the re-finding" of the object (Freud 1920), and, of course, it is the aim of all therapeutic endeavor to promote this kind of creativity. And creativity is not talent—a distinction I will deal with later. It is the proper experience of the developing human being at every level. To develop it in children is the goal of all parents. It is the goal of all therapists for their patients. We must remember, however, that we are not talking about the special child at this point; we are talking about the inner experience of weaving, like Penelope, a fabric whose elements contain inner and outer elements and give to existence a quality of liveness.

Let me comment on how all this starts before we talk about its failures and distortions. Where does it all begin? The root of all play—and for all intents and purposes creativity and play are interchangeable—is unconscious fantasy. And where does unconscious fantasy come from? Loewald (1971), in a discussion of Freud's conception of instinct, suggests that in the newborn the earliest organization of instincts into psychic representation—the movement from only bodily sensation to earliest mental life—is inseparable from the infant's initial experience of the object caring for it. He asserts that the quality of the caring will color, alter, and shape the organization of the instincts themselves, leading to what he calls "mnemic images" (the precursors of memory) which are components of instincts. Upon repetition, over time, these mnemic images, these early psychic representations of instincts as organized by caretaking, are differentiated from the actual experience of gratification. This is the beginning of our mental life, and these images can be seen as the earliest precursors of fantasy. Loewald's formulation is very useful, for it connects the function of fantasy to the earliest biological experience in a developmental scheme. In the larger sense, play and the fantasies underlying play, which are rooted in the earliest bodily experiences of our lives, maintain the separateness of internal psychic reality and the external reality of others and objects. Through play, the two realities create, feed, and locate each other. The intermingling of bits of fantasy and images from inner experience with images and aspects of external life in the act of playing enlivens inner life and enlarges it. It also gives, by projection, a quality of "liveness" to external objects.

According to Winnicott (1971), unconscious fantasy begins at the moment the child is able to use an object. By "use" Winnicott does not mean to exploit but rather the ability to acknowledge separateness from oneself and to surrender the omnipotent sense—initially necessary for creative experience—that created the outer object entirely. The transitional object, the first "not me" possession which contains aspects of internal reality as well as "thingness," is the focus for the child's first use of symbol and first real play. All playing, perhaps psychotherapy itself, takes place in this potential space between inner psychic reality and external reality. Environmental actuality, things out there, and isolated body functioning are bridged by an interdigitation, by projections of internal fantasy which give objects their liveness, and by the taking in, changing, and enriching of internal life by new encounters with external objects. This conceptualization of play permits one to speak of a creative life, a relationship to the outer world, that gives experience its sense of vitality and joy.

It is clear, then, that fantasy, which underlies play and creativity, has different uses. Like the dreams entering through the gate of ivory, inner experiencing can substitute for relatedness to real objects in the world and thus be a means of avoiding or escaping development. In other situations, active fantasies can be adaptive, and we see this, for example, in the enforcedly passive, hospitalized child who either assaults his toys, reversing his sense of his own impotent experience, or invents an imaginary companion who expresses his concerns. By doing this he structures his experience in a way that can ease him through an otherwise traumatic experience.

This moves us into the realm of pathology. There are children who are afraid of fantasy, who cannot play, and in whom fantasy is denied or repressed from fear of the impulses released by it. Other children live in environments with little tolerance for the ambiguity implicit in all fantasy formation and, out of fear, trade off the fluidity and potential for change implicit in all fantasy for the certainty of a fixed reality schema. Hypermature egos, continually traumatized, reveal little capacity for available fantasy. I know of a little boy who imagined that he owned a tame lion which scared others but loved him the most. The reversal of his own and his father's aggression in this fantasy allowed the strength of the lion to be used by him. Fairy tales represent culturally accepted reversals of this sort which nourish children. Adolescents and even adults have their nurturing fairy tales. One function of fantasy is the prevention of the development of excessively rigid defenses. Often adults, whose reality testing is adequate, will first work out new possibilities in fantasy. The next step in development often appears first in the form of a daydream.

If we see the end result or, more modestly, the aim of therapy to be this creative capacity of relating to the external world in such a way that inner and outer energies enrich each other through the activity of the individual, we can look at psychological disturbance from the vantage point of creative function. If the trauma has been to the earliest formation of the self, to its organization and its relationship to reality, in which the spontaneous creative function is barely developed and we have a reactive, compliant, dysphoric individual whose whole relationship to himself and the world is fraught with despair—we are in the realm of narcissistic problems where the capacity to experience life with a sense of self-esteem and authenticity has been undermined from the start. This is a broadly sketched characterization, but for such a grouping of problems—whether we call them narcissistic, borderline, pregenital, or false self—the therapist will function to engender a sense of spontaneous integrated wholeness, perhaps for the first time.

There are, I believe, higher-order problems. Real neurotic conflicts exist where spontaneity can be inhibited or become embedded in psychic conflict requiring dissection and analysis to liberate a creative sense of being in life and work. The fundamental experience has been solidly present but has been strained and blocked.

I would like to share with you some therapeutic interaction during the creation of a drawing by a ten-year-old, barely pubescent, borderline psychotic girl (see fig. 1). I think it demonstrates how the child began a fantasy, revealed, perhaps discovered, aspects of herself in the process of making the drawing, connected the fantasy to other parts of her inner life, and gradually the fantasy changed and developed. These developments emerged out of the interrelationship between the forms she drew, my responses and comments, and her increasing self-revelations until she moved toward an integration of some of the fantasy elements into her self-concept.

She first drew only the jagged dorsal surface of a dragon. Then she asked whether I had any money and said that her family was out of money and that her bank had a little money. There were periodic growls as she turned into bears and lions. (Her conviction that she was a wolf and her physical performance of acting wolflike was what caused her eccentric, intellectual, caring parents to bring her, finally, to treatment.) Then she turned from the drawing and noticed a loosely woven, large wastebasket in the corner of the office. She focused upon it intensely and explained that the basket was beautiful but that it should not be used because little tiny bits would fall out through the holes. I suggested that I could put an inner lining inside the basket for next week and that then the bits would be all right. She talked about this being like "peeing" when it goes all over. Then she came back to the drawing and drew the ventral line and put in the interior dashes and said, "That is fur." Noting her move toward completion of the form and the diminution of her anxiety, I commented that the form was like her, furry and soft but prickly on the outside. She said that she was not going to make the dragon a boy or a girl because mating is all growling and eating; instead it would have babies like snails, with eggs. She

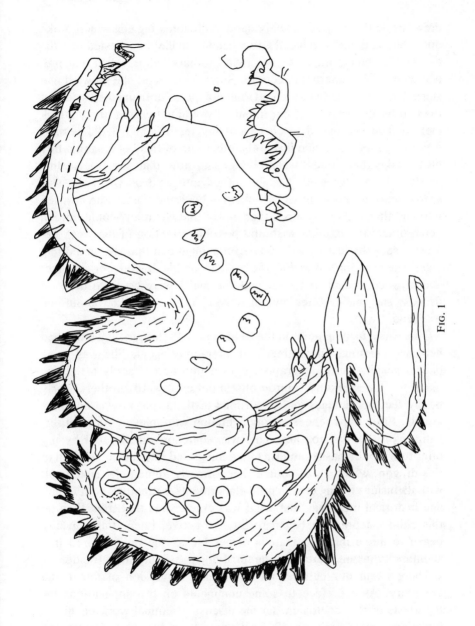

Fig. 1

drew inside the now completely defined dragon a big egg which broke open, hatched, and produced a two-headed snake! I suggested that the two-headed snake might be her twin brothers (whose birth had precipitated major maternal rejection). When I said that, she growled and started to attack me (half pretend, half not quite sure) and then said that the two-headed snake had her initials. I would not permit her to attack me, so then she asked to check out my teeth, which I did permit. Following this, she made inside the other end of this big dragon a tiny little snake that cried "waaah." Sensing now that she was feeling pretty safe, I suggested that she turned into animals when she was scared and did not want to talk about school and home. She crawled into and then out of my lap. I then added that she really could not kill her brothers (an explicit wish and possible intention of the week before). I said she just was not powerful enough and that she would feel bad if she did. She colored all the prickles on the dragon a bright blue; and growled. I said that I thought she and I were going to be good friends; she made softer animal noises. Then we talked about the weekend.

This was a turning point in the treatment with this girl. It established her as a creating, integrating, and interacting agent. She was using paper, pencil, basket, therapist, information about family members, plans for the weekend, murderous impulses toward brothers, early bodily feelings, images and distortions of them, old growls and new growls. Early experiences of fragmentation were played out in observations on the wastebasket. This was somehow ameliorated by my offer to wrap the basket and was then integrated into the completion of this dragon, which is, of course, her formerly vulnerable, naked self with its insides falling out. I could elaborate its instinctual, conflictual, and historical meanings, but what was crucial was that from then on this child's depression began to lift. An active, integrating capacity began to move into other areas of her life as she rediscovered that spontaneity meant more than the terrifying possibility of fratricide.

There is, in our culture, an unfortunate confusion of talent and creativity. As a preface to some comments on the implications for therapists of this confusion, let me discuss a seminal work of the art historian, Ernst Gombrich (1951). We have been discussing fantasy and creativity as they relate primarily to self-object differentiation and the enlivening processes by which living is rich and is a creative act. Gombrich makes a different usage of the same conceptual framework and discusses the act of creation, the creation of external "liveness" as it relates to objects of art. He suggests that originally the child creates the liveness of objects from internal need—that the hobbyhorse is a creation of the child. It is part fantasy and part object (reminiscent of Winnicott's transitional object). He states that all art is the making of images, and all image making is rooted in the creation of substitutions according to the minimum form necessary to match the biological need—the bringing of the inner into the outer world. He then goes on to say that in certain cultures—as in China, ancient Greece, and during the Renaissance—a further development occurs: the image emerges as a "representation" recording a visual experience of external reality, rather than as a substitute for it. But this creates a paradox. For the very belief in this possibility of real representation (that the painting frame is a window to a real image) causes further illusion. Our eye fills in, completes, interacts with, and finishes the form, until, as in Monet's blobs of color, we again create. It is this infusion of fantasy and the completion of perception that gives works of art, external objects, and life their vivacity.

Our state as adults is different from that of the child. Our experience of discovery of our part in the integration of an image in a Van Gogh or Monet painting is not the same as the experience of the child who makes or creates his first hobbyhorse—a broomstick with a towel for a head. To use Gombrich's metaphor. from Genesis 3:24, the way back is barred by the angel with a flaming sword forever barring Adam and Eve from returning. The child cannot return to the undifferentiated state where once he was like God and created the world that he did not know was already there. However, some of this kind of early infantile creativity remains in the imaginative use of fantasy throughout development. And it is this usage that therapists implement and unleash if we are successful at our craft. The kind of creativity I am talking about belongs to everyone. It belongs to the state of being an alive human being.

Who is this creative adolescent being brought to treatment? Is it the young physicist who has problems with his peer groups because he is not adjusted to the peer culture? Or is it the young pianist who has functional paralysis of the fingers or is exhibiting himself in the schoolyard? Is it the problem of the child who simply wants to be like the other kids while his parents have an investment in his special talents—his violin playing, high IQ, or mathematical prowess? Here we have not only a problem of adjustment of the creative adolescent but a simultaneous problem of the parents' living through their child, avoiding marital conflicts, and projecting their own unsatisfied dreams onto their insufficiently differentiated child. Is perhaps the very notion of the especially talented child—the making of him into a special case— not part of the problem? And does our possible seduction into that view undercut our therapeutic effectiveness? Here we have the special connection between narcissism and talent. The patient himself may identify the special talent with a wish or fantasy to be omnipotent—an underlying grandiosity that needs to be worked with and put in perspective. If, perchance, the therapist himself shares that view of creativity, he may be unable to help the patient see that the equation of his talent with his uniqueness—with the resultant fear that to explore the meaning of the creativity is to give up his talent and his identity— may be mere resistance. There is always the possibility that it is not resistance, however, and that a particular talent, of enormous satisfaction to his family and to the therapist, may have been overused and massively overdetermined. The young genius, when finally acquainted with his inner life, desires, impulses, and conflicts—which is our true task—may simply decide he does not want to play the violin but prefers baseball. We must sit back, accept the defeat to our own narcissism, realize that it is his choice, and we may not be the therapist who analyzed Mozart. My language is light, but I am deadly serious. I am suggesting that it is a false notion that we can distinguish between the creative and the uncreative person. That is a countertransference problem of the therapist. I suggest, quite seriously, that all people are potentially creative and that it is this creativity we try to unleash. I am suggesting that a lot about the patient is not our business, including the use he makes of any talent or ability that is not embedded in the conflicts that it is our function to analyze. It is quite possible that the end result of a successful treatment is that a Mozart will have gained the world and the world will have lost a Mozart. And we may be privately bemused, but it can be only in private.

Where do we find creativity in treatment? It seems to me that there are some patients who have unique and special perceptions and perspectives that they use in relationship to their life, comparable to an artistic, intellectual, athletic, or musical talent. As with any way of understanding the world, we try as therapists to feel our way into all our patients and do the same with them. If it is a creative slant, we try to help them use it adaptively. If it is a source of trouble in their world—that is, a special vision may not go so well in some sorts of high schools—we can help the patient understand that this special perception may indeed create the problem. The other creative function that occurs in all therapies is, of course, the transference—that fit of past into present is quite an act of creation, indeed.

Conclusions

A serious problem for therapists is: What use do we make of our patients? Many of us would have loved to be creative artists. The therapist has to resist his grandiose impulse to unleash a patient's unusual talent. What we can appropriately unleash in our patients is only the power to make an authentic choice. The countertransference problems of therapists include a zealous desire to cure and the sense of a power to ruin talent or to create talent. It is our own grandiose fantasies that hinder us in treating the talented adolescent. Therapists have the same problem as Penelope. We are as endangered by the images of our patients that come through the gate of ivory as she was and as the patient is. We too have fantasies of demonic creativity—the power to ruin is, after all, only the obverse of the power to create. And, for us, the creations that come through the gate of ivory are the seductive, dreamlike images of the special patient. And there we join in the defensive or narcissistic use of special gifts, just like parents, teachers, or the patients themselves, and contribute to the hampering of choice, the liberation of which is our true creativity. As therapists we deal with meaning, and that is all we can explore—the meaning to this teenager of his special talent or line of vision. Beyond that, his creativity must be no different than that of every patient we have, that of enlivening and engaging his life.

One of the great creative minds of the twentieth century, Hannah Arendt (1963), argued that the sine qua non of the human is this capacity to begin something new, unprecedented, something unpredictable and surprising. She calls it the spontaneous act. It is what makes the human being human and free. To be deprived of our spontaneity, our freedom, our creativity, is to be isolated and lonely. To recover our creativity, our freedom, is to be able to live in the common world with our fellow humans.

REFERENCES

Arendt, H. 1963. *On Revolution*. New York: Viking.
Freud, S. 1920. Beyond the pleasure principle. *Standard Edition* 18:14–17. London: Hogarth, 1961.
Gombrich, E. 1951. Meditation on a hobby horse or the roots of artistic

form. In I. L. Whyte, ed. *Aspects of Form: A Symposium on Form in Nature and Art*. London: Lund Humphries.

Homer. *The Odyssey*. Translated by Richmond Lattimore. New York: Harper Colophon, 1965.

Loewald, H. 1971. On motivation and instinct theory. *Psychoanalytic Study of the Child* 26:91–129.

Winnicott, D. 1971. The use of an object. In *Playing and Reality*. London: Tavistock.

AGGRESSION REVISITED:
THE VALUE OF ANGER IN THERAPY
AND OTHER CLOSE RELATIONSHIPS

ALLEN J. CAHILL

A long-standing lack of clarity in the basic theory of aggression has occupied clinical thinking about normal development, psychopathology, and the treatment of juvenile delinquency, sociopathy, and violence. The demand for a clear theory of the aggressive drive, occasioned by recent focus on borderline personality organization, separation-individuation difficulties, and self-object confusion, has pressed basic research workers to undertake distinct, longitudinal observations of infants, as well as psychoanalytic work with both mother and child, to clarify the separate stages in the development of the aggressive drive (Parens 1979).

Psychoanalytic and behavioral theorists, Fraiberg (1969), Mahler (1968), Solnit (1966, 1972), Spock (1965), and especially Applegarth (1971), Arlow (1973), Brenner (1971), Eissler (1971), Goodall (1971), and Joseph (1973), Lussier (1972), Rangell (1972), Saul (1976), Stone (1971), have struggled with new approaches to understanding the human aggressive drive. In descriptions of the development of aggression in infants and toddlers by Parens (1973, 1979), the role of aggression as a destructive element in the human personality was questioned. Freud's (1920, 1933) later theory of aggression[1] making destruction the aim of the aggressive drive, even developing a duality in human motivation pitting the life instinct against the death instinct,[2] was largely abandoned. Interestingly, Freud's (1915) earlier theory (mastery as the aims of aggression and other aims, like hostile destructiveness or sadism, appearing more as pathological complications of the drive) has been returned to a position of theoretical primacy.

One cardinal distinction, clinically useful in the treatment of child and adolescent behavior disorders as well as in therapy or counseling with parents or child-care workers involved with teens, is the clear-cut difference (Marcowitz 1973; Parens 1973) between anger and destructive hostility.[3]

As any therapist who has struggled with teenage patients gifted at provoking anger well knows, the manner in which we handle our own aggressive impulses frequently determines the outcome of therapy. In striving to distinguish carefully between angry feelings and hostile impulses, and in employing even our anger for the purposes of therapy, we are but making a virtue of necessity. Would that we were less guilt ridden about our spontaneous anger, less hamstrung by the teen who senses our ambivalence about aggression, more sure that the proper use of anger is a powerful force in establishing intimacy.

The aim of anger is mastery. En route to libidinous objects, if distance, delay, complications, obstacles, or opposition intervene, anger arises to drive the person to persist in the pursuit of the object (Heimann and Valenstein 1972; Hendrick 1942, 1943; Parens 1979; Spitz 1945, 1965, 1969; Waelder 1960; Winnicott 1950).

The aim of hostility is destruction of the object, partial or complete. If obstacles or opposition to attainment of the object prove insurmountable and unpleasure grows to sufficiently extreme proportions (Berkowitz 1969; Storr 1972), both the self and the object[4] may become suffused with an aura of "badness."[5] The frustrating object, instead of being introjected, is projected with much feeling and with a drive to destroy the bad object of the drive. Hostile attack on the mother (or on the self) may be aborted by repression, but the drive remains. Later in life, as unpleasure grows during complications in affectionate relationships, anger arises to master obstacles; if frustration persists, the person "sees red" and begins to deal destructively with the object (lover, parent, child, business partner).[6] The form this hostility takes, in observable behavior, is that of controlling through pain or hurting.

Anger is of great use in overcoming differences and deficits in personalities during the development of intimacies. Uncontrolled hostile drives, however, lead to hurts that accumulate in close relationships and finally bring that alliance to the point of diminishing return. Concrete examples of destructive hostility (in child rearing, in marital relationships, in friendships generally, even in therapy relationships) may help to clarify its difference from anger. Basically, anger operates in the context of a relationship in which the object is trusted and pursued. Hostility implies despair about the object, disappointment, and rejection, and with that a drive to punish or revenge oneself upon the object. In short, disposing of intimacy, one may have settled for painful control, for hurting. Hostility is a manipulation rather than a relationship.

In child rearing, a five-year-old may say in effect, "I won't do it. I don't care what you say (or feel), and I hate you anyway." If the mother believes that the five-year-old could really be detaching from her (instead of just temporarily having difficulty fusing anger and affection in consciousness), the mother may momentarily fear that the relationship is gone and that she can no longer influence the child with her thoughts and feelings. She believes his "I don't care" may be permanent. Therefore, instead of sending the child to his room to cool off and inviting him to come back in fifteen or twenty minutes when he will care about her anger at his behavior, she undertakes to attack and manipulate through hurt, pain, intimidations, spanking, yelling, depreciation, guilt provoking, and most important, threats of abandonment.

There has always been a dichotomy in theory and advice on relationships between spouses versus parent to child relationships. There has been a tendency to treat all aggression as damaging to a child (or patient), leading to a recommendation always to distract the child rather than progressively to confront him with limits backed by the parent's firm anger. In sharp contrast, couples have been urged to "let it all hang out" with no distinctions between aggressive versus destructive drives, fantasies, and feelings. Therapists, in the same category as parents, have been urged never to be angry at a patient. In my opinion, in child rearing, hurting a love object is never helpful. On the other hand, inadequate aggression toward a child, mostly repressed or poorly expressed, robs him of chances for identification with the aggressor and subsequent superego formation.

Hostility of all types, as a drive to destroy (or break or make him do), stimulates resistance in the child. He sees the parent as an enemy attempting to invade his autonomy. If he has sufficient autonomy already, he will stubbornly resist giving in. Even if he does temporarily succumb to control, he will experience the demanded behavior as alien, to be extruded as soon as he is big enough.[7]

In contrast, anger is respectful of autonomy and of the free relationship between mother and child. In essence, the mother says, "I could force you to act properly because I'm bigger. But I don't need to, because I know how attached you are to me. You are perfectly free—I throw away my power. If you wish to continue in a relationship with me, you will want to know what I think about you and how I feel. If you don't do what I wish, I'll be angry. You don't like me angry at any of your behavior, but you have to live with the results of your behavior."

Most parents who have difficulties with aggressive children will have to raise their tolerance for their own aggression. They need to work through their tendency to deny, appease, project, split, get depressed, and withdraw. Dereistic defenses will need to be worked through and anger will have to be tolerated in order for the child to get the full benefit of parental aggression.

Anger discloses that there is a difference of opinion, of perspective, even a difference of purpose between mother and child. Whereas a child might ignore the mother's abstract description of a desired behavior, he cannot as easily defend against the tension created when the other patiently but aggressively awaits his compliance. Though the initial judgment of the child might be a fundamental disagreement, as the mother remains angry, the tension within him leads to a change in thought, "How could she possibly demand such a thing?" And thus he begins to investigate her viewpoint. Though he may not ultimately agree, he does come to understand the terms and possibly the basis of her request. As he begins to try it her way, maybe initially only so that she will not be angry, he may find the home ritual useful to his lifestyle. Tension between them then subsides. If anger and tension does not subside on both sides after a reasonable practice period, the parent needs to reconsider whether the ritual is premature, a useful behavior, or whether it is an outmoded family heirloom.

Anger's usefulness is not confined to parent-child relationships. It is just as useful in developing needed behaviors and skills between lovers, spouses, and between therapist and patient. Distinctions between anger and hostility persist. In angry struggles between spouses, escalation to hostile threats of abandonment (divorce) cause relationships to deteriorate. Anger is a commitment to the relationship and a vote of confidence that we know that the spouse cares about our feelings.

Also the therapist needs his aggression. He may be confronted by an adolescent who brags and lapses into fantasies of great achievements. The first fantasy may be believable, but as the feats multiply the therapist may be compelled to share his skepticism with the teen. Depreciation of the boy and arguing details logically runs the risk of a hostile competition. But the anger of the therapist, who frankly does not enjoy a doubtful conversation, is mild and inescapable. Similarly a droning obsessive recital, or an endlessly blaming or revenge-filled recitation, can be described as painful and irritating to any listener.

Unconflicted hostility, depreciation, threats, or guilt-provoking comments from an unsocialized adolescent are best met with a playback (without depreciatory mimicry) of the unfriendly conversation. Frequently, except for neurotics, there is little to analyze in the hostile attack. Simply describing the conversation as provocative to friends and enemies alike puts the teen on notice that he is undercutting available alliances by such inflammatory speech. Again, the chief penalty is the anger of the other, but, to the degree that the teen is beginning to attach to the other, the calm, controlled anger of the therapist counters the attack and invites the teen to explore solutions to his underlying anger or poorly controlled hostility.

A most notable application for genuine "anger therapy"[8] is in milieu therapy of the aggressive teen (Meeks 1979). Here, particularly, we are but making a virtue of necessity. Effective, dynamic consultation to our child-care workers is focused on first finding the worker with whom the teen forms the tightest bond. Going on then to help the worker be sensitive to the transference-countertransference distortions and to assist the worker in recognizing and interpreting the teen's defenses against relating is of no help if the worker cannot stand the intensity of his own or the teen's aggression. The simplistic distinction between anger and hostility frequently lets the worker off the hook of guilt or shame about his anger, allowing him to persist in a long-term rageful relationship (Masterson 1972; Redl 1966). Picturing aggression to him as a positive, structuring, caring drive helps lighten his taboo against anger at children. Contrariwise, the term "hostility" carries its own taboo against hurtful behavior such as hitting or abandonment. Instead of chuckling at a provocative outburst, meaning, "I can't talk seriously with you," the worker "stays on his case." The personal anger of this worker becomes the principal negative reinforcer; the pleasure and enjoyment of the worker in the teen's success, the positive reinforcer.[9]

Case Example

Tom, age sixteen, the youngest of three and the only boy, was admitted to the hospital because of continuous marijuana use for one year and three years of school underachievement. He had failed ninth grade and, after repeating, was failing tenth. He had subtly begun to under-

543

achieve in sixth grade when his mother became depressed and began drinking heavily, requiring her first hospitalization. The keystone of the family was his father, a high-achieving executive, quite compulsive, controlling, and, in his mid forties, becoming slightly depressed. Mother, also, after ten years of marriage and three children, began to tire of the work and social pace of corporate upward mobility and manifested depression and withdrawal from Tom.

At the time of admission, Tom described a lack of energy, loss of interest in school, and stomach pains. His mother complained of Tom's anger and his "treating me badly." Father talked of mother's alcoholism and depression and of Tom's failure in school and not wanting to do things with him. Treatment included milieu and individual therapy for Tom, individual therapy with each of the parents, and family therapy every two weeks when the parents visited Tom at the hospital.

On the first more restricted unit, he involved himself with an authoritative type child-care worker who supported Tom's guitar playing and continually confronted him concerning his evasion of rules and nonperformance in school. Though he continually sought out the worker, Tom experienced him as a picayune tyrant whom he could never satisfy. Tom dressed sloppily, moved slowly, littering the environment and arriving late for unit tasks, and ignored demands for homework. He verbally and nonverbally communicated, "You can't make me and I don't like you anyway." His worker avoided a power struggle by admitting that he could not make Tom produce, but protested, "I don't have to believe that you don't like me," reflecting on Tom's continual rapprochement.

Later, when Tom met the requirements of the daily routine and decided to try working in school, he was moved to a more advanced unit and set up a relationship with the very aggressive head nurse. While the nurse listened to Tom's music, read his essays, as well as insisting on adherence to rules, Tom again began to view this important staff person as a "pushy, put-down artist" who wanted to entrap him in minor breaches of the rules to keep him in the hospital indefinitely. The nurse continually confronted Tom that Tom's loss of unit privileges and his toying with loss of credits and skills in school was disappointing to staff and that Tom would just have to live with staff anger as long as he was self-destructive. Tom's spoken or unspoken protest that he did not care was met by the observation that Tom always looked like he cared.

In individual therapy, Tom's initial evasion and outright lying was met by the acknowledgment that the therapist could understand Tom's not trusting him and even his fearing him, but that it was annoying to be talking to a boy when you could not always believe what he was saying. Complaints of failure in school prompted, "You must be just as annoyed at these grades as I am. Failure in an associate isn't pretty."

Mother's therapy began in the midst of her intense depression about Tom's hospitalization. She survived a suicide attempt (overdose) precipitated by a conviction that her husband was going to leave her. Mutual hostile threats of abandonment (divorce, travel, suicide) over the years were reconsidered. She declared a nine-month moratorium on discussion of divorce and committed herself to work out the problems of the marital relationship. But primarily she began to organize her own daily routine, to switch from volunteer work to involvement in a part-time job as a survey interviewer. She began going to lunch with a friend and took tennis lessons. Within a setting of living a life of her own, she began talking with father about what she wanted in a marriage with him, angry about the deficits but no longer hostile.

Father was the most defended family member, talking continually of problems and crises in his son's and wife's life. Eventually he began discussing his own work dissatisfaction and his feelings of isolation in his social life and marriage. Basically, he viewed himself as taking care of everyone. If his family were not satisfied with his services or they did not respond to his demands that they grow and be happy, he threatened abandonment. Even in the therapy situation, he concluded most daily sessions by moving reluctantly to the door saying, "I guess we're getting somewhere. Should I come back next week?" He implied a quite tenuous alliance, whereas he was tenaciously involved with the therapist in the work of analyzing his feelings. He began to recognize his denial of how involved he was with his wife and how ready, when angry, he was to threaten abandonment. Progress in unraveling misunderstandings and in negotiating his relationship with her began when he ceased the veiled threats and committed himself to work with her: "I'm not going to divorce you. I'm going to be right here and be angry any time you get drunk."

Family therapy was a kaleidoscope of hostile scenes: raised voices, depreciations, and guilt provoked by tears and implications that father and mother were totally unhappy or dissatisfied in their life because of Tom's behavior. Father was unconsciously using competitive put-downs. Blind to Tom's growing motivation to achieve and holding onto the role of the standard setter, father deprived Tom of his initiative by saying, "I told you that you'd be able to." Sometimes he would even undercut Tom's success by setting new or ever-higher goals, distracting from present gain, and attempting to regain the initiative in the boy's life. Also, threats of abandonment were the stock-in-trade of each. Tom was particularly talented at ignoring and denying the presence of his parents. Focus on the specifics of what each was angry about (as well as direct interpretation of hostile attacks and threats as diversions from therapy and even despair) helped to keep the pressure of their aggression behind the demand of each for change.

The underlying intense attachments rose into consciousness and were increasingly expressed as each became more able to set limits on the other and negotiate differences. Tom continued in school and in inpatient therapy past his seventeenth birthday despite his threat to leave the hospital and home "as soon as I'm old enough." When he was discharged after his eighteenth year, he returned home to finish his last year of high school and prepare for college.

Conclusions

Aggression has been handled ambivalently in the psychoanalytic tradition, much more condemned than treasured. Recent longitudinal observations of infants and therapies with mother-infant have given rise to a distinction between anger (aim: mastery) and hostility (aim: destruction). One practical conclusion from this distinction is to discourage hostile behavior (hitting, yelling, depreciating, blaming, ignoring, or threatening abandonment) in close relationships while encouraging the expression of anger to clarify viewpoints and work through differences.

By valuing gentle anger, we learn to commit ourselves to a relationship, to tolerate intense feelings, to think clearly when angry, to confront the other in a few words with our perceptions and with our feelings before we become too angry to hear, patiently to persist over weeks or months in repetitive confronting interpretations until the friend changes behavior, and to avoid giving up and attacking the other with hostility or at least to apologize and to clarify our intent following those occasions when we have lost control. Valuing anger in human relationships and analyzing and eliminating hostile interchange are preconditions for personal alliances and for intimacy.

NOTES

1. See also Hartmann, Kris, and Lowenstein (1949).

2. Most analysts subsequently did not agree (Bibring 1941; Fenichel 1945).

3. We do not deal here with sadism in the narrower sense—sadism as fused with the sexual drive, a hostile destructiveness aroused as a precondition to erotic arousal (Freud 1905, 1915).

4. The inadequate distinction between self and object in the perception of the three- to eight-month-old infant involves the self secondarily as object of the hostile drive which was primarily directed at the object; both become tainted (see Mahler 1968).

5. Bad: lack of due good (Thomas Aquinas, *Summa Theologiae*, pars. Ia–IIa of XVIII, art. 1), lack of qualities appropriate to a pleasurable object, such as availability or proximity to the reach of the infant.

6. Parens (1979) may be multiplying beings and terms by calling immediate unpleasure discharges "hostility" and delayed discharges (in the atmosphere of pleasurable release) "sadism in the broad sense." Yet this distinction does help to explain in toddlers "unprovoked hurting," hitting or biting stimulated by hostility "left over from yesterday." And, of course, this "delayed hostility," now dubbed "sadism" does offer a bridge to the analytic writings on sadism as linked to or even fused with the erotic drive.

7. Destructive hostility does certainly have its purpose in life, of course—with enemies in war and in criminal situations. Controlling through pain is the only manipulation available in many legal and wartime situations. However, hostility has no place in relationship with family and friends.

8. A so-called anger therapy is currently in vogue in residential programs where children in treatment are humiliated and punished physically. Of course, this is really "hostility therapy" or "destructive therapy."

9. We do not here explore the role of affectionate and even erotic feeling between teen and worker as an even stronger motive to change behavior. But in the early months of inpatient treatment, aggression is the only feeling available.

REFERENCES

Applegarth, A. 1971. Comments on aspects of the theory of psychic energy. *Journal of the American Psychoanalytic Association* 19:379–416.

Arlow, J. A. 1973. Perspectives on aggression in human adaptation. *Psychoanalytic Quarterly* 42:178–184.

Berkowitz, L. 1969. The frustration-aggression hypothesis revisited. In *Roots of Aggression: A Re-examination of the Frustration-Aggression Hypothesis*. New York: Atherton.

Bibring, E. 1941. The development and problems of the theory of the instincts. *International Journal of Psycho-Analysis* 22:102–131.

Brenner, C. 1971. The psychoanalytic concept of aggression. *International Journal of Psycho-Analysis* 39:350–373.

Eissler, K. R. 1971. Death drive, ambivalence, and narcissism. *Psychoanalytic Study of the Child* 26:25–78.

Fenichel, O. 1945. *The Psychoanalytic Theory of Neurosis*. New York: Norton.

Fraiberg, S. 1969. Libidinal object constancy and mental representation. *Psychoanalytic Study of the Child* 24:9–47.

Freud, S. 1905. Three essays on the theory of sexuality. *Standard Edition* 7:123–243. London: Hogarth, 1953.

Freud, S. 1915. Instincts and their vicissitudes. *Standard Edition* 14:111–140. London: Hogarth, 1957.

Freud, S. 1920. Beyond the pleasure principle. *Standard Edition* 18:1–64. London: Hogarth, 1955.

Freud, S. 1933. New introductory lectures on psycho-analysis. *Standard Edition* 21:59–145. London: Hogarth, 1961.

Goodall, J. V. L. 1971. Some aspects of aggressive behavior in a group of free-living chimpanzees. *International Journal of Social Science* 23:89–97.

Hartmann, H.; Kris, E.; and Lowenstein, R. M. 1949. Notes on the theory of aggression. *Psychoanalytic Study of the Child* 3/4:9–36.

Heimann, P., and Valenstein, A. F. 1972. The psychoanalytical concept of aggression: an integrated summary. *International Journal of Psycho-Analysis* 53:31–35.

Hendrick, I. 1942. Instinct and the ego during infancy. *Psychoanalytic Quarterly* 11:33–58.

Hendrick, I. 1943. The discussion of the "instinct to master." *Psychoanalytic Quarterly* 11:33–58.

Joseph, E. D. 1973. Aggression redefined—its adaptational aspects. *Psychoanalytic Quarterly* 42:197–213.

Lussier, A. 1972. Panel on aggression (chairman, M. H. Stein). *International Journal of Psycho-Analysis* 53:13–19.

Mahler, M. S. 1968. *On Human Symbiosis and the Vicissitudes of Individuation*. With M. Furer. New York: International Universities Press.

Marcovitz, E. 1973. Aggression in human adaptation. *Psychoanalytic Quarterly* 42:226–233.

Masterson, J. F. 1972. *Treatment of the Borderline Adolescent: A Developmental Approach*. New York: Wiley.

Meeks, J. E. 1979. Behavioral and Antisocial Disorders. In J. Noshpitz, ed. *Basic Handbook of Child Psychiatry*. Vol. 2. New York: Basic.

Parens, H. 1973. Aggression: a reconsideration. *Journal of the American Psychoanalytic Association* 21:34–60.

Parens, H. 1979. *The Development of Aggression in Early Childhood*. New York: Aronson.

Rangell, L. 1972. Aggression, Oedipus, and historical perspective. *International Journal of Psycho-Analysis* 53:3–11.

Redl, F. 1966. *When We Deal with Children*. New York: Free Press.

Saul, J. S. 1976. *The Psychodynamics of Hostility*. New York: Aronson.

Solnit, A. J. 1966. Some adaptive functions of aggressive behavior. In R. M. Lowenstein, L. M. Newman, M. Schur, and A. J. Solnit, eds. *Psychoanalysis–a General Psychology*. New York: International Universities Press.

Solnit, A. J. 1972. Aggression: a view of theory building in psychoanalysis. *Journal of the American Psychoanalytic Association* 20:435–450.

Spitz, R. 1945. Diacritic and coenesthetic organizations. *Psychoanalytic Review* 32:146–162.

Spitz, R. 1965. *The First Year of Life*. With W. G. Gobliner. New York: International Universities Press.

Spitz, R. 1969. Aggression and adaptation. *Journal of Nervous and Mental Diseases* 149:81–90.

Spock, B. 1965. Innate inhibition of aggressiveness in infancy. *Psychoanalytic Study of the Child* 20:340–343.

Stone, L. 1971. Reflections on the psychoanalytic concept of aggression. *Psychoanalytic Quarterly* 40:195–244.

Storr, A. 1972. *Human Destructiveness*. New York: Basic.

Waelder, R. 1960. *Basic Theory of Psychoanalysis*. New York: International Universities Press.

Winnicott, D. W. 1950. Aggression in relation to emotional development. In *Collected Papers*. New York: Basic, 1975.

35   ANALYSIS OF ADOLESCENTS WITH
DEVELOPMENTAL ARREST

THEODORE B. COHEN

The concept of developmental arrest as used in this presentation stems from the observation that excessive psychological trauma inhibits development of the self and slows psychic growth. Developmental arrest frequently encompasses slow neurological maturation and/or slow psychological maturation, mild ego distortions, and self-pathology. The concept is modeled on the findings of Anna Freud (1965) but is in contrast to Kolansky and Eisner's (1979) theory, which states that developmental arrest does not include ego distortion. They believe arrest is the result of excessive gratification by parent figures, bypassing the healthy conflict necessary for normal development. The Kolansky-Eisner theory, however, coincides with mine in the belief that appropriate parental nurturance can correct development arrest.

Pearson (1955) described the syndrome of slow maturation, as recognized through motor, perceptual, and learning difficulties, and outlined the particular need of such patients for help with their narcissistic development. He stressed that children with low self-esteem and damaged self-perceptions have phobic avoidance defenses against learning which require participation in a therapeutic alliance with a therapist to enable them to want to learn and to be able to face failure. Subsequently the faculties of many special schools offering programs for children with developmental problems included psychotherapists who helped these children to mend their fragmented self-perceptions. It was necessary to decrease their anxiety before they could respond to the special learning tools devised to facilitate their education. Outside of special schools, children who did not respond to tutoring using the newer perceptual techniques were sometimes referred to psychotherapists. Often, if the therapists used faciiitating therapeutic alliances, the result was development of structures and attitudes which encouraged better learning.

In the late 1960s, psychoanalysts such as Colarusso (1973), Kolansky (1979), and Stennis (1972), further elaborated the concepts of developmental arrest as seen in schools. The Bucks County Project was devised, enabling primary school teachers to differentiate ego defective, developmentally arrested, and neurotic or normal children in order to provide differing modes of teaching, with clearly defined strategies, so that children from each group could learn more effectively within the same classroom. Backup supports were essential, including the availability of psychoanalytically oriented psychiatrists. Teachers of over 25,000 children in seven states have used this method. It was discovered that within the normal school population, 5 percent were ego defective, 30 percent were developmentally arrested, and 65 percent were neurotic or normal children. The project further confirmed the theory that developmentally arrested children need and can progress with special help in defining self from others, in healing hurt self-images, and in understanding the rage reactions resulting from the damaged self-images.

From another direction, understanding of developmental arrest was a by-product of work with some children of poverty. Studies by Belmont (1977) and Pavenstedt (1961), both analysts who worked with ghetto children, elaborated how the egos of the children they saw were buffeted by the hostile environment. The children often experienced traumas of overstimulation and/or understimulation, failures of nurturance from unempathic caretakers who, being developmentally arrested themselves, could not support the child through normal developmental cycles. In an ongoing study, Burland and Cohen (1980) describe autistic character disorders in which the primary parent-child defect is the failure to establish the libidinal object; in effect, an incomplete entree into symbiosis. The children they worked with had been subjected to overwhelming stimulation, excessive aggression, early sexual trauma, and they often received erratic care by foster parents. They showed poor reality testing, were unable to develop self and object constancy, and suffered narcissistic fragmentation. The arrested development of intrapsychic structures and/or adequate object relations subsequently resulted in poor school learning patterns.

The special contributions of Mahler's (Mahler, Pine, and Bergmann 1975) concepts of the stages of normal separation-individuation help to clarify our understanding of developmentally arrested children. They consistently have problems in relating to peers and feel lonely and isolated as a result. They usually stick to home, reluctant and fearful of individuation, and they often become depressed if they are forced to leave. In the analyses of children or adults with developmental arrest, it is of the utmost importance to pay closest attention to the feelings around changes in schedule, breaks in the routine of appointments, separation for any reason, and most of all termination. A clear perception of the level of separation-individuation is like having a road map describing the way toward object constancy.

Kohut (1971, 1977, 1978; Kohut and Wolf 1978) has described narcissistic development in adults and children. Tyson (1979) wrote of the analysis of a four-and-one-half-year-old girl using a twinship, narcissistic transference to cure her developmental arrest. Kohut's development of the self is perceived as parallel to the line of oral, anal, and phallic drive development. In my analytic work with adolescents, it has been helpful to use self and drive theory as interrelated. Low self-esteem, rage reactions, failure to develop self-object differentiation, bisexual conflicts, and omnipotent and grandiose defenses which interfere with both reality testing and good object relations are symptoms commonly seen in the developmentally arrested child.

Psychoanalysis and Developmental Arrest

Classically, children with oedipal neuroses are selected for child analysis. Developmentally arrested children have been thought to be more appropriately treated in psychoanalytically oriented psychotherapy. In the past, the presence of developmental arrest in the parents, slow neurological development in the child, or excessive trauma or chaos in the family were all reasons for rejecting a child for analysis. Careful evaluation of a child, sometimes including Freud's (1965) developmental profile, was used to rule out starting an analysis with a developmentally arrested child. However, in spite of careful evaluation, some have been analyzed. Freud (1937) and Hellman (1978) suggested that a trial analysis often clarifies the transference and makes the decision of analyzability sharper. Some analyses of these children have been described as research attempts. Currently, it is possible to hear of analyses of a deaf child by Anthony (1978), an orphan in an institution by Burland (1977), and a borderline child by Kernberg (1975). Cases such as these put us in intimate contact with a degree of chaos of life situation and psyche which is hardly familiar or compatible ground for us.

The introduction of the theories of Anthony (1978), Beres (1974), Blos (1979), Galenson (1976), Kernberg (1975), Mahler et al. (1975), and others have made us more interested in the psychoanalysis of developmentally arrested children. As Kohut's contributions have made our psychoanalytic techniques with the adult narcissistic personality disorders more effective, the same has occurred with children who have major narcissistic defects.

The struggle with this new theory is in process, with Slap and Levine (1978) and others questioning its validity. The fluid state of the art is even greater in child analysis, as we are in a period of a rapidly developing theory of the self in childhood and adolescence. My present attempt at describing the analyses of developmentally arrested children should be considered in the light of beginning research observations.

I would like to outline the analyses of three developmentally arrested adolescents.

John was brought to me at age fourteen with the major symptom of continued soiling. He had few friends, a general immaturity, and was undergoing passive-aggressive struggles with mother and teachers. Parents complained that the patient was sloppy, dirty, and smelled of feces.

Mother and father had both had short analyses before they sought help for John. Mother had been divorced and brought another son, a stepbrother, five years older than John, into the present marriage. During her analysis, which she had undertaken because of chronic anxiety and dead feelings, she had reworked a period of being left in a contagious ward to die when she was five years old. Father, like John, was developmentally arrested, an aloof and detached man who had little to do with John before his own analysis, in which he examined his excessive criticism of his stepson and rage reactions to his wife. Father worked through being abandoned by his father at the age of two. As his rage and hurts were resolved and his parenting relationship clarified, he became successful in business and was able to become an interested and concerned parent, less critical of his wife and stepson.

John's analysis consisted of sessions five times a week for five years. It had many qualities of a self-object merger with slow resolution of his poor self-image. My contacts with the family were rare, but their positive experiences with analysis had helped them to be empathic toward John. During the early phase John was often silent. We examined his passive-aggressive defenses, covering anger with his mother and his twin-like merger with his stepbrother. In the middle phase, the soiling stopped and he became interested in music, playing rock with a group. We struggled together with his low self-esteem, which allowed him to reach out only to peers who were into drugs. As the transference developed further, he was able to work through his rage at his depressed, nonempathic parents of his preoedipal years, which enabled him to deal with them more realistically.

With a new view of his parents and himself, he became closer to his successful father. As his passivity was resolved, he found he could work in school and developed a deep interest in science. He became a leader of his own rock group, composing, making records, and playing concerts. He went on to do well in school and is now a doctoral candidate. It was only in the last phase of his analysis that he worked through his sexual identity. After termination of his analysis, he married a young woman who appears to have had some developmental problems herself. She was adopted and has an illegitimate daughter. It has been a consistent observation that developmentally arrested patients often choose developmentally arrested spouses, likely as nonthreatening objects to their self-esteem. The daughter made this woman especially desirable to John. It seems characteristic of analyzed developmentally arrested adolescents to feel, as John said ". . . safer with dogs and small children than with adults."

In the developmental line of the capacity for making true friends and enjoying empathic experiences, parenting may serve as a transitional stage for those who are narcissistically damaged. Whether they go beyond that stage to loving others is not clear. The capacity to marry and parent does not assure that the person is capable of loving friendships. I continue to see John every six months. To this point he is well and happy; we are reasonably optimistic.

Alan's analysis began when he was thirteen. His symptoms were boredom, no friends, beating his eighteen-months-younger sister, poor school habits, and detachment. His mother had started having affairs with younger men when Alan was two years old. There was much sexual stimulation in the form of nudity, maternal back rubs, and shared bathing. When Alan was five, mother became depressed over the sudden death of her sister. Father, a narcissistic personality, had never separated from his family or the family business. He became depressed over his wife's behavior and moved away from her and the children. Mother has lived with a man ten years her junior ever since. When Alan was fourteen, father went into analysis himself. As he became a more empathic parent, he set up an apartment in which both children could live with him and, with mother's agreement, took them out of the overstimulation of mother's house.

The early part of Alan's analysis dealt with his rage at both parents for not parenting him when he was very young. This was covered by passivity, silence, passive-aggressive struggles with everyone, including the analyst, and active struggles with his sister. As Alan moved away from the fire of living with his seductive mother to the compulsive structure of father's apartment, his symptoms decreased and he gradually thawed and became more active. When the patient was fifteen years old the parents were divorced, and father cut Alan's treatment from five sessions a week to twice a week for financial reasons.

When Alan was sixteen, he recognized that he had attached himself to a girl very much like his mother. That realization motivated him to request analysis five times a week again. Father, who in the course of his own therapy better understood Alan's conflict, agreed. Father's empathy proved decisive in maintaining the working alliance between Alan and me. A stormy time followed, during which Alan worked through his need to repeat his masochistic attachment to the seductive mother with the choice of a girl who alternated between clinging to him and devastating him. Within a few months he tentatively found a more appropriate girl friend and began to make realistic plans to leave home for college, individuating from father, choosing a creative life work, and cutting his ties to the family business. The threat of disruption of the merger between this narcissistic father and adolescent son, however, activated depression and anxiety to both. Analysis of the ensuing struggles between them clarified Alan's bisexual problems and moved him toward establishing a heterosexual identity. Analytic work around the moving away from father and termination of Alan's analysis at age seventeen was crucial in serving to consolidate this adolescent's progress.

Iris is the daughter of developmentally arrested parents. As is often seen with this phenomenon, both Iris and her five-year-older brother were also developmentally arrested. The parents brought her to my office initially at age five, for suspected pseudomental retardation, as she had an IQ test score of between eighty and ninety. Iris fought constantly and violently with her brother and he called her "retard." Her peer relations were poor and her immaturity extensive. In her first hour when I suggested she come into the playroom she urinated on the couch.

Father had been analyzed before marriage, and after marriage he directed his wife to analysis also. That experience helped the parents to be more empathic than they might have been otherwise in supporting Iris's long analysis. The major advances in Iris followed my recognition that traditional defense analysis was not helpful as she was unable to tolerate focusing on libidinal and aggressive conflicts and their defenses. However, when I understood her need to merge before she would be able to define a cohesiveness of self, she blossomed. When we were able to work through her defective self-image and establish a foundation of sublimation, her IQ moved ahead twenty points, she began to learn in school, and she found friends. Rage at her brother became understood as displaced anger and frustration at all the defects in her family.

When she psychologically and physically entered adolescence, the analysis was terminated. She is now seen twice a year. Except for occasional difficulties in math, for which she now calls a tutor, her grades are A's and B's. She has friends and is interested in drama, dance, choir, and playing musical instruments.

Conclusions

The parents of these three patients all recognized that their support and empathic parenting were vitally important to the progress that was made. In response, these young people maintained age-appropriate relationships with the parents. In the long and sometimes arduous and frustrating process, I have furthered my understanding of the ramifications of various treatment models with these seriously damaged individuals.

Prior to our understanding of pathology of the self and developmental arrests, such child patients often experienced relief of symptoms with traditional analysis of defense and conflict. However, we often saw them again as postadolescents with unresolved defects in the self and with narcissistic pathology of depression and identity diffusion. With the new methods, these patients are responding to the analyses of the bipolar transferences described by Kohut (1971). Correct interpretation of narcissistic pathology results in libidinal development and structural growth. Our versatility with patients has been increased as has our effectiveness. Interpretation of narcissistic transferences, as well as uncovering unconscious conflict and the analysis of the transference neuroses, makes analysis a more useful method with adolescents than it was in the past. The integration of our theory is in process, but is far from complete. This is an exciting time for those of us who analyze adolescents.

REFERENCES

Anthony, E. J. 1978. The analysis of a deaf girl. Paper presented before the Mahler Conference, Philadelphia, May.

Belmont, H. 1977. The effect of psychoanalytic concepts on child-rearing practices. Unpublished.

Beres, D. 1974. Structure and function in psychoanalysis. *International Journal of Psycho-Analysis* 46:53–63.

Blos, P. 1979. *Adolescent Passage: Developmental Issues.* New York: International Universities Press.

Burland, J. A. 1977. The syndrome of "mindlessness" in deprived children. Unpublished.

Burland, J. A., and Cohen, T. B. 1980. Psychoanalytic perspectives in prevention and therapeutic approaches with vulnerable and high risk young children. In P. Sholevar, R. Benson, and E. J. Blinder, eds. *Treatment of Emotional Disorders in Children and Adolescents.* New York: Spectrum.

Colarusso, C. A. 1973. *Diagnostic Educational Grouping: Strategies for Teaching Programs.* Doylestown, Pa.: Bucks County Department of Education.

Freud, A. 1965. *Normality and Pathology in Childhood.* New York: International Universities Press.

Freud, S. 1937. Analysis terminable and interminable. *Standard Edition* 23:216–253. London: Hogarth, 1964.

Galenson, E. 1976. Sexual identity. Paper presented before the Lewin Symposium, Philadelphia, November.

Hellman, I. 1978. Assessment of analysability illustrated by the case of an adolescent patient. *Bulletin Hampstead Clinic* 1:65–73.

Kernberg, P. 1975. Object relations in borderline and psychotic children. Presented before the Vulnerable Child Discussion Group, meeting of the American Psychoanalytic Association, December.

Kohut, H. 1971. *The Analysis of the Self.* New York: International Universities Press.

Kohut, H. 1977. *The Restoration of the Self.* New York: International Universities Press.

Kohut, H. 1978. *The Search for the Self.* New York: International Universities Press.

Kohut, H., and Wolf, E. S. 1978. The disorders of the self and their treatment: an outline. *International Journal of Psycho-Analysis* 59:413–425.

Kolansky, H., and Eisner, H. 1979. Psychoanalytic concepts on treatment of preoedipal developmental arrests. Paper presented before the American Psychoanalytic Association, New York, December.

Mahler, M.; Pine, F.; and Bergmann, A. 1975. *The Psychological Birth of the Human Infant. Symbiosis and Individuation.* New York: Basic.

Pavenstedt, E. 1961. A study of immature mothers and their children. In G. Caplan, ed. *Prevention of Mental Disorders in Children.* New York: Basic.

Pearson, G. H. J. 1955. Some developmental problems in children. *Bulletin of the Philadelphia Association for Psychoanalysis* 1 (5):9–14.

Slap, J. W., and Levine, F. J. 1978. On hybrid concepts in psychoanalysis. *Psychoanalytic Quarterly* 47:499–523.

Stennis, W. 1972. *Diagnostic Education Grouping in New Mexico.* Santa Fe: New Mexico Department of Hospitals and Institutions.

Tyson, P. 1979. Some aspects of transference and countertransference manifestations in oedipal and preoedipal children relevant to the gender of the analyst. Paper presented before the American Association of Child Psychoanalysis, New York.

36 COUNTERTRANSFERENCE ISSUES IN A TRANSITIONAL RESIDENTIAL TREATMENT PROGRAM FOR TROUBLED ADOLESCENTS

DAVID HALPERIN, GRACE LAURO, FRANK MISCIONE, JAMES REBHAN, JAY SCHNABOLK, AND BURT SHACHTER

This chapter discusses the countertransference issues that evolve in working with young men in an open transitional residential facility over an extended period of time.[1] It depicts the impact on patients of a multidisciplinary staff who work in close contact, in a setting which may be appropriately described as being close to a "second chance" family.

On admission to the Club, the new resident is confronted with the reality that he has entered a task-oriented society. He works with a staff of social workers, child-care counselors, a nurse, a psychologist, and a psychiatric consultant. The Club requires that each resident work, go to school, or attend some formally structured training program. The residents are also given limited responsibilities for working in the Club. They are expected to adhere to a rather liberal curfew. They must attend a weekly community meeting and meet on a weekly basis with their therapists. Residents who cannot conform to these requirements are eventually faced with a series of curfew restrictions, fines, or even discharge from the Club. All residents are at the Club on a purely voluntary basis. Regression is not encouraged. It is poorly tolerated by the institutional culture. Though the staff must obviously approach each member on an individualized basis, the resident who continually loses jobs or does not attend classes will be confronted with questions about the depth of his motivation or his wherewithal for meeting his contract. Ultimately he may require a more structured facility.

The staff of the Club works in a complex and paradoxical setting. All residents must leave before their twenty-first birthday. The lengthy period of stay encourages a certain tolerance, in staff and residents alike, towards the fulfillment of tasks. Yet, the Club is clearly a transitional program. Tasks are to be accomplished. Aftercare is available for a limited period of time. The population of the Club consists of severely damaged youth who may be poorly equipped initially to undertake work, school, or training, and who often have a rather diffuse attitude toward their futures. The staff, especially the therapists, have been trained in the psychotherapeutic tradition where symptom tolerance and professional detachment are encouraged. Yet, they are working with patients who respond to directness. Thus, the professional staff confronts residents repeatedly with the fact that the Club is not a hotel. "Hanging out" is an expected part of adolescent behavior, but hanging out that prevents the resident from working or attending school is viewed skeptically. It is in this context that attendance at community sessions and individual sessions is required.

Traditionally, attendance at a psychotherapy session is a voluntary act. The patient is expected to have sufficient motivation to attend. Coercion is hardly part of the traditional therapeutic contract. Adolescents often view therapeutic activity as a demand of the adult world towards which they can direct their anger, either actively by acting out or passively by withdrawal. The Club is included in this perception. The psychotherapists must work within a framework in which presence at sessions may be seen as coercive. The psychotherapist may share the patient's discomfort, although attendance at sessions was part of the patient's initial contract preceding his entry into the Club.

The countertransference implications are profound. The therapist may respond by resenting the patients who place him in this quasi-coercive role. He may resent the system which makes him into a coercive figure. At other times the professional may adopt an attitude of rigid expectations of attendance which aligns him with the institutional values of the Club. This alliance can be a tense one because the therapist is adopting an attitude that is uncongenial, and, given the pathology of the Club members, at times quite unrealistic. It is an attitude tainted with the therapist's need to be effective. Or, the therapist may act out his frustration and countertransference by aligning himself with the resident against the Club's work ethic. When the therapist does this, he ostensibly reflects the more permissive psychotherapeutic model. But in actuality, his actions may be counterproductive because then the resident is supported in his unrealistic expectations of work avoidance or a regressive retreat from coping.

The therapist risks becoming inappropriately angry at the resident or the Club. The therapist must strike a balance between rigid expectations concerning the work ethic and the tolerance of a more flexible therapeutic model. The therapist cannot regard the Club in split object terms as being, on the one hand, the all-nurturing, corrective emotional force or, on the other hand, as being a denying therapeutic force. Reconciling and integrating these attitudes are reflected in the work of all the staff at the Club.

The longevity of the therapeutic experience at the Club exacerbates these countertransference issues. It may create an intensity of concern or an intensity of anger. This concern may reflect rescue fantasies. Staff may become aggressively directive when the resident resists being rescued.

In most facilities, the briefness of stay allows the staff to adopt a more disengaged attitude. But, at a facility where involvement continues over the course of two to four years, the staff become real objects to the residents and the residents become real objects to the staff. It is much more difficult for the staff to retain its objectivity. The therapist faces an additional countertransference dilemma in his work with others within the milieu.

In the context of an interdisciplinary staff, there exists the potential for different role delineations which may foster countertransference splitting. The child-care person handles reality problems and must enforce rules, curfews, and work assignments. He is often the recipient of the resident's hostility and negative transference. Thus, he may envy the therapist's more permissive stance. Added to this is the child-care person's sense of lesser status in comparison with the therapist and other professional staff. This may set the stage for the child-care person to act out his competitiveness with the professional staff, to vie for being the recipient of the resident's positive transference. The child-care person may unconsciously encourage the resident's resistance to therapy in order to gain the resident's loyalty and become the sole positive part object. Conversely, the therapist may resent the easy camaraderie that develops between a resident and a child-care person.

Some competitiveness is inevitable in a milieu where each resident works with more than one staff member. Different educational, racial, socioeconomic backgrounds complicate the relationship of professional and child-care staff. This diversity may generate countertransference reactions. It need not lead to insurmountable ones. Such diversity may even be an asset if there is open communication and problem solving within the entire staff.

A review of published contributions on countertransference issues characteristic of residential treatment centers is in order before proceeding with selective case vignettes illustrative of the countertransference issues we seek to emphasize.

Published Contributions

There is increasing attention in the professional literature on the central importance of countertransference. The notion that countertransference can be for either better or worse is in the ascendency. The classical position that the therapist's personal reactions are essentially a hindrance or obstacle in therapeutic work, to be overcome and transcended, is now questioned more frequently. The recent comprehensive collection of articles by Epstein and Feiner (1979) amply attests to this. While countertransference often is countertherapeutic we understand increasingly that our personal countertransference responses can also inform us diagnostically and facilitate our therapeutic objectives.

Writing on countertransference in the treatment of children and adolescents is sparse, in contrast with that focused on adults. Writing dealing with countertransference in residential treatment programs for more disturbed young people is rarer still, though those meager contributions surveyed are quite valuable in enriching our understanding of the role of the personal reactions of residential staff in the therapeutic process. Writing on the still narrower domain of countertransference issues in transitional residential treatment programs is almost nonexistent.

In the literature, definitions of countertransference include many variations on the theme. For the purposes of this chapter, Kernberg's (1976a) reference to two basic concepts of countertransference will be utilized, viz., the "classical" and "totalistic." In the former, countertransference essentially comprises the therapist's unconscious reaction to the patient's transference. The more totalistic definition comprises the total emotional reaction of the therapist to the patient in the treatment situation. This broader conception includes the conscious and unconscious reactions of the therapist to the patient's reality as well as to his transference. This totalistic view allows for positive countertransferential aspects as well as negative ones. In considering

Kernberg's two basic definitions one can justifiably say that the classical form of countertransference is subsumed within the broader totalistic version.

Marshall (1979) observes countertransference to be more intense in work with children and adolescents than is true in efforts with adults. He notes "the intensity of the child's dependence, of his negative and positive transference and the primitive nature of his fantasies tend to arouse the analyst's own unconscious anxieties. The violent and concrete projections of the child onto the analyst may be difficult to contain."

Proctor (1959) wrote about this special countertransference intensity in treating children and adolescents with character pathology. Those in close contact with the patient may regressively identify with his aggression or some constituent of his archaic super ego, his id impulses, or even some psychotic fragment within him. Proctor further cautions that "reality problems are often used by the therapist or therapeutic team in the service of counterresistance or countertransference."

In considering the treatment of borderline adolescents, Masterson (1972), building on Kernberg's (1976a, 1976b) formulations, weights the therapist's management of countertransference heavily. He addresses the range of countertransference responses in the testing, working through, and termination phases. Each phase poses unique problems which heavily involve the conflicts and character structure of the therapist. In the testing phase countertransference problems involve the task of being firm, consistent, and assertive in the face of acting-out behavior. Therapists may minimize the significance of containing the acting out or relating it to expression of affect. Passive-aggressive therapists may be indecisive in limit setting; others may handle anger by withdrawing or handle guilt by appeasing. In the working-through phase, countertransference difficulty may be reflected in the therapist's ability to tolerate intense affect in the form of hostility or depression. Masterson observes that such tolerance is crucial "since the patient, his acting out controlled, is seething within like a tight pressure cooker and must have another outlet for his feelings." In confronting the termination phase some may countertransferentially push too hard and too quickly for autonomy that the patient is unready for. Other therapists with unresolved separation conflicts may have difficulty in letting go.

When one narrows down countertransference to its manifestations in residential programs the literature is meager in quantity but rich in content. It contributes to our understanding of the way in which collective interdisciplinary staff countertransference impinges on the total treatment effort. Stanton and Schwartz (1954) studied the relationship between the progress of schizophrenic patients in a mental hospital and interpersonal relationships among staff. They generally found that staff conflict was strongly correlated with patient decompensation. Conflict among staff that remained unresolved tended to excite regressive behavior. Conversely, effective staff conflict resolution and problem solving was associated with the diminution of anxiety and more effective coping among patients.

Adler (1973), focusing on the hospitalized borderline patient, investigated staff and patient interaction with greater theoretical elaboration. He particularly observed the way the borderline defensive operations of splitting and projective identification impact on residential staff. He noted "the implications of projective identification and splitting are profound. Staff members who are the recipients of cruel, punishing parts from the patient will tend to react to the patient in a cruel, sadistic and punishing manner. Staff members who have received loving, idealized, projected parts of the patient will tend to respond to him with a protective parental love. Obviously a clash can occur between these two groups of staff members, [who] begin to act toward one another as if each one of the them had the only correct view of the patient and as if the part the patient projected onto the other staff members were the only true part of those staff members."

Drawing upon his work with violence-prone youth in correctional settings, King (1976) focused our attention on the immense importance of personal staff reactions. In confronting youth who have records of physically assaultive and homicidal behavior, strong countertransferential emotions are induced. On the spectrum of responses commonly experienced one finds rejection at one end and appeasement or identification at the other. In the former, rage, anxiety, and a sense of helplessness relentlessly pushes staff to rid themselves of the potentially violent youth entirely. Or fearful, lest periods of cooperativeness become upset, necessary confrontations are avoided and reality demands are not pressed. Appeasement exists at the expense of therapeutic progress. In still other instances the acting out of the adolescent may represent a repressed part of the staff member who unconsciously identifies with and encourages disregard for social limits.

In a rather courageous and painstaking scrutiny of case failures in the residential treatment of severely disturbed children at the Southard

School in Topeka, Eckstein, Wallerstein and Mandelbaum (1966) observed a variety of countertransferential patterns. Staff, particularly less experienced younger ones, often invoke fantasies of magically rescuing the children from the wickedness of the child's parents or replacing parents more generically. When the expected change does not appear, bewilderment and frustration ensue. Anger caused by the child's resistance to being rescued can not easily be displaced on the real parents who are not in sight. New displacement objects are sought. They are often found in the cottage parent staff. Similarly, residential staff can project countertransferential feelings on the therapist-child unit. The therapist can be the recipient of the same kinds of love-hate projections as the child himself.

In a population similar to the one considered in this chapter, one of the authors, Shachter (1978), describes the way in which disturbed male adolescents revisit the earlier developmental vulnerability of the unresolved rapprochement crisis in the separation/individuation process. Cycles of intense shadowing and darting behavior reemerge as the possibilities of authentic independence beckon. The objects of the approach and avoidance behavior involve both the real parents back home and the residential staff more readily at hand. Variations on countertransference problems are considered. Shachter observes:

> the availability of the right kinds of transitional parent substitutes (residential staff) facilitates the reality testing process, the loosening and redefinition of ties to real parents as well as the disengagement from more infantile internal objects. To the extent that they (staff) do not play the pathological roles projected for them and to the extent that splitting maneuvers are thwarted, new interim therapeutically useful dependencies arise. As staff permit the modicum of dependency necessary and encourage authentic separateness in more gradual ways, development progresses. . . . When residential staff get too caught up in playing pathological projected roles or when they can't counter the splitting efforts of the adolescent one more often sees failure that is countertransferentially determined.

The notion of positive countertransference cannot be denied. Rescue fantasies or rescuing activity can indeed lead to disillusionment, anger, and divisive displacements so well described by Eckstein et al. (1966). On the other hand, such desire to rescue can energize the rescuer and provide the therapeutic investment necessary to overcome the despair and hopelessness of severely impaired children. Bettelheim (Bettelheim and Wright 1955) in particular long noted the positive value of such countertransference investments of staff in his work with psychotic children.

As we consider this survey of varied manifestations of countertransference,[2] both in positive and negative aspects, we come to the specific question of concern in this chapter. What are the countertransference issues involved in the transitional residential facility for emotionally disturbed adolescents who, for better or worse, must confront the pressures of independent living in the community? And more particularly, how does and should residential staff respond to the kinds of pathologies encountered in this transitional process? Some illustrative case vignettes follow.

Case of Ken T

Ken T is a short, thin, eighteen-year-old boy who because of his diminutive size appears a number of years younger than his chronological age. He has long, dark, wavy hair and a light complexion. Initially, he was verbose with pressured speech. His demeanor was tense, and he often had difficulty sitting still for more than a few minutes at a time. He was boastful, grandiose, and argumentative. He presented certain likeable qualities behind a facade of abrasiveness. During the process of placement Ken initiated a lawsuit against his depriving, self-involved mother. He was suing for his entitlements. Threats to bring suit against perceived injustice became quite characteristic during the course of his stay.

Ken T made his presence felt within his first weeks at the residence. He set himself up as both scapegoat and provocateur. He was boastful, telling stories of various movie stars he knew, musical groups he has seen, and famous people he counted among his friends. At first, this seemed to interest and attract others. But soon the grandiosity and abrasiveness were experienced as weapons, provoking anger, sometimes jealousy and rejection, sometimes retaliation through attempted physical assaults and thefts of his personal property. He was originally placed in a double room. He was transferred to a single room for his own protection as well as the protection of his property.

Staff began to react to the provocation and disbelieved most of the things Ken spoke about. This in turn enraged Ken. The provocative-ness increased. He blamed administrative staff for the behavior of his peers and the lack of protection he experienced. His litigation tendencies emerged. He went to higher administrative staff in the pursuit of justice and, as he put it, "revenge." To add to the provocation, he called staff members at home at all hours of the day or night to complain. Staff found themselves fighting vengeful, angry impulses. Ken eventually brought his protests to the executive director of the large agency complex of which the Club is part. His efforts infuriated, frustrated, and sometimes intimidated staff members, provoking them to retaliation, withdrawal, placation, and acquiescence.

During this stormy period his attendance at his individual therapy sessions was sporadic. He spent most of his time and energy invested in the people with "power." It was decided therefore to endow the therapist with "power" and to promote decathexis from other staff. This was designed to expedite a therapeutic involvement and eliminate diffusion. Contrary to usual procedure the authority to give and to limit was concentrated in the hands of the therapist.

If Ken had a curfew, it was implemented by the therapist. If he needed to speak to a person in "power" on off-hours it was the therapist. If he had concrete wishes (e.g., clothing, paint for his room, advice about a school issue), here too he was forced to turn to the therapist. His attempts to involve other staff were responded to benignly with "speak to your therapist." When he went to still higher echelons of staff they would not be swayed from their administrative duties. He was referred back to his therapist. He began coming to his session, though he often rescheduled appointments during the course of each week in order to test the limits of the therapeutic setting. These sessions were fruitful nonetheless in forcing Ken into a central face-to-face relationship. He was anxious during his sessions. He paced back and forth, often asking about when the session would end. He devalued the therapist's attempts to protect him against his peers. He complained of how he didn't help, of how the therapist was probably incapable of helping.

The therapist experienced many elements of countertransference reactions formerly provoked in Ken's peers, child-care staff, and administrators. Ken's provocative acting out gradually diminished in the environment.

There was a lessening of staff rage, hurt, helplessness, and desire for retaliation. Most importantly, Ken's adeptness at dividing and conquering (of splitting) was unsuccessful. The staff supported the therapeutic effort in a more united way and was rewarded by the diminution of the acting out.

As the therapist continued to set limits (with occasional overreactions in times of anger and underreactions in times of guilt or seduction) Ken's acting out in the environment decreased. The defensive nature of Ken's difficult behavior became better understood. Avarice, seemingly insatiable demands, provocation, and attempts at seduction became progressively clearer in terms of defensive and adaptive purposes. Amidst nurturing and setting limits, the defensive intent of his power struggles, arguments, and devaluation of therapist became more apparent.

As the intensity of his defensiveness decreased, expectations for more appropriate behavior increased. At times humor was used to deflect the impact of defensive behavior. As he felt safer, there was less provocative, acting-out behavior. He came regularly and promptly to sessions and began to struggle with the void in himself and in his life experiences. One saw glimmers of relating on a less defensive and more open and honest way.

The case of Ken T illustrates the difficulties experienced by the staff in attempting to set reasonable limits in the face of provocation and splitting behavior. Intense countertransference feelings were evoked in the process. Coping with these feelings is essential to the therapeutic work.

Sexual orientation problems are also capable of eliciting intense countertransference reactions in an all-male residence. The following two cases show how this issue may present itself within the context of the long-term transitional residential treatment setting. They explore the factors behind the very different treatment outcomes.

Case of Donald W

Donald was a nineteen-year-old black youth who entered placement following a stint of running away from home, influenced by an older youth who introduced him to the world of prostitution. He returned home in a depressed state after his lover left him. Donald's father could not keep him at home because the last few years had been chaotic. Donald did everything possible to drive his stepmother out of the house. Upon admission Donald acknowledged a "confused" sexual identity but his mannerisms and history clearly pointed to his homosexual identification.

The precipitating event in Donald's current emotional difficulties was the death of his mother when he was thirteen years old. Donald was the only boy in the family with two older and one younger sister. He was chosen as his mother's favorite and given special attention. The mother was the life of the family unit as well as its head. The father, a passive man, was a very hard worker who earned a good salary working in a hospital as an X-ray technician.

His mother raised Donald in a strict manner, sending him to a parochial school and dressing him neatly. Being black, she put special emphasis on dignity and created a sense of specialness for Donald. In stark contrast she denigrated her husband whom she viewed as unpolished and beneath her. Indeed, her family, from the northeast, looked down upon him and his southern background. In this family constellation Donald had won an oedipal victory. He had replaced the father as the mother's cherished man. One of the prices he paid for this victory was an intense entanglement with his mother, which, especially due to her unexpected death, left him without a separate sense of self. He could feel special and important as long as his mother was there to reaffirm this through her attentions. When she died he was devastated, since his own individuation had not been encouraged. When his father refused to support his grandiose demands, as had his mother, Donald rebelled through disobedience. When a year later his father remarried, Donald felt that his mother and he were betrayed. He started acting out sexually in the community, poisoned his stepmother's goldfish, and finally ran away from home and prostituted himself. His acting-out behavior was strongly self-destructive. Because of his lack of self-differentiation he was willing to hurt himself in order to retaliate against others. His homosexual activity in the community was unconsciously motivated against others, in part by his desire to humiliate his father and in part to hurt the internalized mother who had abandoned him. His self-denigrating sexual activity was in complete contrast to his mother's grandiose image of him and his "proper" upbringing.

Donald's stay at the residence lasted for eleven months. He was eventually told to leave by the director. It was felt that his prostitution activities in the community were unacceptable. The fear of its contagious impact on the other residents was a factor in the discharge decision. Thus, in eleven months' time, Donald had managed to get himself rejected in the same way that he had been rejected from his home a year earlier. During his stay he stirred up profound countertransference feelings among staff.

Donald split the staff in two ways. He viewed the child-care and administrative staffs as the devalued and rejecting father while he viewed his therapist as the nurturing mother. This was complicated by the fact that his therapist was an intern who was energetic in his own need to rescue and nurture.

In therapy sessions Donald showed his depression and feelings of helplessness. He shared his hopes of graduating high school and going on to college as his mother would have wanted. The therapist was encouraged by this expression of feelings and the desire to improve himself. In fact his expressions of helplessness stimulated the tendency for the therapist to want to rescue him, to take him out of his misery. Here, supervision was helpful in clarifying countertransference feelings. In response to the splitting, his therapist wanted to rescue him while the child-care staff were totally fed up with his provocative behavior and were withdrawing from their investment in helping. He showed his therapist his helpless side while he showed the child-care staff his angry, haughty, and devaluing side. He spoke in superior tones to child-care staff, he broke curfews in open defiance, and he was uncooperative in doing house jobs. Complicating this otherwise classic borderline defense of splitting was Donald's use of his homosexuality. His use of his homosexuality stirred the latent anxieties of many of the staff members, making it more difficult for them to work effectively with him.

He used his homosexuality in a few different ways, stirring up countertransference feelings. During therapy sessions he was seductive. He asked the therapist where he lived, then mentioned that he often walked down that street. He intimated that they might get together socially. In some ways the therapist allowed himself to be seduced. His vulnerability, as an intern who would soon have to find a job in a tight job market, allowed him to identify with Donald's vulnerability. This countertransference initially blocked the therapist from seeing the controlling nature of Donald's seductiveness. Once this was worked through in supervision the therapist could see that Donald was using seductiveness as a defense against extreme feelings of anxiety concerning his impending separation from the therapist, whose internship was soon to terminate.

Donald displayed his homosexuality to the child-care staff in a flamboyant manner. He dressed in clothing which transcended the frontiers of unisex fashion. He pranced around in an affected manner with a feather boa. At these times he was also cold and demeaning in his relationships with child-care staff. He chose the black child-care workers as objects of acting out, replicating his conflict with his father through these interactions. This engendered feelings of anger and disdain in the black child-care workers. The degree of the anger that would often emerge at staff conferences indicated that more was being stirred up than a simple reaction to obnoxious behavior. Donald was an affront to the black child-care workers' masculine identity. Donald was anathema to those of a race which had struggled so hard for equality and dignity and whose men often suffered frustration in masculine assertiveness. When he finally acknowledged that he had been truant from school for three months and that he had been prostituting it was decided that he would be discharged.

This case illustrates how particular forms of homosexuality in combination with borderline and masochistic symptoms can create strong staff countertransference feelings which doom successful treatment. A contrasting illustration of a more successful homosexual adaptation in the transitional residential treatment program follows.

Case of Jamey

Twenty-year-old Jamey was, like Donald W, struggling with sexual orientation problems. His style was of a different mix from that which Donald exhibited. Low-keyed, discreet, he adhered to no homosexual stereotype. He conformed to Club rules. His sexual life was confined to relationships outside the residence. Though a cynical, sarcastic side sometimes surfaced, he was viewed among staff generally as a quietly intelligent "friendly guy who gave trouble to no one." Child-care staff expressed subtly protective attitudes toward Jamey. In their formation of such attitudes, not the least potent ingredient was the impact of his father.

What had been sharply discernible almost from the point of Jamey's entry into the Club were the demanding, intrusive, enveloping qualities of the father's approach to his son. In the beginning, his father's phone calls to the residence had been excessive; they seemed incessant. Jamey was soon viewed, all too readily and all too sympathetically, as something of a victim, struggling to free himself from father's "web." There was plausibility for such a view.

What he had done, in the interim, was to move the arena for the struggle one degree away, into a homosexual relationship with a high school teacher twenty years his senior. This relationship—with all the problems it entailed—came to assume a major role in therapeutic efforts with Jamey.

Collateral meetings with his parents witnessed Jamey's intense conflict in terms of whether—or how—to confront them with the reality of his homosexuality. For their part, his parents—knowing at some level—strenuously maintained their own efforts at denial.

Working in this setting entailed the confrontation of a variety of issues. How, for example, to deal with the whole question of confidentiality? How to navigate appropriate essential bounds when shared staff planning is in order? How to relate to the attitudes of staff and residents, defensively aroused, by Jamey's easy-to-discern homosexuality? As staff confronted issues such as these, we traveled a road which seemed often overgrown with brambles.

Jamey had anticipated derision once staff knew of his homosexuality. Eventually, in one planning conference, the homosexual issue had, of necessity, to be discussed. Aware of that conference, Jamey was surprised when staff continued to relate to him as usual. He had difficulty trusting this, and for a time remained edgy and wary. He related during this period as though expecting something ominous from "on high," or, at the least, for "somebody up there to drop the other shoe." Therapy sessions saw him questioning the trustworthiness of child-care and administrative staff alike. At a housemeeting, on one occasion, he carried on a running, sophisticated putdown of the Club's director.

During ensuing months, Jamey's wariness eventually diminished. Subtle changes became observable. He began to try on roles of responsibility. He tested himself in part-time work situations. He matriculated in a college program. Together with another resident, with staff assistance, he put on an exhibit of photographs at the agency's main office. Through all this, he seemed to grow in self-assurance. Encouraged, staff began to view Jamey as truly experiencing the milieu as supportive, emotionally giving, and flexible.

During the course of Jamey's encounters in therapy, splitting operations involved his female therapist on the receiving end of protective feelings. At other times sarcasm and emotional distancing were also in evidence, particularly during the early phases. Rarer, but rapier-like in the personalized reactions they evoked in her, were Jamey's unconscious projections of a demeaning form of hostility.

In one particular interview he recalled a bitter argument with his adoptive mother in early adolescence. In the heat of that angry interchange, he said she blurted that Jamey's natural mother had been an "Irish whore." Jamey's Irish therapist found herself launching into an involved exposition of Irish history. She also became sheepishly aware of an irrational desire to impress Jamey with her own erudition. By the end of that particular session, Jamey himself had slipped almost out of focus.

Over a period of many months negative transference manifestations subsided. One saw more quiescence with more intense investments in homosexual relations outside the Club.

As his twenty-first birthday approached, so did the termination of Jamey's stay. He had, by this point, begun to engage in some concrete planning on his discharge. Because of earlier signs he had given of a growing maturity, what developed stood out in sharp contrast. As his separation date drew near, there was a resurgence of broken or "forgotten" appointments with expressions of hostility in sessions which were held. There was emotional distancing in contacts with his therapist around the Club. During one of their final sessions, Jamey declared his therapist had "betrayed" him. Moreover, he insisted he did not believe that the Club's director had ever known he was a homosexual. (This, after two and one-half years of daily contacts in the residence.)

How does one explain this development, which seemed to have occurred unexpectedly. Part of the explanation lay in the separation anxiety Jamey was experiencing, and the difficulty he was having leaving the Club in a responsible way.

But there was another part. This had to do with his relationship with Andy, his lover. Andy and Jamey had been planning to enter into an apartment-sharing arrangement after Jamey's departure from the Club. One day, Andy had pulled out the stops. A practicing church member, Andy informed Jamey that he was going into a monastery—that any sharing they might do could not extend beyond the next six months.

In a subsequent therapy session, Jamey defensively denied his own anger and frustration toward Andy. He displaced those feelings onto the therapist. The therapist, in turn, experienced an intense, self-righteous sense of outrage at Jamey's failure to recognize her own long-standing therapeutic input.

Jamey could not confront the tensions of termination and the uncertainties of his new gay life in the community. He could not terminate other than by a precipitous break off and flight into his postresidence world. In follow-up contacts Jamey discussed finding his way in his gay life without excessive difficulty, despite a residue of unresolved problems.

In contrast with the more flamboyant, provocative homosexuality of Donald W, the countertransference responses evoked by Jamey were more subtle, less disruptive of the therapeutic work. Staff accommodations and tolerance prevailed for the most part. Staff attitudes were corrective and benign in the face of the judgments and betrayals projected by Jamey.

The Case of Bernie O

When a patient at the Club becomes acutely ill, it sometimes evokes an intense response from the staff. Some of these responses reflect the staff's long-term investment collectively and individually in the particular patient. When people have worked with a patient over a period of years, their investment in his progress is obvious. Even when the patient has resided at the Club only briefly, the staff response may also be intense and concerned. Countertransference issues emerge along with appropriate human concern.

The patient's regression becomes more than simply an acute illness. It may be perceived as a defeat for the caretaker. The patients at the Club are often very damaged. Progress is necessarily slow, hesitant, and faltering. Indeed, only after a long process may meaningful change become apparent. Nonetheless, the staff may work with the conviction that with sufficient tenacity progress will come. A resident's acute illness which requires hospitalization and/or transfer to a more structured facility challenges one sustaining myth of the Club. The staff's countertransference is in part a response to their being deprived of a sustaining group fantasy and in part a response to a narcissistic injury. Responses elicited will include denial, displacement, and change in intensity of therapeutic activity. Let us examine these in context of a case:

Bernie O, an eighteen-year-old male, was transferred from another facility. He had resided there since age thirteen. That facility referred Bernie because it recognized that he had already been institutionalized for five years. They felt he should have the opportunity to prepare for his inevitable deinstitutionalization in a less structured setting. Everyone recognized that transfer would be difficult because of Bernie's dependence on the referring institution. Within two weeks after his transfer, Bernie became grossly disorganized—presenting all the major and minor signs of a florid schizophrenic illness. Yet, the staff was very ambivalent about pursuing the obvious disposition of hospitalization. Why?

The initial response at both facilities was denial. Bernie was not really that sick. His symptoms were just an acute exacerbation of his chronic illness. Some regression had been anticipated. Examination at both facilities showed the presence of a flight of ideas, loosening of associations, and inappropriate affect. These symptoms were dismissed as symptomatic of the expected separation anxiety. Other signs of clinical and prognostic importance were denied. Bernie had received some five years of treatment. There clearly had to be more in the way of positive change for this investment of time and energy. Ergo, he was not really sick, just overanxious because of separation.

The staff's countertransference may manifest itself by its displacement of anger onto a referring institution, or onto its own institution, that is, the administrative staff. Or, a split may develop between the professional and paraprofessional components of the staff. The staff felt coerced into accepting an inappropriate patient; others had somehow manipulated the Club into admitting a patient who should not have been admitted. The staff's own unrealistic assessment of Bernie or even its grandiosity in accepting a young man who was still clearly not suited for a nonstructured setting was hardly mentioned. It was the fault of the referring agency rather than the responsibility of the accepting agency.

Countertransference anger is expressed in the change of intensity of therapeutic activity. The staff became very angry at Bernie because he was getting sicker despite all its efforts. He was aggressively started on medication, with some staff passive-aggressively making little effort to see that he took it. Or the staff would get into battles with Bernie to ensure that he act in a more suitably mobilized manner. This alternating activity and passivity was not constructive. It delayed the necessary hospitalization. It reflected the staff's adherence to an institutional culture which implies that residents should not require medication. It reflects staff's narcissistic investment in proving that all patients can fit this model. The therapeutic hopefulness which works so well for many patients may approximate therapeutic delusion in the case of a patient like Bernie O.

In working with the acutely ill patient, the question of hospitalization is, of course, an important one. As the example of Bernie shows, some staff are often reluctant to hospitalize because of overidentification with the patient and the narcissistic injury experienced at perceived failure. But, the staff members are not alone in their ambivalent perception of hospitalization. Nowadays, it is extremely difficult to hospitalize anyone. It is not surprising for staff who have waited in an emergency room only to be told by an inexperienced emergency room physician that the patient in question is not sick enough to pass the muster of a utilization review committee or a patient rights attorney. The road to hospitalization is understandably paved with a great deal of ambivalence.

Conclusions

This chapter deals with a range of countertransference issues which emerge in one kind of long-term residential treatment facility for disturbed adolescents. The four case vignettes presented represent some of the variations on personal staff reactions so vitally a part of the therapeutic process. Primitive mechanisms like splitting, projective identification, and intense displacements are common elements experienced by the staff. The feelings that would be dissipated or avoided in brief treatment are manifest and intensified here. Expectations, disappointments, and gratifications assume a more intense cast. Staff burn out is much greater if countertransference problems are not recognized and dealt with collectively. Individual management of countertransference often becomes the essential ingredient in therapeutic payoff in this kind of interdisciplinary setting. The long-term residential treatment facility is currently in disfavor because of financial limitation, budgetary cutback, and, as we suggest, because of the intensity of the countertransferential issues one must address. It should be recognized that the work of rehabilitation and growth with the kind of troubled adolescent population involved takes time. Short-term models may be neater, cheaper, and less demanding on staff but one must question whether they truly do the job that needs doing. If not, what price to society and the individuals concerned?

NOTES

1. The Stuyvesant Residence Club of the Jewish Board of Family and Children's Services is a transitional residential facility for the New York metropolitan region. It provides a residence for thirty youths between the ages of sixteen and twenty-one for an average stay of two to three years.

2. The authors remind the reader that a totalistic definition of countertransference is used for purposes of this chapter. As restated by Kernberg (1976a) this comprises the total emotional reaction of the therapist to the patient in the treatment situation. It includes the conscious and unconscious reactions of the therapist to the patient's reality as well as to his transference. It allows for positive countertransferential aspects as well as negative ones.

REFERENCES

Adler, G. 1973. Hospital treatment of borderline patients. *American Journal of Psychiatry* 1:25–32.

Bettelheim, B., and Wright, B. 1955. Staff development in a treatment institution. *American Journal of Orthopsychiatry* 25(4):705–719.

Ekstein, R.; Wallerstein, J.; and Mandelbaum, A. 1966. Countertransference in residential treatment of children. In R. Ekstein, ed. *Children of Time and Space of Action and Impulse*. New York: Appleton-Century-Crofts.

Epstein, L., and Feiner, A. H. 1979. *Countertransference*. New York: Aronson.

Kernberg, O. 1976a. *Borderline Conditions and Pathological Narcissism*. New York: Aronson.

Kernberg, O. 1976b. *Object Relations Theory and Clinical Psychoanalysis*. New York: Aronson.

King, C. 1976. Countertransference and counterexperience in the treatment of violence prone youth. *American Journal of Orthopsychiatry* 46:43–52.

Marshall, R. J. 1979. Countertransference with children and adolescents. In L. Epstein and A. H. Feiner, eds. *Countertransference*. New York: Aronson.

Masterson, J. F. 1972. *Treatment of the Borderline Adolescents: A Developmental Approach*. New York: Wiley.

Proctor, J. T. 1959. Countertransference phenomena in the treatment of severe character disorders in children and adolescents. In L. Jessner and E. Pavenstedt, eds. *Dynamic Psychopathology in Childhood*. New York: Grune & Stratton.

Shachter, B. 1978. Treatment of older adolescents in transitional programs: rapprochement crisis revisited. *Clinical Social Work Journal* 6:293–303

Stanton, A. H., and Schwartz, M. S. 1954. *The Mental Hospital*. New York: Basic.

THE AUTHORS

E. JAMES ANTHONY is Blanche F. Ittleson Professor of Child Psychiatry and Director of the Edison Child Development Center, Washington University School of Medicine, St. Louis, Missouri.

IRVING H. BERKOVITZ is Clinical Associate Professor of Psychiatry, University of California at Los Angeles Center for the Health Sciences.

ALLEN J. CAHILL is Clinical Instructor of Psychiatry, University of Texas Health Science Center, Dallas.

ROBERT A. CAPER is Assistant Clinical Professor of Psychiatry, University of California at Los Angeles School of Medicine, and Instructor and Supervisor, Reiss-Davis Child Study Center, Los Angeles.

GABRIELLE A. CARLSON is Assistant Professor of Child Psychiatry, University of California at Los Angeles Center for the Health Sciences.

THEODORE B. COHEN is Clinical Professor of Psychiatry and Human Behavior, Jefferson Medical College, Philadelphia, and Consultant to the National Institute of Mental Health, Washington, D.C.

ADRIAN D. COPELAND is Clinical Professor of Psychiatry and Chief, Adolescent Psychiatry, Jefferson Medical College of Thomas Jefferson University, Philadelphia.

LOREN H. CRABTREE, JR., is Director, Young Adult Program, Horsham Clinic and Hospital, Ambler, Pennsylvania.

SHELLEY DOCTORS is Attending Clinical Psychologist, Adolescent Medicine Division, Montefiore Hospital, and Instructor in Pediatrics

579

and Psychiatry, Albert Einstein College of Medicine, Yeshiva University, New York.

SHERMAN C. FEINSTEIN is Clinical Professor, Pritzker School of Medicine, University of Chicago; Director, Child Psychiatry Research, Psychosomatic and Psychiatric Institute, Michael Reese Hospital and Medical Center; and Coordinating Editor of this volume.

SUSAN FISHER is Professorial Lecturer, Pritzker School of Medicine, University of Chicago.

PETER L. GIOVACCHINI is Clinical Professor of Psychiatry, Abraham Lincoln College of Medicine, University of Illinois, Chicago.

LEE H. HALLER is Assistant Clinical Professor of Psychiatry, Georgetown University Hospital, Washington, D.C.

DAVID A. HALPERIN is Assistant Clinical Professor of Psychiatry, Mount Sinai School of Medicine, and Medical Director, Stuyvesant Residence Club, Jewish Board of Family and Children's Services, New York.

LILY HECHTMAN is Associate Professor of Psychiatry, McGill University, and Clinical Director, Department of Psychiatry, The Montreal Children's Hospital.

ADELE D. HOFMANN is Associate Professor of Pediatrics, and Director, Adolescent Medical Unit, Bellevue Hospital–New York University Medical Center.

HARVEY A. HOROWITZ is Director, Adolescent Coordinate Program, The Institute of Pennsylvania Hospital, Philadelphia.

JOAN B. KELLY is Director, Northern California Mediation Center, Greenbrae, California.

GRACE LAURO is a psychotherapist, Stuyvesant Residence Club, Jewish Board of Family and Children's Services, New York.

NANCY R. LEWIS is Child and Adolescent Life Therapist, Bellevue Hospital–New York University Medical Center.

THE AUTHORS

LILI LOBEL is Clinic Coordinator, Division of Child-Adolescent Psychiatry, Albert Einstein College of Medicine, Yeshiva University, New York.

JOHN G. LOONEY is Director, Department of Child and Adolescent Psychiatry, Timberlawn Psychiatric Hospital, Dallas, and a Senior Editor of this volume.

ROBERT MARTIN is Professor of Psychiatry and Chief, Section of Behavioural Science, Department of Psychiatry, University of Manitoba, Canada.

DEREK MILLER is Professor of Psychiatry and Director of Adolescent Psychiatry, Northwestern University School of Medicine, Chicago.

THOMAS MINTZ is Associate Clinical Professor of Psychiatry, University of California at Los Angeles Center for the Health Sciences.

FRANK MISCIONE is a psychotherapist, Stuyvesant Residence Club, Jewish Board of Family and Children's Services, New York.

MICHAEL L. PECK is Director of Youth Services, Institute of Destructive Behaviors and Suicide Prevention Center, Los Angeles, California.

TERRYE PERLMAN is Psychoeducator, Department of Psychiatry, The Montreal Children's Hospital.

SUE V. PETZEL is Assistant Professor, Program in Health Care Psychology, University of Minnesota School of Public Health, Minneapolis.

HARRY PROSEN is Professor and Head, Department of Psychiatry, University of Manitoba, and Chairman, Specialty Committee in Psychiatry, Royal College of Physicians and Surgeons of Canada.

VIVIAN M. RAKOFF is Professor of Psychiatry and Chairman, Department of Psychiatry, University of Toronto, and Director and Psychiatrist-in-Chief, Clarke Institute of Psychiatry.

HAROLD A. RASHKIS is Attending Psychiatrist, Institute of Pennsylvania Hospital, Philadelphia.

SHIRLEY R. RASHKIS is Assistant Professor of Psychiatry, Hahnemann Medical College, and Attending Psychiatrist, Institute of Pennsylvania Hospital, Philadelphia.

JAMES REBHAN is a psychotherapist, Stuyvesant Residence Club, Jewish Board of Family and Children's Services, New York.

MARY RIDDLE is Research Associate, Psychology Laboratory, University of Minnesota Medical School.

DONALD B. RINSLEY is Clinical Professor of Psychiatry, University of Kansas School of Medicine; Senior Faculty Member in Adult and Child Psychiatry, Menninger School of Psychiatry; Fellow in Interdisciplinary Studies, Department of Education, Menninger Foundation; and Associate Chief for Education, Psychiatry Service, Topeka Veterans Administration Medical Center.

MAURICE J. ROSENTHAL is Senior Psychiatric Consultant, Institute for Juvenile Research; Associate Clinical Professor of Psychiatry, Abraham Lincoln School of Medicine; and Assistant Clinical Professor in Psychiatry, Rush–Presbyterian–St. Luke's Medical Center, Chicago.

PERIHAN ARAL ROSENTHAL is Associate Professor of Child Psychiatry, University of Massachusetts Medical School, and Associate Clinical Professor of Psychiatry, Tufts Medical School, Boston.

JAY SCHNABOLK is a psychotherapist, Stuyvesant Residence Club, Jewish Board of Family and Children's Services, New York.

ALLAN Z. SCHWARTZBERG is Associate Clinical Professor of Psychiatry, Georgetown University School of Medicine, and a Senior Editor of this volume.

BURT SHACHTER is Professor of Social Work, New York University School of Social Work, and Director of Clinical Services, Stuyvesant Residence Club, Jewish Board of Family and Children's Services, New York.

JON A. SHAW is Associate Clinical Professor, Georgetown University Medical School; Professor, Uniformed Services, University of the

582

THE AUTHORS

Health Sciences; and Chief, Department of Psychiatry, Walter Reed Army Medical Center, Washington, D.C.

BERTRAM SLAFF is Associate Clinical Professor of Psychiatry, Mount Sinai School of Medicine, City University of New York, and Director, Adolescent Psychiatry Clinical Service, The Mount Sinai Medical Center.

ARTHUR D. SOROSKY is Associate Clinical Professor of Psychiatry, Division of Child Psychiatry, University of California at Los Angeles Center for the Health Sciences, and a Senior Editor of this volume.

NORMAN TABACHNICK is Clinical Professor of Psychiatry, University of California at Los Angeles, and Training and Supervising Analyst, Southern California Psychoanalytic Institute.

JOHN TOEWS is Associate Professor of Psychiatry, University of Manitoba, Canada.

DAPHNE TUCK is Research Assistant, Department of Psychiatry, The Montreal Children's Hospital.

GABRIELLE WEISS is Professor of Psychiatry, McGill University, and Director, Department of Psychiatry, The Montreal Children's Hospital.

CONTENTS OF VOLUMES I–VIII

591

595

NAME INDEX

SUBJECT INDEX